THE COMPLETE WRITING GUIDE TO NIH BEHAVIORAL SCIENCE GRANTS

THE COMPLETE WRITING GUIDE TO
NIH BEHAVIORAL SCIENCE GRANTS

Edited by
LAWRENCE M. SCHEIER, PH.D., & WILLIAM L. DEWEY, PH.D.

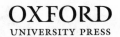

OXFORD
UNIVERSITY PRESS

2008

Oxford University Press, Inc., publishes works that further
Oxford University's objective of excellence
in research, scholarship, and education.

Oxford   New York
Auckland   Cape Town   Dar es Salaam   Hong Kong   Karachi
Kuala Lumpur   Madrid   Melbourne   Mexico City   Nairobi
New Delhi   Shanghai   Taipei   Toronto

With offices in
Argentina   Austria   Brazil   Chile   Czech Republic   France   Greece
Guatemala   Hungary   Italy   Japan   Poland   Portugal   Singapore
South Korea   Switzerland   Thailand   Turkey   Ukraine   Vietnam

Published by Oxford University Press, Inc.
198 Madison Avenue, New York, New York 10016

www.oup.com

Oxford is a registered trademark of Oxford University Press

Library of Congress Cataloging-in-Publication Data
The complete writing guide to NIH behavioral science grants / edited by
Lawrence M. Scheier & William L. Dewey.
p.   cm.
Includes bibliographical references and index.
ISBN: 978-0-19-532027-5
1. National Institutes of Health (U.S.)—Research grants. 2. Social
sciences—Research grants—United States. 3. Psychology—Research grants—United States.
4. Psychiatry—Research grants—United States. 5. Medical sciences—Research grants—
United States. 6. Research grants—United States. I. Scheier, Lawrence M. II. Dewey,
William L. III. Title: Guide to NIH behavioral science grants.
[DNLM: 1. National Institutes of Health (U.S.) 2. Behavioral Sciences—
United States. 3. Financing, Organized—United States. 4. Research Support—United
States. 5. Writing—United States. WM 20 C736 2007]
RA11.D6C65 2007
362.1079—dc22   2007012367

9 8 7 6 5 4 3 2 1

Printed in the United States of America
on acid-free paper

This book is certainly a tribute to the numerous grant review panels on which all of us have participated. Many unnamed colleagues helped to shape this book, and we are deeply grateful for their dedication to science and contribution to the valuable peer review process. Most of us play a dual role regarding grant reviews, having served on committees and having submitted grants that undergo peer review. Our fundamental belief in how the system works helps to shape our own scientific pursuits as well as to give form to the charge we bear when reviewing.

To the individuals that helped shape our lives with critical but unfettered review ...

My daughters Kyley Johnna Ann and Shane Jodie Ann

—LAWRENCE M. SCHEIER, PH.D.

My wife Pat and our six children, all of whom have suffered and benefited from all sides of the grant process for many years

—WILLIAM L. DEWEY, PH.D.

Behavioral scientists are often characterized as having a burning desire to conduct research. Otherwise, the time, trouble, and (sometimes) tedium of pursuing funding for research would drive most would-be scientists toward other, easier or more lucrative endeavors. Furthermore, they are usually expected to learn about how to get funding through osmosis, usually by proximity to someone who already has funded research, or by observation. Rarely is there a systematic teaching tool available to behavioral scientists that can provide a step-by-step guide to selecting a type of research grant to pursue and developing a research proposal with a sufficient amount of detail to tip the scales in favor of getting funding. As NIH funds are becoming dear, and NIH instructions for grant proposals are becoming more labyrinthine, a practical guide to writing NIH grants is critical. This book is such a guide.

The chapters in this book generally reflect four areas of interest: research and grant mechanisms targeting junior or emerging researchers, grants and awards for established researchers, alternatives to typical NIH funding mechanisms, and practical but important considerations in developing research proposals.

Chapters 1, 3, 5, 6, 7, 11, and 12 are aimed primarily at junior researchers. These chapters identify NIH funding mechanisms and considerations that relate to research training and career development. Chapters 5 and 11 also cater to researchers who are shifting from one research area to another, or who have research ideas that are in an incubation phase rather than a phase that entails systematic testing. Collectively, these chapters are also relevant to a new, emerging cohort of scientists who will become the next generation of interdisciplinary researchers. This new cohort should be better prepared to pursue the NIH cultural, roadmap, and gene–environment initiatives.

Chapters 2, 8, and 9 are of particular interest to established researchers. These are researchers who could gain "added value" to their current work by considering how to leverage and extend their research ideas and resources. Chapters 13 and 14 cater to researchers who may be approaching a dissemination or diffusion stage in their research. In this respect, they are ready to create a product out of a previous research study outcome, to move evidence-based research findings into practice, or both.

Chapters 4, 15, 16, 17, and 18 address the practical considerations in developing, submitting, and revising research proposals. With periodic changes being made by NIH in grant requirements and the submission process, these chapters benefit both new and senior researchers.

In summary, this book addresses two key questions that may seem at opposite ends of the research spectrum or, at the very least, contrary. One is "What is it like to submit an NIH research proposal today?" The other is "Should I be careful of what I ask for?" Answers permeate throughout the chapters. My first real NIH project officer, Dr. Thomas Glynn, helped me to navigate the waters of NIH and to answer these questions. Readers of this book will get the answers right here.

MARY ANN PENTZ, PH.D.

When we envisioned writing this book, we hoped that it would be useful for investigators from the scientific community who were starting out writing and submitting their first NIH grants. During a brief lunch meeting at an NIH grant review held in Washington, DC, the main contributors engaged in a lively discussion over the book's utility, in effect sizing up the market, given the proliferation of grant writing books (a Google Internet search shows more than two million hits on "how to write successful grants," quite a number of books covering "successful writing," and a fair number of online tutorials that capitalize on this burgeoning market). After careful consideration, we considered expanding the focus to include additional materials that might be useful to individuals affiliated with community-based or nongovernmental organizations and smaller research enterprises also seeking to break through the barrier regarding receipt of federal funding.

Another concern as we sized up our potential audience was how to make the book useful to an entire community of researchers, clinicians, and educators submitting grants to the NIH. A good number of contributors to this book both are seasoned researchers themselves and have participated as grant reviewers for various federal agencies and private philanthropic organizations. Their professional acumen brings to the table both positive stories about successful grantees and horror stories painting a grim picture of seasoned investigators with excellent track records of extramural funding periodically receiving very poor priority scores (below the funding pay-line).

The general consensus among the contributors is that poor scores derived simply from two concerns: (1) the investigators did not follow certain specific guidelines and adhere to generally accepted conventions when submitting grants, and (2) the investigators failed to follow the "unspoken" or unwritten conventions expected by their respective review committees. A picture emerged from this meeting suggesting we include a broader focus for the book and organize it in such a manner that all readers would be able to glean important information that could help them construct highly successful grants. The end result was a more protracted discussion of the mental algorithms used by reviewers as they sift through their respective grant materials. In a sense, if we could address the different grant review criteria designated as both "expected" and "unspoken," the book would potentially capture the essence of successful grants and have greater utility for a wider audience.

Another important feature of this book is the inclusion of seasoned investigators from a wide range of physical and behavioral science disciplines. We did this intentionally so that individuals reading the book would feel comfortable preparing and streamlining their grants according to an appropriate yardstick. In this respect, we invited researchers with track records in funding from neuroscience, psychiatry, psychology, health sciences, and education, although we acknowledge that this body of contributors does not cover the full gamut of persons submitting to the NIH. It is our hope, however, that their shared and collective experiences conducting reviews, submitting their own grants, and participating in the peer review process over many years will "trickle down" to inspire all potential grant applicants who read this book.

The end result of this arduous effort and collective spirit is a virtual "cookbook" specifically outlining the appropriate measures needed to construct successful grants. The design of the book moves chronologically from early career awards (i.e., fellowships), small grants, and exploratory grants to independent investigator, senior career, and training awards. We also included a chapter on center grants, highlighting smaller scale "core" or NIH P30 funding mechanisms as well as the larger P50 Center grants through which many investigators develop junior faculty and build pilot research projects. As an added benefit to our readers, we also include three very important chapters written by key personnel from within NIH. These chapters provide key insight into the machinations inside NIH, emphasizing the need for new and junior investigators to communicate with program staff, learn the ropes of grant submission and grants management, and overall to keep invested in the peer review process. Given the recent introduction of electronic grant submission, we also thought it prudent to include a chapter of great instructional value attending to the new SF424 electronic submission guidelines.

In keeping with the entrepreneurial spirit of many investigators, we also include a thoughtful chapter on Small Business Innovative Research (SBIR) awards, which help shape many research programs into commercial products available for wider public consumption. Since SBIR grants usually consist of a series of integrated projects for commercial use, the chapter skillfully takes the reader from the early developmental phase to more extensive commercialization stages that involve full-blown field trials and product testing. Added to these very important chapters are a chapter on power and one addressing budgetary concerns. Together, these chapters and those addressing specific grant mechanisms make it possible for investigators to grapple with the finer points of grant writing. It would be a Herculean task to include all of the different NIH funding mechanisms in a single book. Notwithstanding, much of the material embedded in each of the chapters should have broad application. At the very end of the book, we have included appendices detailing the NIH and institutional Web sites that help grantees during the submission process. Accessing these URLs provides extensive information on protocols for obtaining federal grant submission forms, filing instructions, human subjects, and technical support that ensure the applicant has attended correctly to all the necessary paperwork required for federal grant submissions.

    This book is truly a collaborative product owing to its nascence on the back of a Marriot Hotel napkin that came to life during a lunch meeting (see figure P.1). In addition to expressing our heartfelt thanks to the many contributing authors, we thank the people at Oxford who brought the idea of this book to press, particularly Mallory Jensen and Abby Gross, editorial assistants at Oxford who held our hands during the process and made publishing a book seem relatively easy. Joan Bossert was the presiding editor at Oxford, and we are thankful

Figure P.1. Outlining the Content of *The Complete Writing Guide*

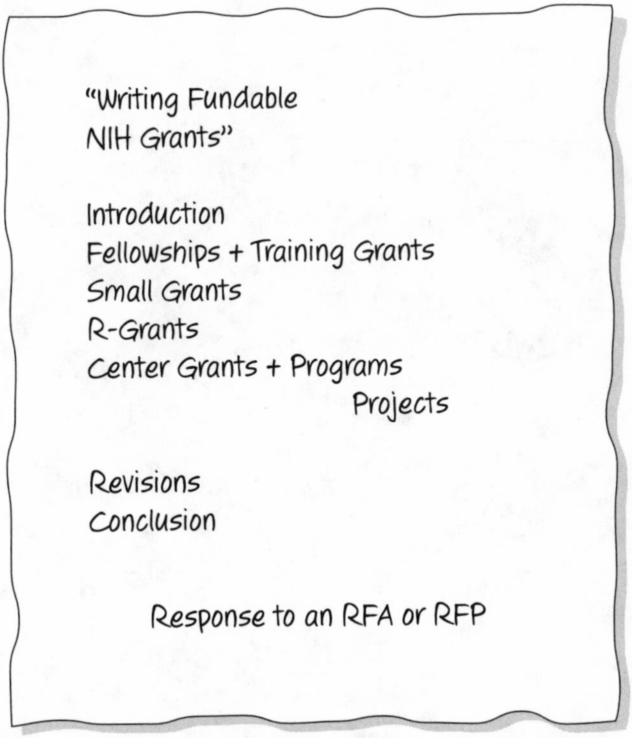

"Writing Fundable
NIH Grants"

Introduction
Fellowships + Training Grants
Small Grants
R-Grants
Center Grants + Programs
                Projects

Revisions
Conclusion

    Response to an RFA or RFP

for her candor, inspiration, and support. We now recognize the truth that no grant gets funded without internal support and various lobbying efforts by program staff. Likewise, book proposals benefit from inside support and ardent lobbying by editors and their staff.

Finally, we would be remiss not to thank all the respective program personnel and project officers inside the NIH and its various institutes and centers who really made this book possible. Their continual zeal and thirst to keep abreast of the latest research findings, their compassion for the lives of the scientists whose work they shepherd, and their commitment to a fair grant review process all help make the peer review process work. It is one thing to write a grant guided by personal impetus to solve the missing piece of a puzzle. It is another thing, however, on a much grander scale, to plan the broader agenda of how to solve the myriad of social and health problems that affect our lives. Regardless of whether the significance of a grant addresses cancer, mental health disease, alcoholism, drug addiction, educational dropout, crime, or any of the other salient problems that fall under the purview of the NIH, we are truly grateful for the financial support received through the NIH grants and contracts. Clearly, the rope that binds us all together has a common thread tethering us all to the pursuit of knowledge.

Overview

Lawrence M. Scheier & William L. Dewey

Some books are to be tasted, others to be swallowed, and some few to be chewed and digested.
—Francis Bacon, *"Of Studies"*

It goes without saying that organization is a key principle and sine qua non of successful grants. From the very first word of the abstract to the very last word on the last page (usually Human Subjects), a grant needs thematic integration and stylistic organization. The power of integration offsets any comments you might receive from reviewers such as "I just don't get it," or verbiage reading along the lines that "the applicant failed to link their aims to their analytic plan." An investigator's job when writing a grant is to be convincing, to make sure the reviewer obtains a complete picture regarding the explicit goals of the grant. This consistency should be apparent from the abstract, which provides an overview of the proposed research, through the Specific Aims section and eventually through a final summary encapsulating the grant objectives (we discuss the importance of including a summary paragraph later in the book). Even in the last section detailing Human Subjects considerations, the investigator must come to grip with all the details required to address patient or subject contact, handling animals if that is the case, and treatment of concerns related to privacy and personal information. Seamless integration is the cornerstone of well-written grants.

It also is important to consider that a reviewer chosen specifically to read your grant may not share an identical substantive training and expertise but, for some quirky reason, has been chosen for this particular review cycle. It is not uncommon, especially during special review cycles (i.e., special emphasis panels) that cross boundaries between unique areas of science, to encounter reviewers who bring a host of different skills to the review table. One reviewer may research the clinical pathology of anxiety disorders, for instance, whereas another reviewer is trained as a quantitative psychologist with expertise in measurement and psychometrics. A particular grant submitted during this review cycle may highlight developing a new measurement tool in mental health research to fill a specific void, and thus each reviewer's relative expertise comes into play. Despite exhortations from each reviewer citing they are ranging outside their professional acumen in conducting the review, the essential bottom line to any reviewer is whether the grant is logically coherent and makes sense from a scientific point of view.

In this respect, a critical requirement for any successful grant is the underlying logical train of thought pervading the writing and the style of presentation. In the interest of placating reviewers and helping them to better appreciate your proposal (does the reviewer "get it?"), your grant, like this book, has to be seamlessly packaged, clearly defined, and convincing. Attending to these three areas alone can often be the difference between receiving an "outstanding" score in the 1.0–1.5 range and otherwise dropping below this critical cut-point, where funding may become more difficult to obtain (as you will find out later in the book, the different NIH institutes invoke different pay-lines or cut-points that factor into which grants are ultimately funded).

It is not uncommon to find, particularly during the review process, that grant applicants (from this point forward, we will use the word "investigator" interchangeably with "applicant" to mean the individual or team of scientists submitting a proposal) become so attracted to their own thoughts, ideas, and expressions that they contract a myopic and limited vision of their scientific pursuits. Further exacerbating this point, investigators become upset after receiving news that their grant may not have fared well during review or even become irritated (and maybe even agitated) after reading the actual "pink" sheets or summary statements that contain the reviewers' comments and critique. Summary statements contain only a synopsis of criticisms (or positive regard) that reflect the overall tenor of the conversation that took place during the actual review. The process of boiling down multiple reviewers' comments to a more concise set of seamlessly integrated ideas is conducted by a team of experts working in-house for NIH. Given the leap from reviewer's pen (or laptop) to that of the scientific review administrator inside NIH, this makes the process of distilling reviewer comments into the summary sheet reflect more "art" than "science." The way to offset this process, the quintessential preventive antidote, involves writing logically coherent, grammatically correct, picture perfect, well-defined grants (more on this subject later!).

We took this focus to heart in designing this book, knowing that no single individual could accurately write and competently organize a book of this scope. First, there are so many diverse funding mechanisms available at the various NIH institutes and centers that it is hard to find a single investigator or reviewer with broad enough experience in the many different grant mechanisms. Table O.1 shows many of the different funding mechanisms that were available at different research career stages. Again, a careful reading of the careers of many of the contributors to this book will show they have chosen only a few of the many possible funding mechanisms on their career path. There are so many that it

TABLE 0.1 Research Training and Development Opportunities by Career Stage	
Career Stage	Frequently Used Mechanisms—Program Title
High School/ Undergraduate Students	• R25—NIMH Career Opportunities in Research (COR) Honors High School Research • T34—NIMH Career Opportunities in Research (COR) Honors Undergraduate Research Training Grant • R25—Mental Health Education Grants • RPG—Research Supplements for Underrepresented Minorities
Postdoctoral Clinical Residency	• T32—NRSA Institutional Research Training Grants • T32—Underrepresented Minority Fellowship Programs in Mental Health • F32—NRSA for Individual Postdoctoral Fellows • K01—Mentored Research Scientist Development Award • K08—Mentored Clinical Scientist Development Award • K23—Mentored Patient-Oriented Research Career Development Award • R25—Mental Health Education Grants • RPG—Research Supplements for Underrepresented Minorities
Independent Scientists: "Early," "Middle," "Senior"	• R03—NIMH Small Grants Program • R03—Behavioral Science Track Award for Rapid Transition (B/START) • R25—Mental Health Education Grants • RPG—Research Supplements for Underrepresented Minorities • K01—Scientist Development Award for New Minority Faculty • R01—Investigator-Initiated Research Project Grant • R24—Minority Research Infrastructure Support Program • K02—Independent Scientist Award • K24—Midcareer Investigator Award in Patient-Oriented Research • K05—Senior Scientist Award
Graduate/Medical Students	• T32—NRSA Institutional Research Training Grants • T32—Jointly Sponsored NIH Predoctoral Training Program in Neurosciences

(*continued*)

TABLE 0.1	Research Training and Development Opportunities by Career Stage *(continued)*
Career Stage	**Frequently Used Mechanisms—Program Title**
Graduate/Medical Students (*continued*)	• T32—Underrepresented Minority Fellowship Programs in Mental Health • F30—Individual Predoctoral NRSA for M.D./Ph.D. Fellowships • F31—NRSA for Individual Predoctoral Fellowships • F31—NIH Predoctoral Fellowship Awards for Minority Students • R03—Dissertation Research Grants • R25—Mental Health Education Grants • RPG—Research Supplements for Underrepresented Minorities

Note: For additional programs and links to specific program announcements, please go to www .grants.nih.gov/index.cfm and for the OER listserv on grant opportunities go to www.grants.nih .gov/grants/guide/listserv.htm.

would be hard to write them all, let alone know about each and every type of mechanism in great detail. Along these same lines, those working within the confines of NIH may see a bevy of grants submitted in response to different funding mechanisms; however, reviewers themselves may be familiar with only a few of the many potential mechanisms. Thus, reviewers are provided "cheat" sheets that help them become familiar with a particular funding mechanism, and these guides can be useful in scoring and understanding any specific requirements that accompany a particular grant mechanism.

All of this goes a long way toward saying that no one individual could feasibly be proficient in all the different funding mechanisms available at NIH. For instance, a seasoned P50 Center investigator should have experience writing R01 applications but may not have entertained thoughts about submitting R03 or R21 applications (though junior investigators at the center may choose these mechanisms to jumpstart their careers). Likewise, many R01 investigators with long track records in funding have never considered the benefits of R13 conference grants, which can showcase their cumulative research efforts, or R43 Phase I or R44 Phase II Small Business Innovative Research (SBIR) initiatives, which can bring to market and help commercialize health-related interventions or products that have benefited from years of sponsored research.

In order to pull together the many disparate types of funding mechanisms under a single umbrella for this book, we chose the tactic of soliciting participation from several authors and respective teams of authors, each of whom provided a chapter covering their specific grant writing expertise. Moreover, most if not all of the contributors have at one time or another served in the capacity of reviewer for NIH or a related sister government agency. For providing advice on constructing center applications, we sought the advice of individuals with excellent track records procuring center funding, and likewise, for fellowship applications, we sought investigators and reviewers who had mentored more than their share of graduate students and postdoctoral fellowship applicants. The overall design of the book is intended to benefit a wide range of potential investigators who may be seeking different angles on improving their grant writing skills and, in this respect, are searching for slightly different pieces of advice and guidance.

When we set out to write this book, we also felt compelled to organize the book along defined lines (as every grant should be!). Contributors needed to be experts not only in their respective field, but also recognized by NIH and other federal agencies as top-notch reviewers, having strong records in training and mentoring. Once we selected a cadre of expert grant writers and seasoned reviewers, the book's thematic integration surfaced quite nicely (the chapter on P50 grants extols the virtues of letting thematic integration surface independently!). In fact, the book addresses a wide range of substantive expertise and provides a large umbrella covering different strategies and grant writing tactics. This was no easy task, given the penchant for different investigators to use different writing styles and formats for their grants. Imagine writing a center grant consisting of four projects, thematically integrated and sharing a common data pool but nonetheless each individual grant under the center possessing somewhat different substantive focus. For example, a P50 Center examining drug etiology could include studies of risk-taking in youth and also involve studies of risk-taking in *Rattus norvegicus* (a common strain of laboratory rat). One program project could be tendered by an experimental psychologist, whereas another project is written by a methodologist with expertise in longitudinal data analysis. Their diverse professional training could promote different views on drug etiology but needs to coalesce to support the center's thematic integration. Even further exacerbating this daunting task, each investigator decides on his or her own statistical analysis approach to examine the stated research hypotheses. A team of reviewers with this application has to decide first whether the grant is really "centered" and second whether the full breadth of research hypotheses will appropriately push the field to the next event horizon. This example showcases how difficult grant construction can be as well as the challenging task a reviewer or expert panel faces when deciding on the scientific merit of an application.

Using the "Center" framework as a structural foundation to this book, we decided a more optimal learning tool would coalesce into a single opus the expertise of several reviewers and grant writers, each possessing polished grant writing skills coupled with an excellent track record of service to the field. As a result, the blend of scientists writing the different chapters should provide a full range of highly stimulating ideas and cover substantial ground when it comes to essential grant writing skills. Given the wide purview that exists under the NIH funding umbrella, we have taken special care to include scientists with different research foci. In this respect, no matter what your individual area of expertise (e.g., neurochemistry of schizophrenia or psychological treatment of mental disorders), we hope that you find some value in reading this book as you prepare your next NIH grant submission.

In addition to the individual chapters covering grant funding mechanisms, we have included a few extra chapters attending to grant scholarship issues, the necessary art behind communication with program officials at NIH, constructing revised submissions (after your first grant gets trashed, what to do next), budgetary and administrative concerns, estimating power, and the sensitive albeit important topic of human subjects. The book also includes appendix materials that point you in the right direction for obtaining all the necessary information on filing grants, appeals, contacts at the NIH institutes and centers, grant scoring, submission timelines, the new electronic review system, and a host of Web sites that "make you smart." Speaking of electronic submission, we have included a chapter devoted to explaining this new submission process. For members of smaller grassroots community organizations who read this book, we also included information that fills in the knowledge gap so that you, too, may fill out applications with confidence and assure yourself that no paperwork or required form is missing. For yet another audience, we have included specific grant submission instructions in several chapters that help new investigators learn the ropes as you grapple with NIH grant requirements.

One final comment worth noting with respect to the book's organization regards our decision to frame the progression of chapters dealing with different funding mechanisms from small grants to larger independent scientist awards and center initiatives. Using this approach should map nicely to an investigator's career if you bite off small pieces first using a series of pilot or "exploratory" grants as a point of embarkation to get your foot in the door at NIH and then developing broader visions seeking more sustained funding. It is a rare phenomenon that a postdoctoral fellow working in some laboratory fresh out of graduate school will, as part of his or her first encounter with an NIH grant, construct a massive five-year R01 and receive funding immediately following its first submission. While there are rare instances of this happening, the norm is that young investigators need several rounds of review before they fare well and obtain funding. Grant writing, like any other professional skill, takes time to develop, and paired with this progressive, if not stage-sequential, movement is the need to incrementally hone and refine the skills of scholarship.

A CHAPTER-BY-CHAPTER ANTHOLOGY

As a brief introduction to the contents of this book, chapter 1 by Mark Swieter, Chief of the Training and Special Projects Review Branch, Office of Extramural Affairs at NIDA/NIH/DHHS and himself a long-time scientific review administrator for NIDA (and member of the NIH Review Policy Committee), provides a framework for the book's remaining chapters, discussing at length the intricate nature of the peer review process. His discussion outlines what happens to an application along the road to becoming a grant. This knowledge, including the machinery of peer review, assignment of grants to review committees, and scoring procedures, all should be quite helpful to both seasoned and new applicants. Additional components of this chapter provide an organizational overview of the NIH, a frank discussion regarding opportunities for interaction between investigators and program staff, and an insightful look at what steps applicants may take to increase the likelihood of a favorable grant review. The detailed information on various activity and assignment codes, review procedures, and information from inside NIH make this chapter an indelible feature of the book.

Chapter 2 by William J. Bukoski and Wilson M. Compton is a real treasure for this book owing to the fact that both individuals work at the NIH and possess the "inside" information that helps differentiate a solid, well-written grant from less meritorious submissions. Where most of us have wondered who dictates the "science" and determines the directions for the NIH, Bukoski and Compton spill the beans and provide an inside view of who is steering the boat. They particularly exemplify NIDA as one institute that has closely followed the NIH mandate for science. With this in mind, their chapter also highlights how investigators need to shepherd their resources and open clear lines of communication with the NIH program staff to increase their face recognition as well as gain a clearer picture regarding funding lines and news inside the NIH. These types of conversations with the NIH program staff lead to increased investigator visibility and can help channel a grant to the proper review committee, whether it is submitted in response to a specific RFA or represents an extension of existing empirical research. Either way, knowing what goes on at the NIH, how funding decisions are made, and the role of council can all make a difference in the long run.

A central goal of this book is to prepare potential applicants for the rigors of NIH grant review. As a result, we want readers to become more familiar with the procedures and "mentality" underlying the review process and the requirements for grant submissions. Given this stated goal, we have devoted the first part of the book to a discussion of generally accepted guidelines for research applications and coupled these materials with the essential points of scholarship and review criteria considered mandatory for reviewers. (Appendix 1 shows you how to gain access to information on review criteria so that you can begin to shape your applications according to the reviewers' mindset.) Chapter 3 by Lawrence M. Scheier provides an overview and discussion of the requisite scholarship needed to write effective grants, addressing issues related to general format, and scoping out their essential ingredients. Included in this chapter is a discussion of the standard NIH review criteria for research-based grants, how they are bundled together during review, and how things get mangled in a grant application. Style and format, presentation, grammar, and brevity are all major components of scholarship, and the chapter is rife with tips and strategies to make your grant "sexier" and sell like you were a used car salesman.

The reading and learning process gets a little more tortuous in chapter 4 on power estimation by David M. Murray. Power represents a critical stopgap for many grants, and the inability to correctly compute power or estimate sample size hinders many investigators. The truth is that a good portion of grants are chock full of great scientific ideas and are based on truly innovative thinking. The problem is that even with a modicum of zeal for an application, major bones of contention expressed by reviewers resonate around a poorly constructed analytic plan, shoddy experimental designs rife with problems, and paying short shrift to power. The absence of these critical ingredients helps reviewers sift through the mound of applications in order to create distinctive piles for the "unscored" applications (applications in the lower half of the pool that will not receive priority scores but do receive summary statements). In contrast, rigorously de-signed applications with adequate power analyses usually are stacked in a pile deserving higher merit (and receive priority scores). Regardless of in which pile the application ends up, if the sample is too small to detect significant group differences or infer stable program effects, the science will evaporate and not curry favor among reviewers. That said, we felt obliged to include a chapter attending to design and power issues up front, so that junior faculty, novice grant writers, or those with less formal education in statistical analysis and meth-odology will realize the importance of including this information in their grant. Murray provides the necessary background and supporting formula to help in-vestigators prepare power analyses for a wide range of clinical trials and ran-domized experiments (including group randomized trials). Perhaps the most compelling piece of advice in this and related chapters is to seek outside advice if your own expertise falls short of the stated required criteria for a successful grant.

Subsequent chapters detail the "do's and don'ts" for different grant funding mechanisms. Kenneth W. Griffin delves into the requirements for small grant mechanisms (R03) and developmental/exploratory (R21) grants in chapter 5. These two mechanisms can be used to help spawn a successful research career, providing a jumpstart for young investigators to conduct small manageable and cost-effective projects. Even more seasoned investigators can benefit from these funding mechanisms, using them to mine existing data or conduct small pilot projects that help fuel new, but untested, research ventures. The materials in this chapter can also be useful for mentors searching for outlets that help promote careers of junior investigators. By necessity, both mechanisms must trim from the 25-page application certain essential materials. This is because many institutes and centers require no more than 10 pages for R03 grants and R21 grant applications mostly skirt including preliminary findings. Griffin attends to stylistic components used for these applications and provides a wealth of data showing funding success rates should you choose this particular route for funding.

The now infamous book by Richard N. Bolles, *What Color Is Your Parachute?*, helps people come to grips with hefty career decisions and match their personality affinity with professional employment aspirations. Likewise, the fellowship grant mechanism (F31) does a nice "Myers-Briggs" job of matching professional interests, acumen, and academic training with career goals, adding to this fray a touch of mentorship. In chapter 6, Jennifer Weil, Susanna Nemes, and Kelly Munly artfully outline the goals of fellowship grant applications, highlighting the tremendous need for mentors to actually sit down and pen a portion of the application. Reading this chapter is exceptionally enlightening, especially if you are curious about why a fellowship application from one of your graduate candidates might get "trashed" at review. Highlights of the chapter include an in-depth examination of the historical precedence that led to fellowships as well as a step-by-step guide on how to construct successful fellowship applications. The authors include sample training plans and instructional materials that help prospective candidates build successful fellowship applications.

This chapter is seamlessly followed by chapter 7 attending to minority and international funding opportunities, written by Jenny N. Karp, Ida K. Namur, and Susanna Nemes. Health and behavioral science research can be successful only when the full range of human problems is examined across a wide swath of people regardless of race, ethnicity, gender, and citizenship. To address these concerns, and the fact that minorities are underrepresented in behavioral science research, the authors provide a comprehensive review of funding outlets for minority and international researchers that encompasses educational and training activities, fellowships, and research opportunities. This detailed compendium of grants, scholarships, and fellowships goes considerably beyond the federal horizons and includes public and private foundations, thereby opening additional doors for landing research dollars. The chapter is neatly arranged to showcase funding opportunities, uses a notational format detailing eligibility requirements, and provides Web site addresses to locate funding information (all are more expansively covered in appendix 1).

As a seasoned grant writer and longstanding NIH reviewer, William L. Dewey, with the assistance of his graduate student Michelle R. Hoot, presents in chapter 8 a careful examination of grant construction and critical insights for independent research grant (R01) applications. This chapter provides a useful overview appropriate for the novice as well as seasoned grant writer who wants to learn more about the "unspoken" factors that often surface and reflect the human side of peer review. Independent scientist research awards tend to be funded over longer period of times, although that is not a necessity by NIH standards. Given longer periods of funding, and the more advanced stages of research outlined in R01 grant applications, it is inevitable the research is scrutinized more carefully. In many respects, R01 applications represent a peak of excellence and scholarship, thus making these applications harder to come by. In this respect alone, Dewey and Hoot encapsulate a good deal of wisdom, owing mostly to a lengthy career bent on scholarship and mentoring.

When a critical mass of scientists can cobble their research interests under a single thematically integrated umbrella, you have the making of a center grant. Steven Sussman, Jennifer B. Unger, and Alan W. Stacy landed one such behemoth at the University of Southern California and in chapter 9 provide some interesting insight as to how P50 Center grants can and should be structured to accomplish the myriad of research goals incorporated under a single roof. Some of the highlights of this chapter (kernels of truth) showcase that management style of the center director goes a long way toward establishing the effectiveness and longevity of the center. If that is not enough to make you sweat beads of perspiration from your forehead, there are any numbers of different types of centers, including those accentuating dissemination, research, and even to collectively establish cores that support different program projects. Chapter 10 by Robert J. Pandina and Valerie L. Johnson augments the P50 Center chapter and discusses the different routes a group can take when establishing smaller developmental centers. These highly successful researchers with a long track record in funding deftly articulate the possible administrative headaches (strengths?) and financial machinations that accompany P20 and P30 centers. A big part of their chapter highlights the essential contribution smaller scale centers make to advancing science through training, providing funding and support resources that can auger small developmental pilot projects, and the beauty of collective thinking among a group of scientists.

As Frances R. Levin points out in chapter 11, the transition from early to mid-career and even later to more senior career positions can be accompanied by a host of career recognition awards that take shape as NIH grants. One such mechanism is the senior scientist award (K05), which is accorded to top-flight scientists seeking freedom from administrative duties and who wish to pursue a career entirely devoted to research, training, mentoring, and empirical study. In addition, Levin showcases a litany of other K awards appropriate for behavioral or mental health clinicians seeking to jumpstart career transitions when they adopt more rigorous empirical practices. Included in this chapter is a timely explanation of K grant mechanisms that may be appropriate for physicians seeking to blend scientific inquiry with their clinical skills in an era of heavily sponsored pharmaceutical and biobehavioral research. This chapter should excite an entire army of clinicians to pursue more advanced graduate studies while engaging in small research projects funded by NIH.

Linda B. Cottler's chapter 12 on constructing T32 National Research Service Award Training Grant Awards emphasizes the critical importance of including specific training information in these highly specialized applications. Consistently, reviews of NIH training grants harp on weaknesses in T32 applications involving the proposed mentoring and methods of didactic training. The concept of mentoring resonates throughout any number of chapters in this book and refers directly to the pedagogical arm of an institute or academic center. As numerous authors point out in this book, scholarship can be taught, and the T32 mechanism clearly embodies this viewpoint. The chapter fully embraces mentoring as a core feature of training grants, showcasing the importance of detailing specific training experiences, their contribution to a high level of scholarship, and the role of training in the ethical conduct of scientific research as a staple component of NIH T32 funding mechanisms. As Cottler points out, it is worth noting that any small deviation from the expected conventions in grant writing, and especially for T32 grants, will tip the balance and move a score from the "Outstanding" category to a less favorable priority score.

While most grants focus on empirical research as a means of promoting scientific discovery, grant funding mechanisms exist that focus on commercial development of products, interventions, or training materials that share a dual scientific and commercial market purpose. To address these specific mechanisms, in chapter 13 Jeffrey A. Hoffman, Susanna Nemes, and William B. Hansen cover the role of SBIR grants showcasing the procedures for Phase I and Phase II applications as well as providing an overview of successful strategies that blend empirical research with commercial marketing strategies. If that is not enough, the chapter also delves into the Small Business Technology Transfer (STTR) funding mechanism and shows the clear lines that separate who should apply for STTR and SBIR mechanisms. This entire chapter is entrepreneurial in flavor but encased wholly in the premise that scientific methods fuel all human discoveries.

As mentioned above, the NIH is only one source of federal dollars for scientific enterprise. Additional avenues exist within the federal government, and grant funding expenditures from other agencies surpass the $23.4 billion spent in FY 2005 on research by the NIH (the Department of Education alone spent $38.6 billion on grants in FY 2005). Thus, chapter 14, in which Karol Kumpfer and Julia Franklin Summerhays highlight additional federal dollars available for grants, dovetails nicely with the focus of this book. Even more compelling, Kumpfer is one of the leading drug abuse prevention researchers in the field and at one point headed the Center for Substance Abuse Prevention, an arm of the Substance Abuse and Mental Health Services Administration. The chapter industriously outlines the way to procure funding for contracts and grants outside of NIH but inside the beltway.

A book on grant writing would not be complete unless it pays some attention to budgeting and cost accounting for scientific grants. Michelle A. Lewis has produced more budgets than most of us collectively have produced grants, and her expertise in financial systems management for NIH grants is invaluable. In chapter 15 on cost accounting and budgeting scientific grants, Lewis points out that science must dictate costs, so her initial level of preparatory involvement rests with the investigator, while at some later point in time she liaisons between contracts and grants, the investigator, and university departments to ensure a seamless integration of everyone's view on financing science. This chapter is replete with examples of budgetary information and key formulas for computing costs, salary, percentage time, and finalizing budgets. All of us wish this information had been part of our own education a while back.

Descriptions of the use of human (or animal) subjects are the bane of a grant writer's existence and cause a good deal of havoc during review. While the rules and regulations regarding use of human subjects (or vertebrate animals) are quickly being revised, there are still some mainstream diehard policies that must be met in order to experiment with "real live people" as part of scientific inquiry. Equally important, HIPAA (Health Insurance Portability and Accountability Act of 1996) is here to stay and has changed the landscape of how grants must attend to personal health information and how this information will be collected, managed, stored, and even destroyed. Consent and assent forms are slowly being modified to address the HIPAA Privacy Rule, and data safety and monitoring plans are becoming a staple ingredient in training, fellowship, and research-based programs. Danny R. Hoyt brings to chapter 16 years of experience from participating at institutional review board (IRB) meetings, writing large-scale center and investigator-initiated grants, and now chairing a university IRB where he slams down the gavel in mock irony at investigators not adhering to HIPAA privacy regulations. Since the Human Subjects section appears at the tail end of an NIH grant application, it naturally dovetails with the final portions of the book, seamlessly and effortlessly bringing together the loose ends of a grant into a coherent whole.

You can pay your bills online, purchase books and other sundries at amazon .com, and order plane tickets electronically from the Internet, so why not submit a grant electronically? That is what the NIH decided in some fitful state of mind and then developed and implemented the electronic SF424 Research and Related (R&R) application system. Thankfully, Mark R. Green, Deputy Director of the Office of Extramural Affairs at NIDA, has taken the time to outline the electronic submission process before we all prematurely gray. Chapter 17 is included to assuage our readers' fears, but also as an educational tool to help applicants streamline their grants and eliminate mistakes. Thankfully, the NIH is looking out for its applicants as part of the kinder and gentler national credo.

Unlike cats that supposedly have nine lives, applications submitted to the NIH have a mere three mortal lives. These entail an initial submission plus two subsequent revisions. An initial piece of advice before you turn the page is that you should not gamble with revisions. Increase your odds of getting funded by carefully recrafting your application according to specific criteria and guidelines. Chapter 18 by Thomas N. Ferraro and Lawrence M. Scheier covers revisions and resubmissions, outlining the specific language to use for revised introductions, and highlights the importance of connecting with program staff at the respective NIH institute or center to learn more about what actually occurred during review of the application. It is likely that things were said during the review that were not fully incorporated into the summary statements but are worth considering prior to resubmission. Members of the various institute program staff are notorious for having the capability to listen and "hear" review comments that complement nicely the actual written reviews. If you are looking for a cookbook on how to write revisions, this chapter has the right recipe.

Okay, enough said, enjoy your reading, and feel free to contact us if you have questions (www.larsri.org).

Contents

THE COMPLETE WRITING GUIDE TO NIH BEHAVIORAL SCIENCE GRANTS

1   Peer Review at the National Institutes of Health

Mark Swieter

The future ain't what it used to be.

—Yogi Berra

THE NATIONAL INSTITUTES of Health (www.nih.gov) is a component of the U.S. federal government whose mission is "science in
pursuit of fundamental knowledge about the nature and behavior
of living systems and the application of that knowledge to extend
healthy life and reduce the burdens of illness and disability" (www
.nih.gov/about/). The NIH is one of the leading providers of funding for biomedical and behavioral research in the United States and
currently spends about $21 billion a year to support roughly 50,000
research grants involving more than 200,000 researchers in every
state and in numerous countries throughout the world.

The majority of the research grants that NIH awards are for
multiyear projects. Thus, in any given year, most of the NIH budget
(about 70% goes) toward maintaining research grants that were
awarded in the previous year or earlier and that have not yet
reached the end of their funding period (grants1.nih.gov/grants/
award/research/rgmechact9905.pdf). The remaining 30% of the

grants budget is made available to create new grants or continue existing grants that have reached the end of their funding period. Maintaining a reasonable balance in numbers between these three types of grants—continuing, new, and renewal—in order to ensure that the extramural research enterprise continues to thrive represents an important aspect of NIH's stewardship.

Getting a research grant from NIH requires, first and foremost, that outstanding research be proposed, yet there are other important factors that operate, as well. Accordingly, decisions to fund research grants are based not only on the quality of the research proposed but also on the number of outstanding applications received, on the availability of funds, and on programmatic needs (for more on how funding decisions are made, see chapter 2). The NIH budget presents a relatively inconsistent variable affecting success rates. For example, between 1999 and 2003, the NIH budget doubled. As a result, in 2001, times were more favorable for getting a research grant, and one in three applications was funded. However, by 2005, after the budget doubling had ended and the budget had remained relatively flat for a couple of years, only about one in five applications was funded (grants1.nih.gov/grants/award/success/Success_ByIC.cfm). Of course, budget alone is not solely responsible for success rates. Each year the number of applications NIH receives increases (up to nearly 80,000 applications processed in 2005), as does the average cost per grant. Thus, at times when the budget is less favorable for higher success rates, investigators are confronted with deciding whether and how to economize on the research proposed. Likewise, NIH staff must decide whether to reduce the size of at least some of the grants so that more may be funded overall (this tremendous battle over limited resources may portend whether centers are funded at all).

Since the latter half of the 1940s, NIH has used a two-tiered peer review system for evaluating the scientific and technical merits of grant applications and for identifying outstanding research: an initial peer review for scientific merit and a subsequent National Advisory Council or National Advisory Board review to concur (or not) with the peer review. Council also considers portfolio balance, policy directives, and other issues. A favorable outcome of the peer review process is practically a requirement for an application to become a grant. Therefore, knowledge of the workings of the peer review machinery is essential. In addition, the entire grants enterprise at NIH is currently undergoing a number of changes, and more changes are expected in the near future, with even more changes being planned beyond this.

This chapter addresses those changes that have already been instituted and that are germane to this book. Overall, the chapter is intended to provide insight into the peer review process at NIH by which outstanding research is identified and to give context to other chapters in this book. This chapter begins with an orientation to the organization and functions of NIH, and then it provides an overview of the route by which an application becomes a grant. This material is then followed with a more thorough examination of the peer review and referral processes at NIH. Also included are some tips, hints, and guidance about when and how to check to ensure that an application submitted to NIH has been properly assigned and is moving through the grant review process as it should. The aim of this chapter is to provide useful information to both novice and experienced grant writers alike that might aid in ensuring that the value and impact of their applications are not diminished by procedural and/or administrative ills that could have been prevented.

GENERAL ORGANIZATION OF NIH

The NIH consists of the Office of the Director of the NIH and 27 institutes and centers, of which 24 fund grants (refer to table 1.1). Operationally, the Office of the Director of the NIH is responsible for making NIH-wide policy, for providing overall direction, and for ensuring that the NIH as a whole functions as it should. This means that the various institutes and centers throughout NIH have, for the most part, the same set of operating rules and that, as a consequence, there are vast similarities in how business gets done. However, there are also some differences in how the various institutes and centers interpret and operationally define the common rules. This is important to understand because it is actually the individual institutes and centers that make grants and contracts, not corporate NIH. Accordingly, because the individual institutes/centers have different research missions and agendas, they do not all support the same types of grants and they do not all use the same types of grants in the same ways.

In an effort to make clear what their research interests and directions are, the institutes and centers provide this type of information on their Web sites. And to simplify finding this information, there is a common format for institute and center Web site addresses: www.IC.nih.gov, where the letters "IC" represent the three- to five-letter acronym for the institute/center, such as "nida" for the National Institute on Drug Abuse (www.nida.nih.gov) or "nigms" for the National Institute of General Medical Sciences (www.nigms.nih.gov). Another valuable resource for obtaining this kind of information is institute/center staff, particularly those directly involved in making funding decisions (program staff). Establishing good working relationships with institute/center staff can be a valuable tool in the grantsmanship armamentarium (chapter 2 goes into detail on this important tool). Staff names and contact information are usually available at the institute and center Web sites. For an NIH staff member whose name is known but it is not known how to get in touch with them, contact information may also be found in the NIH Enterprise Directory (ned.nih.gov/). This is a really useful search tool because it will search the entire NIH or a designated institute/center. It will search by first name only, last name only, full names, or parts of names (two letters are all that are needed to initiate a query). Once you reach

TABLE 1.1	**NIH Institutes and Centers**
CC*	NIH Clinical Center
CIT*	Center for Information Technology
CSR*	Center for Scientific Review
FIC	John E. Fogarty International Center
NCCAM	National Center for Complementary and Alternative Medicine
NCI	National Cancer Institute
NCMHD	National Center on Minority Health and Health Disparities
NCRR	National Center for Research Resources
NEI	National Eye Institute
NHGRI	National Human Genome Research Institute
NHLBI	National Heart, Lung, and Blood Institute
NIA	National Institute on Aging
NIAAA	National Institute on Alcoholism and Alcohol Abuse
NIAID	National Institute of Allergy and Infectious Diseases
NIAMS	National Institute of Arthritis and Musculoskeletal and Skin Diseases
NIBIB	National Institute of Biomedical Imaging and Bioengineering
NICHD	National Institute on Child Health and Human Development
NIDA	National Institute on Drug Abuse
NIDCD	National Institute on Deafness and Other Communication Disorders
NIDCR	National Institute of Dental and Craniofacial Research
NIDDK	National Institute of Diabetes and Digestive and Kidney Diseases
NIEHS	National Institute of Environmental Health Sciences
NIGMS	National Institute of General Medical Sciences
NIMH	National Institute of Mental Health
NINDS	National Institute of Neurological Disorders and Stroke
NINR	National Institute of Nursing Research
NLM	National Library of Medicine

*Does not fund grants

this site, the search tool provides whatever contact information that staff member has allowed to be provided.

MAJOR NIH STAFF ROLES: PROGRAM, REVIEW, AND GRANTS MANAGEMENT

For those who are not fully aware of how NIH institutes and centers are organized, it can be a daunting task to figure out who to contact to get answers to questions (how to get in touch with them is addressed in the preceding section). Program staff in each institute/center who are involved in grants administration have one of three roles: program official, scientific review administrator, or grants management specialist. As depicted in table 1.2, program officials (sometimes also referred to as program directors or project officers) are scientists responsible for helping set scientific priorities for the institute/center in their areas of scientific expertise, recommending which applications are to be funded, how much money they should get, and managing a portfolio of grants that includes ensuring that appropriate progress is being made.

There is typically more program staff in an institute/center than any other type of employee. They are the most appropriate institute/center source of information about the research interests of the institute/center and should be consulted before submitting an application. Program officials not only may be able to provide advice on the interest of the institute/center in the research an investigator is considering doing, but they also should be able to help select the type of grant mechanism most suited to the needs of the research and the investigator. Since program staff make funding recommendations, it would also be appropriate to contact them after an application has been through the peer review process to learn whether there is any intent to fund it.

Responsibilities of scientific review administrators are outlined in table 1.3. As depicted, these individuals are scientists who manage peer review committees. They are responsible for determining whether applications are suitable to be sent to review, for forming peer review panels with sufficient and appropriate expertise and experience to review a batch of applications, for ensuring that each

TABLE 1.2	Program Officials
Sets scientific/programmatic priorities	
Provides information on program priorities, grant process, application submission, research issues	
Sets funding levels/recommends funding	
Administers grants and contracts	

TABLE 1.3	Scientific Review Administrator

Evaluates applications for appropriateness for review by a scientific review group (SRG)

Recruits SRG members

Assigns applications to SRG members

Manages SRG review

Approves release of priority scores and percentiles

Writes and approves release of summary statements

application gets a fair and appropriate review, and for making certain that the results of the peer review panel deliberations are made available to institute/center staff, to applicant organizations, and to investigators. Once a grant application has been submitted to NIH and throughout the duration of the review process, NIH rules stipulate that all communications by investigators with NIH staff about that application should be with the scientific review administrator to whose review committee the application has been assigned.

Table 1.4 shows that grants management staff is involved in making the money flow from the institute/center to the grantee institution. They ensure compliance by grantee organizations with applicable federal rules and regulations and keep track of budgets.

THE UNIVERSAL AVAILABILITY OF THE INTERNET AND THE eRA COMMONS: WHAT THEY MEAN TO THE GRANTS ENTERPRISE AT NIH

Now that the World Wide Web is available to essentially everyone, NIH is in the process of modifying how it does business to take advantage of the wealth of resources made possible by email and the Internet. The initial deployment of some changes has already occurred; others will be coming soon, and still others are being planned. Much of the information about researchers and their grants

TABLE 1.4	Grants Management Specialist

Initiates and implements funding process

Sends notice of grant award

Watches over budgetary issues

Ensures compliance of grantee with institute policies and regulations

and applications that is kept in the NIH database can now be accessed by principal investigators and their institutions through a Web-based portal called the electronic Research Administration Commons (www.commons.era.nih.gov). The eRA Commons is a Web site, and it is a requirement for principal investigators on grant applications to have a Commons account. Account holders have access only to information about themselves, including any grants and applications on which they are the principal investigator. Access to such information is not granted to co-investigators or collaborators. In general, NIH provides master accounts to institutions and institutions create individual user accounts for investigators they employ. Thus, most researchers get the NIH eRA Commons accounts through their institutional business or grants offices and not directly from NIH.

It is now expected that principal investigators and their institutions will keep contact information in the NIH database up-to-date, because they are best suited to do this and because they should have a keen interest in ensuring that NIH can effectively communicate news about their grants and applications with them. Such information include their name, degree, institutional affiliation, academic rank, departmental affiliation, email address, phone number, and fax number. The importance of maintaining up-to-date contact information, in particular, is that NIH will use this information as a primary means to communicate with researchers and their institutions. For example, documents that used to be sent to principal investigators and their institutions concerning the outcomes of peer review are no longer being mailed; instead, they can be viewed in electronic format via the eRA Commons. To alert principal investigators and their institutions when new information becomes available, email notifications are sent to them using the contact information in the database. Letters containing priority scores and mailings containing summary statements (more about these two topics below), which used to be sent to principal investigators, are now things of the past. Researchers are expected to get this information via the Commons. With the Commons, researchers have access to information in real time, as soon as it comes available, instead of needing to wait the weeks or even months that it used to take to receive hard copy via regular mail. This allows them to make decisions earlier about the need to rewrite and resubmit their applications or to proceed otherwise.

At present, NIH is converting from paper-based grant application forms to electronic application submissions that, rather than come directly to NIH, are submitted via a Web site called Grants.gov (www.grants.gov). It is expected that this method will obviate the need for, or at least expedite the process of, reviewing applications by NIH staff for conformity with formatting and page limitations because these will be determined by electronic means, and noncompliant applications will simply not be allowed through the electronic portal (i.e., Grants .gov). These types of changes and others as well may allow for more expedited review of applications, shortening the time between review and submission of revised applications. Soon, the official grant file will be electronic rather than paper and contents of the "grant folder," the official NIH file on each application and grant, will be made available to principal investigators and their institutions via their eRA Commons accounts, as well. The World Wide Web represents a boon to peer review, allowing for the use of Internet-assisted review. With Internet-assisted review, access to applications and other meeting related materials is given to reviewers, who also have the opportunity to submit their own reviews of applications and view those of other reviewers in advance of a review meeting.

FUNDING OPPORTUNITY ANNOUNCEMENTS: PAs AND RFAs

The NIH institutes and centers are required by law to advance the frontiers of science in the interest of the public health. To help in this endeavor, they make their research interests available to everyone by way of publicly available documents referred to as program announcements (PAs) and requests for applications (RFAs). These documents are posted at a common location known as the *NIH Guide for Grants and Contracts*, which is publicly available at all times at grants1.nih.gov/grants/guide/index.html. The institutes and centers also make links to these announcements available at their individual Web sites. PAs are used primarily for one of two purposes: (1) to inform the research community of areas of scientific research that are of interest to a particular institute/center and (2) to provide information about the types of funding mechanisms that a given institute/center uses to make grants.

In effect, one should consider that PAs are not solicitations, but rather documents intended to provide information useful to applicants as they contemplate composing and submitting an application. In contrast to PAs, RFAs are truly solicitations. They are used by institutes/centers to stimulate research in areas that are considered important to the institute/center and that the institute/center either does not have any grants examining this substantive area or does not have a large enough portfolio of grants to push the frontiers of science far enough and fast enough. Unlike PAs, RFAs have a specified amount of money attached to them targeted by the institute/center to fund grants. The prospect of money often generates a number of applications in response to an RFA, thereby providing the issuing institute/center with the potential for filling a research gap that previously existed.

HOW AN APPLICATION BECOMES A GRANT: AN OVERVIEW

Figure 1.1 shows that the entire process of grants management begins with the submission of an application by an investigator. All applications submitted to NIH are received and processed by the Division of Receipt and Referral at the

Center for Scientific Review. During processing, the applications are logged into the NIH database, assigned to an institute or center for possible funding, given an assignment number that includes the type of grant mechanism being sought, and assigned to a review committee.

Scientific review groups are composed of individuals with the expertise and experience to review the applications assigned to them. For each application, review committee deliberations result in a numerical rating called a priority score indicating the committee's judgment of the scientific and technical merits of the application and a written summary statement detailing the application's strengths and weaknesses. Other chapters in this book deal effectively with how to read summary statements that are produced during initial reviews and subsequent revised resubmissions.

NIH staff use the priority scores and summary statements to determine which applications should be considered for funding. They also use the priority scores and summary statements to provide advice and guidance to investigators on how to improve their applications for future reviews and future funding considerations.

NIH rules require that all grant applications receive two levels of review before funding decisions are made. The purpose of the second level of review is to ascertain whether a fair and appropriate review had been conducted by the scientific review group during the first level of review. For most grant applications, the second level of review is provided by the National Advisory Council or National Advisory Board for the institute or center. A grant cannot be funded unless the second level of review concurs with the outcome of the scientific review

Figure 1.1. Review Process for a Research Grant

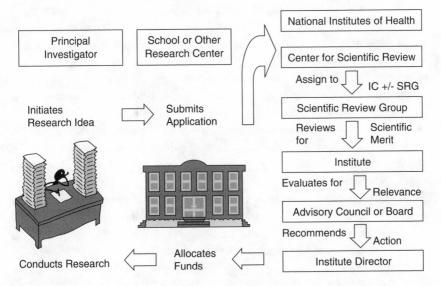

There are three overlapping cycles per year:

FEB	MAR	APR	MAY	JUN	JUL	AUG	SEP	OCT	NOV	DEC	JAN	FEB	MAR	APR	MAY	JUN	JUL

Cycle 1

◄— Receipt —►   ◄— Review —►   ◄ Council ►   △
    ◄— Referral —►   Award

Cycle 2

◄— Receipt —►   ◄— Review —►   ◄ Council ►   △
    ◄— Referral —►   Award

Cycle 3

◄— Receipt —►   ◄— Review —►   ◄ Council ►   △
    ◄— Referral —►   Award

Figure 1.2. Time from Submission to Award

group. Once the second level of review has taken place, the institute or center director authorizes funding; a grant application that is funded becomes a grant.

The Cycle or Round

The processes outlined in figure 1.1 from application submission to funding decision constitute a cycle or round of activity at NIH. Each round is bounded at the outset by application receipt dates and at the end by the council recommendation date, with review dates occurring in between. Awards are made following council deliberations, but the precise start date for a grant is determined by a number of factors, some of which are unique to individual grants. Each round lasts approximately nine months, though most investigators who submit applications know soon after the results of the review meeting are released whether they need to revise and resubmit their application. Nevertheless, it is recommended that investigators wait until they get the written results of the review meeting (the summary statement) before undertaking revisions, lest unnecessary revisions be made and necessary revisions be overlooked.

The workload involved in each round is sufficiently arranged that it has been possible for NIH to schedule three overlapping rounds per year (figure 1.2). Thus, while the applications from the first round are being reviewed, applications from the second round are being received, and after the summary statements from the first round have been released, the applications from the second round are being reviewed, the applications from the third round are being received, and so on. Although the schedule is somewhat complicated for NIH staff to keep track of, such an arrangement does provide three different periods each year when in-

TABLE 1.5	Mechanisms/Activity Codes

Research Grants

R01 Research Project Grant

R03 Small Research Grant

R21 Exploratory/Developmental Grant

P01 Program Project Grant

P50 Specialized Center Grant

Career Development Awards

K01 Mentored Research Scientist Career Development Award

K02 Independent Scientist Award

K23 Mentored Patient-Oriented Research Career Development Award

K24 Mid-Career Investigator Award in Patient-Oriented Research

Individual Fellowships

F31 Predoctoral Individual RLK National Research Service Award

F32 Postdoctoral Individual RLK National Research Service Award

vestigators can submit grant applications. As a result, this rolling schedule helps to fuel the engine of research, allowing it to race forward and drive the frontiers of science further into the future.

Submitting an Application: Mechanisms and Activity Codes

All grants are not alike (and several chapters in this book are devoted to helping distinguish them from one another). Some are small, some are large, some are intended to be used to obtain mentored training, some are intended to move research ideas into business applications, and there are a host of other kinds of grants, as well, depending on the needs of the investigators and the needs of the institutes and centers. To help keep the different kinds of grants separate and easier to identify, each one has its own designation (called a "mechanism"), and each mechanism is represented by a three-character set or "activity code" (one letter of the alphabet and two numerical digits). Table 1.5 lists a handful of the more commonly used mechanisms and their activity codes among the more than 70 mechanisms/activity codes that NIH uses (grants2.nih.gov/grants/funding/phs398/instructions2/p3_general_info_mechanisms.htm).

The R01 is the most versatile of the funding mechanisms and is the most commonly sought mechanism for funding research. It can be used to request any amount of money and any period of support up to five years. Many of the other chapters in this book provide more detailed information regarding specific funding mechanisms.

Each of the mechanisms has its own set of guidelines regarding what can be requested in a grant application, including level of support (dollars), years of support, and number of pages the research plan can take up in the application. For this reason, it is important for applicants to know what the various mechanisms allow and to apply for the appropriate mechanism that will provide them with the amount of time and money they will need in order to succeed. Reviewers also need to know what mechanisms are being pursued in grant applications they are reviewing so that they understand the constraints and limitations that applicants faced composing the application. And as stewards of the grants enterprise, NIH staff needs to know what mechanisms are being sought and funded because they must maintain balance among the various areas of their research portfolios.

With activity codes such as R01 and P50 and F32, it is not intuitively obvious which mechanism might be the best one to apply for or what the features of that mechanism include. In addition, the same mechanism may be used for different purposes by different institutes/centers, and the same mechanism may even be used for different purposes in different research programs within the same institute/center. For these reasons, it is usually advantageous to contact institute/center staff to discuss appropriate funding mechanisms before submitting an application.

The Application Form (PHS398 vs. SF424)

Until very recently, NIH has used a paper-based application process. For this procedure, there have been two standard application forms, the PHS398 and the PHS416-1, with the former being the most commonly used form and the latter being used exclusively to apply for individual fellowship grants (Ruth L. Kirschstein [RLK] National Research Service Award fellowships). Both of these forms are still being used to apply for most types of grants, although plans are progressing to slowly phase these paper forms out by the end of 2007 and replace them with a single electronic application form called the Standard Form 424 or SF424. Until the phase-out is completed, paper application forms and their instructions will continue to be used for some types of applications, and they can be downloaded from the NIH Web site found at grants1.nih.gov/grants/forms.htm. Completed paper applications must be sent to the Center for Scientific Review at NIH for processing.

The SF424 is a set of forms used by several government agencies for research grant applications, which can be obtained and submitted at the Grants.gov Web site (see discussion above). NIH applications submitted to Grants.gov are appropriately routed electronically to the Center for Scientific Review at NIH for processing. More on the SF424 and electronic applications can be found in chapter 17.

Since December 2005, only a few mechanisms have been switched to using the SF424. However, NIH will continue to transition mechanisms from paper applications to the SF424 throughout 2006 and into 2007. The R01 (the most commonly used mechanism at NIH) converted to electronic format in February 2007. All R01s must now be submitted using the SF424 via Grants.gov. The transition of all other mechanisms is expected to be completed by the end of 2007. Once a mechanism has been switched to electronic submission (SF424), applications will from that point on only be accepted as electronic submissions, and paper applications for that mechanism will no longer be accepted. For guidance in knowing when the various mechanisms are expected to transition to electronic submissions, see figure 1.3 (which also can be accessed at era.nih.gov/ElectronicReceipt/files/Electronic_receipt_timeline_Ext.pdf).

A good rule of thumb when putting an application together is that application forms and instructions should be downloaded shortly before they are to be used rather than using ones that were obtained months or years earlier. This is because NIH considers its application forms and instructions to be "living" documents and modifies them whenever they need to be updated. When major changes are made, there is usually a lot of fanfare, with a notice placed in the *NIH Guide* and consideration given to the timing of the changes since the changes are likely to affect applicants and reviewers alike. When minor changes are made, alerts are posted to appear when application forms and instructions are accessed from the Web sites informing the viewer as to what the changes are. In any case, there is an expectation at NIH that the latest version of the application forms will be used.

The Cover Letter

It is often useful to accompany an application with a cover letter containing information relevant to assigning the application to an institute/center for possible funding and/or to assign the application to a specific review committee. NIH staff appreciates and encourages the inclusion of cover letters with this type of information. For example, if the scientific focus of the application clearly lies within the domain of an institute or center and/or if the investigators have worked with staff in a particular institute or center to shape the application more toward the mission of that institute/center, that information is pertinent in making assignments and is reasonable to include in a cover letter. Similarly, if the focus of the application is more in line with the scientific area of a particular review committee, explaining this in a cover letter would also be helpful and appropriate. If an application is sent in after a receipt deadline, an explanation as to why it is late should be included in the cover letter (see next section).

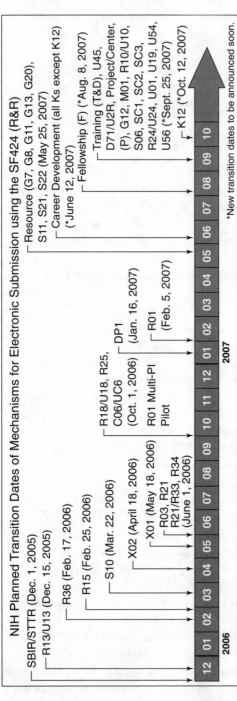

Figure 1.3. NIH Planned Transition Dates of Mechanisms for Electronic Submission Using the SF424 (R&R)

Receipt Dates

There are deadlines by which applications must be received or submitted to NIH or they will not be reviewed. These deadlines are officially called receipt dates. Applications using the SF424 form and applications submitted in response to an RFA have to be *received* by the receipt date; most applications using the PHS 398 and PHS 416-1 forms (other than those sent in response to an RFA) have to be *submitted* by the receipt date. For most applications, what determines the receipt date for an application is whether the application is being sent in response to an RFA or in response to a program announcement with special review (PAR), or whether an unsolicited application is sent to NIH. Receipt dates for applications sent in response to an RFA or PAR are included in the RFA or PAR.

Since most applications received by NIH are unsolicited, NIH has established standard receipt dates for them, and these dates do not change from year to year. Standard receipt dates for the most commonly used mechanisms are listed in table 1.6. For a listing of all standard receipt dates, go to grants1.nih.gov/grants/funding/submissionschedule.htm. Staggered receipt dates provide for a measured influx of applications and allow staff at the Center for Scientific Review time to process one batch before the next batch arrives. As indicated in table 1.6, standard receipt dates for the various types of applications recur every four months. This means that if a particular receipt date is missed, the next available receipt date is four months later. For those with the luxury of time, this is good news. For those with more pressing schedules, this is not good news. Most departmental chairs and deans would probably regard preparing applications early enough so that receipt dates are not missed to be an indication of good grant writing preparation and skills.

There are situations in which applications fall into more than one receipt date category, and it may be confusing as to which receipt date applies. In these cases, the rule of thumb on what the appropriate receipt date would be is that mechanism is the primary determinant in all areas except HIV/AIDS. That is, if a new R01 is being sent in unsolicited, it must arrive by February 5, June 5, or October 5 (beginning in 2007), and an unsolicited revised R01 must be sent in by March 5, July 5, or November 5, unless the preponderance of science in the applications is HIV/AIDS. In contrast, if an unsolicited F31 (a predoctoral individual RLK National Research Service Award fellowship application) is being sent, it must arrive by April 8, August 8, or December 8, unless the preponderance of science in the applications is HIV/AIDS. Because federal regulations require that HIV/AIDS applications have expeditious reviews, HIV/AIDS applications have the latest receipt dates of any applications: May 1, September 1, and January 2, and these dates apply regardless of whether an HIV/AIDS application is new, revised, or competing continuation or whether it is an R01, F31, T32, and so forth. As it turns out, these dates may change somewhat in the near future. The current

TABLE 1.6 Standard Receipt Dates			
Mechanism	Cycle 1	Cycle 2	Cycle 3
Ts, Ps, Gs, Ss, Other Rs (R18, R24, R25)	Jan 25	May 25	Sept 25
R01s – new	Feb 5	June 5	Oct 5
Ks – new	Feb 12	June 12	Oct 12
R03s, R21s – new	Feb 16	June 16	Oct 16
AREA – all	Feb 25	June 25	Oct 25
R01 – renewal, revision, resubmission	Mar 5	July 5	Nov 5
Ks – resubmission, revision	Mar 12	July 12	Nov 12
R03s, R21s, R34s – resub., renew., rev.	Mar 16	July 16	Nov 16
New Investigator R01 resubmission	Mar 20	July 20	Nov 20
Small Business – all	April 5	Aug 5	Dec 5
Fellowship – all	Apr 8	Aug 8	Dec 8
Conference – all	Apr 12	Aug 12	Dec 12
AIDS – all	May 1	Sept 1	Jan 2

transition from the paper PHS 398 application to the electronic SF424 application is being viewed at NIH as a reasonable time to spread out standard receipt dates in order to avoid having so many applications received at the same time.

There are a variety of circumstances that prevent investigators from submitting grant applications by the receipt deadlines. Some of these are considered valid by staff in the Division of Receipt and Referral at the Center for Scientific Review, and they will accept late submissions when they occur. Weather is one such type of valid circumstance that happens not uncommonly, including blizzards, hurricanes, and floods. When one of these occurs, NIH usually publishes a notice in the *NIH Guide* (grants1.nih.gov/grants/guide/index.html) informing the extramural research community that it views the weather phenomenon to be a valid reason for late application submissions and apprising all of the procedures to follow to pursue extensions of the deadlines. Another valid reason to seek an extension of the receipt deadlines is service as a reviewer on NIH review committees, an exception that can be found at grants1.nih.gov/grants/guide/notice-files/NOT-OD-05-030.html. This helps ease the stress of trying to write and submit a grant application while at the same time participating in a review. No matter what the reasons are for seeking an extension of an application receipt deadline, they need to be explained in the cover letter that accompanies the application in order for staff in the Division of Receipt and Referral at the Center for Scientific Review to accept a late application.

Resubmissions

Given that far fewer than half of all research grant applications submitted to NIH are funded, most need to be revised and resubmitted (see chapter 18). Planning for this eventuality is a hallmark of good grantsmanship. In the case of unsolicited applications, NIH permits up to two revisions. Revisions must respond to the comments of the previous review, and the text must be marked in such a way that the revisions are obvious to the reviewers. Moreover, revised applications must contain an introduction detailing how the application was modified in response to the previous review and how the new text was highlighted. Failure to follow these rules may result in the scientific review administrator determining that the application is incomplete and returning it to the principal investigator without review.

Applications that are submitted in response to RFAs are exempt from the two revision rule (grants2.nih.gov/grants/guide/notice-files/NOT-OD-03-041 .html). If an application submitted in response to an RFA is not funded and the principal investigator decides to resubmit it as an unsolicited application on a regular receipt date, the application must be composed as a new application. It must not contain any responses to the RFA review, must not contain marked up text showing how the application has been modified, and must not contain an introduction explaining the changes.

THE ROLE OF THE PRINCIPAL INVESTIGATOR IN THE PROCESS BY WHICH AN APPLICATION BECOMES A GRANT

No one should be more interested in ensuring that a given application is processed through the NIH system appropriately and in a timely manner than the application's principal investigator. Therefore, principal investigators may want to give serious thought to examining institute/center and review committee assignments to determine whether they appear to be appropriate. If there are any questions or concerns about the assignments, NIH staff should be contacted. Staff within the Division of Receipt and Referral at the Center for Scientific Review should be contacted if either no information is available by six weeks after submitting an application or if some aspect of the assignment number is incorrect or in question and the application has not yet been assigned to a review committee. If it has been assigned to a review committee, then the scientific review administrator of that committee should be the person to contact. If assignment information is not available in eRA Commons within six weeks of submitting an application, this may be an indication that the application may have gotten misplaced or lost. Given that the Center for Scientific Review processes tens of thousands of applications every year (about 80,000 applications in 2005), there is a reasonable likelihood that a few applications may not end up where they should and in the time frame they should get there. In addition, there have been occasions in which principal investigators have been asked by NIH staff to provide all or parts of applications because the parts have gone missing. Accordingly, it would seem prudent for principal investigators to keep copies of everything submitted to NIH in the event something unforeseen occurs.

PROCESSING AN APPLICATION BY REFERRAL STAFF AT THE NIH

One of the 27 institutes and centers that comprise the NIH is the Center for Scientific Review. Its two main functions are to provide services to all of NIH regarding (1) receipt and referral and (2) review. The Center for Scientific Review is uniquely positioned to perform its referral functions because, unlike most of the other institutes and centers at NIH, it does not fund grants. This allows it to serve as an unbiased assessor of the most appropriate institute or center to refer applications to for possible funding. The second vital service the Center for Scientific Review provides is to review the majority of the applications that are submitted to NIH. Thus, approximately 70% of all the applications that are submitted to NIH are reviewed by the Center for Scientific Review, whereas the other 30% are reviewed by review offices in each of the other institutes and centers at NIH that fund grants. The applications reviewed by institute/center-based review committees are those that have special review considerations, such as those submitted in response to RFAs, those for large, multicomponent operations known as program projects and research centers, those for RLK National Research Service Award Institutional Training Grants, and those in areas of research restricted to an institute/center's mission.

The Division of Receipt and Referral at the Center for Scientific Review serves as the central receiving and referral operation at NIH charged with the responsibility of logging all applications into the NIH database so that they can be tracked. Once applications are logged in, staff at the Division of Receipt and Referral assign each application to an institute/center for possible funding and determine the grant mechanism that is being applied for. These bits of information, as well as a serial number, are also logged into the NIH database and provide a unique identifier for each application, which is referred to as the "assignment number" (more about assignment numbers below). Referral staff at the Center for Scientific Review also determine whether an application will be reviewed by a review committee at the Center for Scientific Review or by a review committee based in one of the institutes/centers. If an application is to be reviewed by a committee based at the Center for Scientific Review, referral staff at the Center for Scientific Review assign the application to the committee. However, if an application is to be reviewed by a committee based within one of the institutes/centers, referral staff based in the individual institute/center makes the assignment. In either case, once the assignments to the institute/center for possible funding and to the review committee are complete and after the assignment number has been completed, that information is made available to the principal investigator's eRA Commons account (see below). Under normal circumstances, this occurs within six weeks of receiving an application. If these bits of information are not available in the Commons within six weeks, there may be a problem with the processing of the application. The principal investigator may want to check with the Division of Receipt and Referral at the Center for Scientific Review (phone 301-435-0715, fax 301-480-1987) to see if something needs to be done.

DECIPHERING THE ASSIGNMENT NUMBER

Assignment numbers are given to applications that have been logged into the NIH database. They are 14–16 characters in length, and they carry several important pieces of information. As shown in figure 1.4, the first character is a number from one to nine indicating the type of application it is. For example, a type 1 application is one that has never been funded before; a type 2 application is one that has been funded before (is or was a grant) and a continuation of funding for additional studies described in the current application is being sought. The second set of three characters in the assignment number (one letter and two numerical digits) indicates the activity code of the mechanism being pursued. The next set of two letters indicates the institute or center to which the application has been assigned for possible funding.

The next set of five numbers is a serial number. The next set of two numbers indicates what year of funding is being requested. An application that has never been funded before must have 01 as this character set, whereas an application to continue an existing grant must have a two digit-character set greater than 01 (i.e., anything but 01). The last set of two characters (one letter and one number) is present only on applications that were reviewed previously and were not

Figure 1.4. Deciphering the Assignment Number

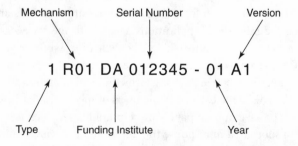

funded. Two revisions of an application are allowed at NIH. The last character set indicates which of the two revisions the current application represents. If any of information contained in the assignment number is incorrect, it would be appropriate to contact either staff at the Division of Receipt and Referral at the Center for Scientific Review or the scientific review administrator of the review committee to which the application has been assigned.

ASSESSING THE SCIENTIFIC AND TECHNICAL MERITS OF AN APPLICATION: THE FIRST LEVEL OF REVIEW

Standing Study Sections and Special Emphasis Panels

Most applications are logged into the NIH database within three weeks of receipt at NIH; by six weeks, most have been assigned to review committees, and an array of information about the application and its assignments is made available to the principal investigator's account in the eRA Commons. A component of this array is the review committee (a.k.a. scientific review group or study section) assignment. The information is written in NIH shorthand; nonetheless, the assignment will be of one of two types since there are two types of review committees at NIH. All review committees whose designation begins with the letter "Z" are called special emphasis panels, whereas all review committees whose designation begins with any letter other than "Z" are referred to as standing study sections. Regardless of what type of review committee it is, its designation can be used to access the roster of the participating reviewers at era.nih.gov/roster/index.cfm.

Standing study sections are review committees that meet regularly (usually three times a year) and that have a core of reviewers, referred to as permanent members, who have agreed to serve on a regular basis for one to four years. This provides continuity in review from meeting to meeting and, for an application that did not get funded the first time it was submitted, it often assures that at least one reviewer who reviewed an application previously will be available to review the application after it has been revised and resubmitted. NIH rules require the permanent membership on a standing study section to be balanced not only on the basis of scientific and technical expertise, but also on the basis of gender, ethnic/racial diversity, and geographical distribution. Ad hoc reviewers (nonpermanent members brought on for a single meeting) are used on standing study sections when the number of applications assigned to the review committee is more than the permanent membership can handle or when the expertise needed is outside that covered by the permanent membership.

Special emphasis panels are usually formed to review applications at a single meeting and then disbanded. Thus, all members of special emphasis panels are ad hoc reviewers. Special emphasis panels are commonly used to review applications that have been submitted in response to an RFA and to review applications that have been submitted in response to a PA with special review considerations. They are also commonly used when an application is submitted on which one or more members of a standing study section plays a key role and the research proposed in the application falls within the scientific domain of the member's own study section. To avoid any conflict of interest or perception of a conflict of interest, the application must be reviewed by a panel other than the standing study section. This is because all permanent members of a standing study section are considered to have a close working relationship, and close working relationships are considered to represent one type of conflict of interest in the peer review process. Such special emphasis panels are often referred to as member conflicts committees.

Another potentially useful bit of information about special emphasis panels is that their designation also reveals the NIH component responsible for constituting the review committee. As already mentioned, all special emphasis panel designations begin with the letter "Z." The "Z" is always followed by a two-letter code denoting the institute/center that the special emphasis panel belongs to. For example, the two letters DA refer to the National Institute on Drug Abuse, CA refers to the National Cancer Institute, and RG refers to the Center for Scientific Review (which until October 1, 1997, was known as the Division of Research Grants). Thus, ZDA1 would designate a special emphasis panel organized by NIDA; ZCA1 would designate a special emphasis panel organized by NCI; and ZRG1 would designate a special emphasis panel at CSR.

If an application does not get assigned to the review committee recommended by the principal investigator in a cover letter sent in with the application or if no recommendation was made, the principal investigator would be well advised to assess the review committee assignment for appropriateness and contact the scientific review administrator if any concerns arise.

The Roles of the Scientific Review Administrator in the Review Process

Peer review committees at NIH are managed by scientific review administrators. It is the scientific review administrator's responsibility to oversee all aspects of the peer review process and to ensure that every application assigned to his/her review committee receives a fair and appropriate review. Accordingly, if an investigator has any comments, questions, or concerns about any aspect of the review of his/her application, those issues should be taken up with the scientific review administrator to whose review committee the application was assigned. Scientific review administrators have plenty of work to do. Nonetheless, they are usually more than willing to help resolve concerns, especially those that occur prior to the meeting of the review committee, and particularly if it involves helping move the application to a more appropriate review committee. Contact information for the scientific review administrator should be available in the principal investigator's eRA Commons account.

A scientific review administrator's duties for those applications assigned to a given meeting are divided into premeeting, meeting, and postmeeting responsibilities, and each of these divisions is associated with deadlines. The vast majority of premeeting tasks are undertaken after the applications are submitted to NIH and are subsequently assigned to the review committee. All premeeting responsibilities must be concluded by the meeting date, and many of them, including identifying an appropriate cadre of reviewers, assigning the applications to reviewers, and mailing of the applications and other meeting-related documents to the reviewers, must occur several weeks before that. The day or days the review meeting actually takes place are when applications are discussed by the entire review committee and scores representing reviewers' judgment of the scientific and technical merits of the applications are assigned. Although the review committee's chairperson runs the review meeting, the scientific review administrator is present to ensure that applicable law, policy, and practice are followed. Within a few working days after the review meeting ends, scores for every application reviewed are calculated and released, under the authority of the scientific review administrator, into the NIH database where they are made available via the eRA Commons to principal investigators. The postmeeting period ends at the date the National Advisory Council or National Advisory Board meets. As soon as possible, which usually means within six to eight weeks of the end of a review meeting, summary statements for each application reflecting the deliberations of the review committee are prepared and released into the NIH database. As with the scores, this process makes the summary statements available via the Commons to principal investigators. It is important to have applications available to reviewers several weeks before the review meeting takes place in order for them to have sufficient time to read and properly evaluate each of their assignments. So, too, summary statements must be available several weeks before the council meets to allow council members adequate time to determine whether a fair and appropriate review occurred.

One of the first tasks a scientific review administrator undertakes for every batch of applications is to determine whether each application should be reviewed. All review committees have a scientific purview, and applications assigned to a review committee must fall within that area or be reassigned to another review committee with more appropriate expertise. Another consideration is eligibility— whether the applicant organization or investigative team is eligible for the type of grant being pursued. For RFAs, scientific review administrators evaluate applications for responsiveness because applications must sufficiently meet the aims and intentions of the RFA or they are considered nonresponsive and are returned without review. Scientific review administrators also check to see if each application meets the format, page limitations, and budget restrictions of the grant mechanism. If a scientific review administrator finds that some part of an application is either missing or in error, he/she may contact the principal investigator.

After performing an administrative review of the applications assigned to a review committee, the scientific review administrator determines the areas of scientific expertise needed to appropriately review each application. Once the range of expertise needed to review the entire batch of applications is known, reviewers who will participate in the review meeting are identified and the roster is made available (era.nih.gov/roster/index.cfm). For standing study sections, many if not most of the reviewers who will participate are already known. However, all ad hoc reviewers must be recruited. For special emphasis panels, this means the entire review committee must be recruited, and this process often takes several weeks. Each application is assigned to specific reviewers to read in detail, provide written critiques for inclusion in summary statements, and present to the rest of the review committee at the review meeting. Because scientific review administrators must ensure that all applications receive fair and appropriate reviews and because there are limitations to how many reviewers ought to be involved in a review meeting, efforts are made to enlist reviewers who have broad expertise rather than expertise specifically tailored to the precise details of every application. Also, because there are limits to the number of applications that can be assigned to reviewers and because some reviewers have broader expertise than others, applications may be assigned to reviewers who have adequate knowledge of the subject matter rather than to reviewers who have the most specific knowledge in a given area. Yet another factor affecting assignments is the increasing use of multidisciplinary research teams on applications. Appropriate review of these types of applications may require broad rather than more targeted expertise. Finally, committee deliberations are the result of all members discussing and scoring each application and not just a few selected individuals. Thus, all reviewers with relevant expertise have the opportunity to express their views about each application at a review meeting.

From time to time, investigators realize that errors were made in composing an application but these errors are not discovered until after the application is submitted to NIH. Such errors include mistakes in budget entries or calculations, missing reference citations, and the absence of a key word such as "not" in a sentence. If allowed to remain unchanged, these types of errors may negatively affect the review of their application. Also from time to time, investigators may acquire additional information that is relevant to the review of their application but that was not available at the time the application was submitted. Such information includes preliminary data for experiments proposed in the application or manuscripts described in the application that have since been published. In these cases, it is reasonable to contact the scientific review administrator of the review committee to which the application has been assigned to ask if he/she will allow supplemental information to be provided, especially if it will be sent to reviewers. Scientific review administrators are more likely to allow supplemental information if it is sent earlier in the process rather than when it is closer to the meeting date.

CONFLICTS OF INTEREST AND CONFIDENTIALITY

Critically important to a fair and appropriate review of applications, and to the integrity of the review process itself, is the assurance that all reasonable steps will be taken to preserve the confidentiality of the documents and other information provided by investigators, that conflicts of interest will be avoided, and that it will not be possible to attribute specific review comments or scoring recommendations to individual reviewers. For these reasons, all meeting related documents, including applications, appendix materials, supplemental materials, emails, and conversations are treated as confidential, and all persons involved are instructed these materials are not to be shared with anyone other than NIH staff with a need to know or review committee members who do not have a conflict of interest. It is also important to note that because of confidentiality rules, NIH staff will communicate information about an application only with the application's principal investigator. Information will not be communicated to a co-investigator, a mentor, a department chairperson, or a dean.

Conflicts of interest are of two types: real and apparent. Real conflicts exist when a reviewer or a close relative or professional associate has a financial or other interest in an application that is know to the reviewer, when a reviewer has a long-standing scientific or personal disagreement with the applicant, when a reviewer feels unable to provide an unbiased review, or when a reviewer is a salaried employee of the applicant institution. An apparent conflict of interest occurs when the relationship between an application/investigators and a reviewer would cause a reasonable person to question the reviewer's impartiality. A reviewer who works in the same area of science as that proposed in an application does not have a conflict of interest with the application merely because of this.

Some conflicts of interest are not easy to identify and would not be identified were it not for reviewers, investigators, or other NIH staff pointing them out. Examples include family members with different last names, close associates who have not published together, personal friends, and individuals involved in antagonistic relationships. Sometimes investigators include this type of information in the cover letter they send with their application. However, directly contacting the scientific review administrator is a more effective approach.

REVIEW CRITERIA

There are five standard review criteria for mechanisms whose designation begins with the letter "R" (e.g., R01, R03, and R21): significance, approach, innovation, investigators, and environment. Chapter 3 goes into significant detail on each of these five criteria. Other mechanisms, such as those for career development awards, institutional training grants, and individual pre- and postdoctoral fellowships, all have different sets of review criteria, which are clearly enumerated in the PAs for each of the mechanisms. What is important about making the review criteria available for all to know is that it helps make the review process fairer. Scientific review administrators ensure that reviewers use the appropriate set of review criteria, and knowledgeable investigators prepare their applications with the review criteria in mind.

Priority Scores and Percentiles

At a review meeting, all applications are rated by all reviewers participating in the review. In general, applications may be either scored or unscored. Scored applications are discussed at review meetings; unscored applications are not. In either case, summary statements are composed for every application containing written comments of at least two reviewers. In the case of scored applications, summary statements also contain a resume and summary of the discussion of the application that took place at the review meeting. The resume is written by the scientific review administrator and usually contains an explanation of those issues that led the review committee to score the application as it did.

NIH rules hold that reviewers are to determine which applications should be considered more meritorious and which are less meritorious. Those that are less meritorious do not receive a score. More meritorious applications are generally scored in a range from 1.0 to 3.0, where 1.0 represents the highest quality and 3.0 represents an application with substantive weaknesses. Within a few days of the end of the review, the individual reviewer scores are entered into the NIH database. The database then adds all the individual scores for an application, divides that sum by the number of scores used to calculate it, and multiplies the result by 100. The resultant value is called the "priority score." Once the accuracy of the input scores is verified, the scientific review administrator releases the system-generated priority scores so that they may be viewed by other NIH staff and by principal investigators using their eRA Commons accounts.

Percentiles are values used with standing study sections to indicate how a particular score ranks among others given by the same study section over a three-review-meeting period (usually one year). That is, all the scores that a standing study section has given during the current review meeting and the two meetings previously are amassed. Then an individual priority score is fit into that range, and the score's relative ranking in the range is computed, which in essence indicates what percentage of all applications reviewed over the three-round period the current score was better than. For example, an application that receives a priority score of 150 and a percentile of 4.2 indicates that that application was one of the most meritorious applications reviewed by that study section, since only 4.2% of the applications reviewed by that study section over the past year had a priority score better than 150. In this way, any score can be compared with others given by that study section over a one-year period. Also, however, percentiles allow NIH staff to compare scores given by different standing study sections. Thus a priority score of 150 may represent one of the most meritorious applications evaluated by one study section and have a very low percentile, whereas a 150 given by another study section may be only one of many similar scores given by that study section and have a higher percentile.

There is no uniformity across NIH concerning the number and types of mechanisms used to compute percentiles. Each institute/center determines which mechanisms will be used for its applications. In some institutes/centers, essentially only R01s are percentiled, whereas in others essentially all mechanisms are included, and still other institute/centers include some and not other mechanisms. In addition, because the computing of percentiles requires scoring behavior by a review committee over a three-meeting period, percentiles are computed only for applications reviewed by standing study sections and not for those reviewed by special emphasis panels, which meet only one time. Regardless of how they are computed, percentiles are used by NIH staff along with priority scores to help determine which applications to fund.

Summary Statements

Scientific review administrators assign each application to be reviewed to at least two reviewers to read in detail, who are also expected to prepare written comments and to present the application to the rest of the review committee at the review meeting. The written comments of the reviewers are collated into a document called the summary statement, which is prepared by the scientific review administrator before being made available to institute staff and the principal investigator. Summary statements are the official documents of the outcome of the review and contain, in addition to reviewers' critiques, the priority score the application received, a roster of the reviewers and federal review staff who participated, and the name and contact information of the program official to whom the application was assigned for funding determinations. Questions about the possibility of receiving funding and how to respond to the comments contained in the summary statement should be directed to the assigned program official.

Summary statements are made available as soon as possible after a review meeting, usually within six to eight weeks. Every application reviewed receives a summary statement, whether the application was scored or not. The only difference between the summary statements of scored and unscored applications is that the summary statements of scored applications also contain a paragraph called the Resume and Summary of Discussion, which appears near the top of the summary statement, that is written by the scientific review administrator and that describes the major strengths and weaknesses discussed by the review committee that led to the priority score the application received.

APPEALS

From time to time reviewers make errors of fact that substantially affect the priority score an application receives. It is therefore important for investigative teams to carefully read over the summary statement for their application to determine whether such errors may have occurred and, if any are found, to bring those to the attention of the program official to whom the application was assigned. If he/she concurs that the summary statement contains substantive factual errors that likely influenced the outcome of the review, the scientific review administrator should be contacted. If the scientific review administrator agrees that the application was unfairly judged, he/she will likely seek to have the application re-reviewed without any further action by the principal investigator. Should there be enough time before council review, the application may be re-reviewed the same round. If not, the application will be deferred to the next round for review. In those circumstances in which institute/center staff do not agree with a principal investigator as to the outcome of the review, there is still a path of redress that the principal investigator may pursue. It is called an appeal, and there is an official appeals process to follow (grants2.nih.gov/grants/guide/notice-files/not97-232.html). If an appeal is successful, the application will be re-reviewed and the existing summary statement will be withdrawn. If the appeal fails, the original review stands. Regardless of how a re-review is initiated, the application is reviewed in the same form and with the same supporting documents as were used by the original review committee. Principal investigators are not permitted to respond to reviewers' comments (since officially they no longer exist), and no new documents or supplemental information may be provided.

Seeking a re-review is not always the best course of action to take because of the delay it may cause. A re-review may merely push back the date when a revised application can be submitted. The advice and guidance of the program official to whom the application was assigned may be quite valuable in helping the principal investigator arrive at the decision to seek a re-review.

CONCLUDING REMARKS

NIH continually strives to make more and more of its operations transparent and to make available to investigators information about their grants and applications that is stored in the NIH database. With the amount of information that is currently available to investigators, there is little reason that the grants enterprise should be a black box to them or to their colleagues. The NIH staff, including program, review, and grants management officials, is available to interact with the extramural research community and should be contacted when questions, comments, or concerns arise. Establishing a network of contacts at NIH may prove, after all, to be beneficial to the health of an investigator's research grant portfolio.

2 Drug Abuse Research Collaboration in the Twenty-first Century

WILLIAM J. BUKOSKI & WILSON M. COMPTON

Challenge is the core and mainspring of all human activity. If there's an ocean, we cross it; it there's a disease, we cure it; if there's a wrong, we right it; it there's a record, we break it; and finally, if there's a mountain, we climb it.

—CLIMBER AND HISTORIAN JAMES RAMSEY ULLMAN

THE NATIONAL INSTITUTE on Drug Abuse (NIDA) has a long and rich tradition of partnering with the research community to formulate sound research programs, policies, and practices. This collaborative process has become even more important in today's complex research environment emphasizing team science, interdisciplinary research, and behavioral genomics. In order to meet the increased scientific demands encountered when studying complex diseases such as drug abuse and addiction, NIDA has expanded research management strategies by providing enhanced support for interdisciplinary research and scientific teams that have complementary expertise from a wide spectrum of genetic, behavioral, social, and medical research disciplines. In addition, NIDA has developed exciting new research opportunities and scientific forums for scientists to provide meaningful input into the research planning process. One key feature required to support dynamic interaction between members of the scientific community requires active involvement and discussion with NIDA program staff about emerging trends and future needs in science. Finally, the formation of the next generation of research scientists resides in the very capable hands of senior scientists who actively and effectively develop and implement high-quality scientific mentoring programs. Given this investment of time, talent, and inspiration, the future of research at NIDA appears promising given the prospects of exciting new scientific discoveries and the application of scientific findings to improve health through more effective prevention and treatment interventions.

TWO RECENT EXAMPLES OF RESEARCH COLLABORATION AT NIH

In an ideal world, partnerships between scientific leadership at any one of the NIH institutes or centers and independent research scientists across the nation lead to prudent and wise investment of limited research resources, increased viability of the nation's research infrastructure, enhanced opportunities for significant scientific discovery, and improved translation of science into practice. The key to actualization of scientific success in all of these areas is teamwork among the communities of federal, private sector, and university-based academic scientists.

To facilitate and promote these important collaborations, NIDA has fostered interdisciplinary research by participating in efforts to reengineer the fundamentals of research development, review, and research management currently underway at NIH. For example, NIDA actively participates in the NIH Roadmap for Medical Research initiative (nihroadmap.nih.gov; see appendix 1 for a brief description of key NIH Web site addresses) and the NIH Blueprint for Neuroscience Research initiative (neuroscienceblueprint.nih.gov). Both of these programs advance interdisciplinary biomedical research in basic, clinical, and translational sciences and promote team-oriented science. The NIH Roadmap is a trans-NIH initiative launched in 2004 with the purpose of deepening our understanding of the role that biology plays in various diseases, stimulating creation of interdisciplinary research teams, and reshaping clinical research to accelerate medical discovery and improve the nation's health. The roadmap consists of three major themes: New Pathways to Discovery, Research Teams of the Future, and Reengineering the Clinical Research Enterprise. The NIH Blueprint for Neuroscience Research initiative aims to develop new tools, resources, and training opportunities that can accelerate the pace of discovery in neuroscience research. The NIH Blueprint initiative was launched in 2004 and involves the NIH Office of the Director and 15 NIH institutes and centers that support research on the nervous system.

The Roadmap initiative was crafted after considerable exchanges between scientific leadership at NIH and the best scientific minds in the country, further assisted by special planning conferences, individual consultations, public review, discussion, and debate of the premises and concepts underlying this innovative new approach in NIH scientific management. Based upon a thorough review and discussion, the subsequent program planning process was acted upon by teams of NIH scientists who then developed a wide variety of Roadmap research program announcements (PAs) and requests for applications (RFAs) that address specific components necessary to advance the stated goals of these initiatives. To foster quick response by the scientific community, NIH provided set-aside research funds to pay for outstanding research projects that emerge from the peer review process tailored for each NIH Roadmap and Blueprint research activity.

Preliminary indications gleaned from the number of highly creative grant applications reviewed and funded thus far clearly indicate that both the Roadmap and Blueprint initiatives are outstanding success stories due in large measure to the collaborative and deliberative nature of the partnership between NIH and the scientific community at all stages of implementation. In order to accomplish the goals of the Roadmap and Blueprint initiatives, NIH recognizes the importance of developing scientific capacity that can address a variety of diseases and has sponsored *targeted research training grants* as part of both the Roadmap and Blueprint programs. As part of this portfolio of research activities, NIH also recognizes the importance of creating teams of scientists with diverse yet complementary skills spanning a wide array of medical and behavioral disciplines with an explicit goal of investigating complex diseases, such as substance use disorders. Toward this end, NIH held a two-day symposium on the topic of scientific collaboration that was sponsored by the Bioengineering Consortium (BECON). Focal topics included opportunities that might stimulate team capacity building, as well as perceived barriers that might hinder creating collaborative networks. BECON was created in 1997 by then NIH Director Harold Varmus as an effective means of linking all bioengineering activities at NIH. BECON is administered by the National Institute of Biomedical Imaging and Bioengineering under a federal mandate (www.becon2.nih.gov/becon.htm).

Many of the keys to effective teamwork in science discussed in this chapter are highlighted in a report issued by BECON. For more information on NIH team science and the recommendations for the field, see the published report located at www.becon.nih.gov/symposium2003.htm.

PUBLIC HEALTH SCIENCE FOR THE TWENTY-FIRST CENTURY AT NIDA

Several key principles for substance abuse research supported by NIDA were derived from the leadership at NIH and are related specifically to interdisciplinary research and scientific teamwork. Consistent with the NIH objectives outlined in the Blueprint initiative, a cornerstone for the NIDA research planning process in the twenty-first century heralds collaboration between the institute's scientific leadership and the scientific community. These collaborations will help foster seminal scientific discoveries, create research partnerships, promote active participation in NIDA-sponsored science symposia, and encourage ongoing dialogue with NIDA's scientific leadership at the division, branch, and working-group levels.

Investigators interested in the research portfolio at NIDA are encouraged to explore several basic steps that will help them become more informed and involved. First and foremost among these steps is widening grant and funding opportunities through expanded personal contacts at NIDA (this holds true for many of the NIH institutes and centers). These efforts should then be coupled with a more effective use of electronic Web sites to ferret out additional information. Appendix 1 lists many of these and related NIH Web sites, and this readily accessible information should become a staple part of any investigator's efforts to improve their operative knowledge of funding mechanisms and submission protocols.

Expansion of personal contacts serves investigators well by helping open new channels of communication with appropriate institute scientific staff. Potential applicants are encouraged to proactively contact scientific program staff in their area of research to discuss recent research findings; explore possible new directions for knowledge development, for example, hypothesis-driven research, interdisciplinary studies, translation research, and technology transfer; learn more about upcoming NIDA-sponsored scientific meetings, symposia, special tracks, or satellite meetings at annual conferences (e.g., Society for Prevention Research or the College of Problems of Drug Dependence); become aware of changes in NIH policy (e.g., the shift to electronic grant submission and the conversion from form 398 to form 424 [R&R]); and keep abreast of emerging research funding opportunities as described in NIH/NIDA PAs and RFAs. While these remain only a handful of the possible points of discussion, they are well within the purview of scientific staff to provide assistance and commentary to potential applicants.

REVIEW OF DRAFT SCIENTIFIC CONCEPTS

One of the most important conversations that can aid an applicant prior to formal peer review involves two integrated components: (1) holding preliminary discussions with program staff regarding a proposed research project, and (2) sharing with program staff a draft concept paper. The former component provides a two-way street for applicants to learn about how they can focus their research interests to better meet the institute's funding priorities. Likewise, these conversations open doors and help generate a wealth of ideas that enhance a proposal's strengths prior to submission and formal peer review. NIDA's division and branch scientific staff are well aware of the gaps in current research and can offer insight as to how newly released PAs and RFAs were crafted to attract specific types of innovative and meritorious studies that address current or perceived future deficits in scientific knowledge.

It goes without saying that all of the NIH institutes and centers also cherish applicants' specific research ideas regardless of whether these ideas specifically address current PA or RFA foci. The scientific leadership at the various institutes and centers recognize that ideas generated by applicants may bridge stated gaps in science, address a cornerstone notion required to advance the field, or proffer conceptually novel, albeit untested, areas of science. In this respect, applicants' knowledge of the scientific literature, their appreciation of any noted gaps in empirical findings, and their identification of critical new areas of study are essential to advance a division or institute's research portfolio and promote new horizons for their respective funding agenda. In many respects, the language of a PA or RFA is quite general and provides only suggested areas of future study. The PA and RFA announcements do not spell out specific study questions, nor do they endorse one research design over another. Likewise, funding announcements do not showcase a particular analytic framework that should be developed or implemented by the scientific community. Rather, these funding announcements make recommendations for further scientific inquiry based on what is known in the field and what might hold potential for the field given our current knowledge base. The choice of approach, technique, analysis, and conceptual orientation rests with the individual grant applicants and their respective scientific teams. By exploring new research opportunities suggested by PAs, the scientific community, by the very nature of the grant process, obtains new insight into untested waters. In this regard, individual applicants and their respective research teams collaborate with an institute's scientific leadership to jointly shape and enhance the future research agenda.

With respect to the second component, applicants may want to circulate a concept or draft paper that outlines their research interests. Draft papers often provide needed stimulus inside an institute and permit program staff to further scrutinize your ideas to see if they are consistent with the current research climate. Certainly, it does not hurt to find out prior to the huge commitment of time required to submit an application whether the research ideas are favored. Many times, center directors will draft a conceptual paper that outlines the focus of a new center or discusses how individual projects are intended to be linked together under the umbrella of a center prior to actually constructing the center application. If centers are not in favor at the time, or funds are severely limited, it pays to find out before the painstaking effort involved with constructing such a large and detailed application. Program staff may recommend that a P50 center be scaled back to a P30 with projects linked through cores or that R01 applications will fare better under the current climate of funding. Either way, the draft paper will help an investigator sort out the best grant writing strategy prior to engaging formal review.

If a draft paper does not fit with the current research climate, it can always be referred to another institute or center or sent to a different federal agency (education, justice, transportation, and mental health, to name a few examples). You can be assured that program staff will prepare a critique identifying strengths and/or weaknesses from the perspective of a potential institutional review group. Program staff will also suggest revisions to increase the application's competitive level, making sure that the research uses state-of-the-art instrumentation, contains a rigorous research design, uses innovative and appropriate data analytic methods, passes muster with regard to human subjects issues, and contains a high level of significance that will raise the eyebrows of reviewers.

FEEDBACK ABOUT NIH AND NIDA PEER REVIEW

The scientific program staff at the NIDA attend and listen carefully to the reviews of grant proposals submitted for evaluation under the NIH/NIDA peer review system. Because program staff attend many peer review committee meetings in person, they are in a unique position to share with applicants the review committees' concerns and expectations as expressed in the summary statements provided to applicants. These issues include reviewers' views of what makes an application competitive, what are the critical ingredients that advance current theory, what types of approaches contain methodologically rigorous research designs, and what kind of data and statistical analyses are considered state-of-the art in each of the core areas of the institute's science portfolio (e.g., basic, behavioral, treatment, epidemiology, services, prevention, and HIV/AIDS research).

As a result of observing the review committees' discussion of a specific application, members of program staff are able to provide meaningful elaboration to the written summary statement, particularly addressing points that may have adversely influenced a priority score. Moreover, program staff can offer insightful interpretation when select components or sections of an application are regarded as scientifically meritorious but the overall priority score is somewhat dampened by other prominent concerns. Interpretation of summary statements by program staff offers important insight on the nature of the review process and promotes a more thorough understanding of what generated any criticism or was responsible for any lingering concerns with a specific application. Other chapters in this book go into great length on how to handle revisions if necessary and also highlight the importance of contacting program staff prior to resubmission.

At another level, program staff can reflect on the research problems raised during the review and help inform subsequent research program planning initiatives by highlighting the complexities of some types of studies that may have not faired well during review. Problematic review outcomes across several grants may indicate to staff that a different strategy or tactic may be needed in order to address a particular gap in research. When this occurs, and several grants addressing a critical gap do not fare well during review, program staff may subsequently release a revised PA or develop a new research program to build institutional infrastructure, for example, through a research center mechanism. As a result of their internal analysis of peer review outcomes, coupled with the volume and content of submitted applications, the scientific community and program staff work together as they continually shape an institute's next generation of research programs.

FEEDBACK FROM REVIEW STAFF AT NIDA

Another very valuable NIDA resource includes members of NIDA's scientific review staff located in the Office of Extramural Affairs (OEA). This group of drug abuse scientists plans and manages the review process by organizing a variety of peer review committee meetings that target specific program areas at NIDA such as services research, research training, and proposals submitted in response to RFAs.

NIDA's review staff can provide information about the standards of review, procedures for review, disciplinary composition of review committees, and policy issues that crop up during review. In many cases, applicants want to know more about specific issues that arise during review, including recurring problems in assessment of human research protections, bars to funding, and the institute's handling of possible conflicts of interest between reviewers and the applicant undergoing grant review. Applicants are encouraged to direct specific questions on these and other similar types of topics to the appropriate OEA staff member. The same holds true for addressing specific questions to the scientific review administrator (SRA) selected to preside over the review committee. The SRA has a significant interest in preserving the integrity of the review process from start to end and can attend to important issues regarding compliance with NIH grant review policies.

In addition, NIDA's OEA staff serves as liaison to peer reviews conducted by the numerous study sections organized and administered by NIH's Center for Scientific Review (CSR). For example, in response to an applicant's question, NIDA's OEA staff may refer an investigator to a specific scientific staff member at CSR who could appropriately respond to such an inquiry. Likewise, OEA could refer an investigator to the CSR Web site where detailed information exists that can adequately address the applicant's information request.

SERVING ON A PEER REVIEW COMMITTEE AT NIH OR NIDA

An excellent opportunity to actively help shape any institute's research agenda involves serving as an ad hoc or charter member on any one of a variety of NIH peer review committees. Work of this nature can be time consuming; however, it provides a very important venue to exchange points of view with scientific peers concerning innovative and timely research studies that come before the committee for critical review. To explore this possible opportunity, investigators are encouraged to indicate their interest in serving as a peer reviewer and provide their qualifications to the OEA scientific staff member most related to the investigator's own substantive expertise. It goes without saying that each applicant's work as a peer reviewer can help shape the future direction of research funded by NIDA. Moreover, participation as an ad hoc or charter committee member can surely serve to expand an applicant's own scientific horizons. For example, during the review process, applicants may meet and establish working relationships with future collaborators, leading to sustained research activities addressing both current and future innovative research.

PARTICIPATION IN SCIENTIFIC MEETINGS AT NIDA

Another avenue for helping to shape the research agenda at NIDA involves participation as a presenter or as a member of the scientific audience in a variety of NIDA research meetings that occur over the course of the year. One approach is to discuss with NIDA program staff any forthcoming scientific meetings that might be of interest to you and your colleagues. The major purpose of scientific meetings at NIDA is to review and discuss the status of research findings in a given area of science and to explore possible new research directions to address gaps in the knowledge base. For example, over the past year, NIDA has sponsored scientific meetings on a variety of emerging topics such as HIV and drug abuse, children in foster care, application of social network analysis to the prevention of substance use and delinquency, health disparities, enhancing practice improvements in community-based care for drug prevention and treatment, and the role of faith-based groups in drug abuse research. Of importance here is that the scientific papers presented at NIDA meetings and the resulting discussions they prompt help program staff identify key research themes that may lead to new research initiatives in the near future. NIDA scientific meetings provide challenging and productive opportunities for the research community to offer input, guidance, and consultation addressing the current state of drug abuse science and the need for innovative research across a wide range of topics in drug abuse research.

NETWORKING YOUR WAY THROUGH THE NET

In order to more effectively network with scientific program staff at NIDA, potential applicants need to be well informed about the mission and research programs operating in the larger arena of science (NIH), within their specific institute (e.g., NIDA), and at the divisional level (e.g., the NIDA Division of Epidemiology, Services, and Prevention Research).

A number of federal Web sites provide a clear perspective of the mission, current scope of research sponsored by NIDA, summaries of the scientific knowledge base, new directions planned for future research, important policies and practices, and emerging changes in research administrative and management practices (appendix 1 showcases several of these Web sites at each level mentioned).

The starting point for networking at NIH is www.nih.gov/, and the NIDA Web site can be found at www.drugabuse.gov. These Web sites provide up-to-date information on the mission statements and organizational structure for different research divisions and offices, contact points for key scientific staff, descriptions of new research programs and information about research training opportunities, lists of forthcoming scientific meetings, press releases summarizing significant research findings and access to publications, tips on writing competitive research grants, a listing of current clinical research trials, abstracts of currently funded projects (available on CRISP, a public access database), data on NIH awards and success rates (see also chapter 1), and a variety of other important research application topics that can be directly accessed from these Web locations.

A very helpful Web site is the Research Assistant (www.theresearchassistant .com/), which provides a comprehensive array of tips, tools, and information to navigate the NIH world of behavioral research, from formulating research questions to writing competitive research grants. A second and more recently created NIH Web site, the New Investigators Program (grants.nih.gov/grants/ new_investigators/index.htm), targets new investigators and provides very informative links to research Web sites, and special resources that help jump-start careers. For example, NIH recently announced a new funding mechanism for new investigators titled Pathway to Independence Award. It combines a mentored K award (K99) with a research grant (R01). More information on this new NIH program and others of interest for new investigators can be found at the New Investigators Program Web site.

Vigilant monitoring of Web sites at NIH and NIDA serves to expand an applicant's knowledge base regarding the various interests and funding directions at NIH and NIDA. In addition to federal Web sites, prominent scientific journals have Web sites that frequently provide invaluable guidance to early career scientists who are seeking information and guidance on a variety of training and career development topics such as competing for prestigious postdoctoral training, getting hired, obtaining funding, research grant resources, publishing, and a wide range of logistical concerns including time management vis-à-vis workload, laboratory protocols and procedures, personnel opportunities, teaching, tenure and other professional issues, immigration requirements, and tips on joining scientific networks and various listservs to promote interaction between potential future research collaborators (senior and peer level). For example, the American Association for the Advancement of Science sponsors a very helpful Web site for postdocs and junior faculty that provides timely articles on advancing one's scientific career (sciencecareers.sciencemag.org/). The Academic Scientists' Toolkit, can be found at sciencecareers.sciencemag.org/career_development/.

FORMATIVE DEVELOPMENT OF THE NEXT GENERATION OF NIDA RESEARCHERS

The basic building block of team science and science in general is the fundamental professional relationship that gets established between a senior scientific mentor and predocs, postdocs, trainees, students, junior faculty members, and professional colleagues. To a large degree, science is based upon meaningful and time-honored collaborations between senior colleagues and pre- and postdoctoral students who embody the future of the scientific enterprise. Essential to this collegial team building process is mentoring. So important are these topics that several chapters in this book are devoted exclusively to K-series mentored research awards (chapter 11), F31 and F32 fellowships (chapter 6), and T32 training grants (chapter 12).

NIH has recognized that mentoring is a key component to accelerate scientific careers to reach professional independence signified by the award of a scientist's first R01 grant. A recent National Academy of Sciences (NAS) report[1] indicates that the average age to reach scientific independence at NIH is 42 and that fewer than four percent of research awards at NIH in 2002 were granted to new investigators. The NAS report stresses the importance of increasing opportunities for new investigators at NIH and providing research-training programs that enhance scientific mentoring in order to address this problem. Toward this end, NIH recently announced a pilot program to expedite review of grant applications submitted by new investigators. More information on this program for new investigators can be found at grants.nih.gov/grants/guide/notice-files/NOT-OD-06-013.html (see appendix 1).

ESSENTIAL STAGES IN THE MENTORING PROCESS CONDUCTED BY SENIOR RESEARCHERS

As mentioned above, the role of mentoring cuts across several important grant mechanisms and is covered elsewhere in this book. Mentoring is such a crucial element of successful grant writing that it is worth mentioning from a different vantage point and is thus covered in some detail in this chapter, as well. A number of well-established and recognized stages in the mentoring process include (1) finding a high-quality scientific mentor who is committed to a new investigator's career development, (2) becoming a scientific mentor to early career scientists just entering the field or to well-qualified scientific peers from an allied discipline who represent potentially new collaborators on an interdisciplinary or multidisciplinary research study, and (3) creating a systematic mentoring program by recruiting and training highly promising pre- or postdoctoral fellows and early-career scientists as part of an existing research laboratory or designated center. This latter effort can be conducted under the rubric of an NIDA Research Training Center using the T32, T90, or K12 NIH institutional grant mechanism to train groups of highly promising pre-/postdoctoral fellows and mentored scholars (for more on this particular mechanism, see chapter 12).

What better way to influence the research agenda of NIDA (or, for that matter, any institute or center) than to be integrally involved in shaping the hearts, minds, and motivations of the next generation of drug abuse research scientists. Graduates of mentored research training programs experience significant advancement in their careers, including visible achievements in research, teaching, business and industry, and research administration at the federal level. Mentoring of the next generation of research scientists by senior researchers is one of the most important keys that can effectively shape and influence the future research agenda, promoting ongoing collaborative studies and inculcating expansion of future funding and career development opportunities for future research scientists.[2] Of all of the critical choices that graduate students can make about their academic training and preparations for a career in public health research, none is more important than identification, selection, and cultivation of a mutually beneficial mentoring experience with a senior scientist.[3]

One important feature that characterizes high-quality mentoring involves promoting a student's networking with other scientists who can fill in vital gaps regarding knowledge, experiences, and career opportunities. Good mentors introduce their students to other key scientific faculty within their department, institution, and at other centers of excellence. This process leads to expansion of career opportunities and additional and specialized training to meet the needs and interests of the student and provides for meaningful connections with other scientists who share the same or similar research interests. Good mentors build a community of scientists who can benefit their students not only during their training but also in the years to come.

GIVING BACK TO THE FIELD OF SCIENCE BY MENTORING NEW INVESTIGATORS

Becoming a scientific mentor to pre- or postdoctoral fellows, junior faculty members, or accomplished scientists from other disciplines who are collaborating on a multidisciplinary research project is a hallmark of professional development as a senior scientist. Nevertheless, an even higher level of giving back to the field requires organizing and managing a formal interdisciplinary/multidisciplinary research training program at your institution by becoming a training director and principal investigator under the aegis of an NIH T32, T90, or K12 institutional training mechanism. There are a number of research-training funding opportunities at NIH. For example, a recent NIH Roadmap research-training program provides support for senior scientists to establish institutional predoctoral training in clinical and translational science. This PA can be found at grants.nih.gov/grants/guide/notice-files/NOT-RM-06-008.html.

For detailed information on standard, Roadmap, and Blueprint research training funding opportunities, applicants should consult the appropriate sections of the NIH home page. Under a variety of research training awards, including Ruth L. Kirschstein National Research Service Awards for pre- and postdoc fellows (F30, F31, F32) and institutional training centers (T32) and or Mentored Career Development Awards (K01, K08, K23, K12), a senior scientist takes the responsibility for establishing high-quality academic training opportunities and superior lab or field research experiences for the next generation of research scientists at NIDA. To obtain additional information, see the NIH research training Web site at grants2.nih.gov/training/extramural.htm.

The task of mentoring requires dedication, commitment, and sacrifices in that extensive quality time and attention are required by a senior mentor to ensure that each scientist in the training program receives the necessary technical preparation to successfully compete and contribute to science and subsequently become an independent research scientist in drug abuse research.

Over the course of time, not only has it been repeatedly demonstrated that high-quality scientific mentoring leads to outstanding scholarship from graduates of these programs, but also history shows that high-quality mentoring leads to significant scientific discoveries and forward progress in a given field of research. Likewise, time has shown that graduates of high-quality scientific mentoring programs provide outstanding leadership to the field and in numerous ways have shaped the research agenda of NIH and its constituent institutes. Generally speaking, research scientists who have received high-quality mentored training have become today's influential scientists and frequently are also those senior mentors who take on the additional professional responsibility of training the next generation of scientists. Thus, the circular effect of receiving high-quality mentoring and eventually becoming a high-quality mentor reinforces the strengths of this program to achieve scientific promise for the individual and benefit society as a whole.

SUMMARY AND CONCLUDING REMARKS

NIDA facilitates scientific collaboration with the scientific community to shape and advance basic and public health substance abuse research through a variety of approaches. This chapter has (1) described how NIDA encourages the scientific community to help formulate the research agenda at NIDA, (2) illustrated how NIDA advances innovative new science through technical assistance and guidance to researchers who are developing research ideas, (3) delineated a number of Web-based resources that assist researchers to effectively participate in sponsored research programs at NIDA, and (4) described the essential role of senior scientists to train the next generation of researchers whose funding is part of the research portfolio at NIDA.

A Brief Guide to the Essentials of Grant Writing

Lawrence M. Scheier

The whole of science is nothing more than a refinement of everyday thinking.

—Albert Einstein, *Out of My Later Years*

This chapter focuses on three cardinal issues related to successful grant writing and grant production skills. In the first part of this chapter, I review the five essential review criteria used specifically for research-based grants (e.g., R01, R03, and R21). Many of these review criteria permeate reviewers' mindsets and are used as a template to evaluate and critique a wide range of grants. The five review criteria have come to represent a "schema" that underlies the mental process by which reviewers assign a score to a grant. Taking readers inside the peer review process should be very helpful to investigators and applicants new to the grant submission process and help formalize review criteria even to the more seasoned reader. Grant reviews are not a "crapshoot" as one of my esteemed colleagues once said. Rather, grant reviews illustrate quite nicely how scientists formulate their view of the future and regard scientific progress.

Following the section examining review criteria, I then present materials examining Specific Aims, which receive a lion's share of attention during peer review. Poorly constructed aims can portend the death knell for a grant, given their centrality to the overall research synthesis presented in a grant. Many a reviewer painstakingly searches a grant to see whether investigators have linked their research plan to the aims. Questions surface during review regarding whether applicants tied their aims to the analytic plan and whether the research design permits addressing the specific aims. Reviewers will pose the question of whether addressing the stated aims scientifically provide a means to acquire new knowledge and accrue significant findings. It is therefore prudent to spend some time querying whether the aims are tethered to the science outlined in the grant application and whether the aims adequately highlight the significance of the research.

A third and final section provides additional detail examining specific features of successful grants and also attends to the more salient reasons why some grants fail. Wrapped up into this section is a discussion of the ardors of scholarship, the latter concern hindering some grants from receiving better priority scores. As a piece of advice, this last section on scholarship should permeate the reader's mindset when examining the remaining chapters in this book. Scholarship, as you will find out, provides a springboard from which to embark on all your writing efforts, whether you are a novice grant writer or a more seasoned professional with storage cabinets full of publications. Regardless of style and acumen, scholarship is central to the process of making headway in science, since scholarship is tethered to the process of communication and is the fundamental means through which we share our knowledge. Lacking written (or, for that matter, oral) communication skills, a grantee is doomed to failure or at least to play a minor role in a laboratory. Poor scholarship can jettison a career faster than any single contributing factor, and if you look around at successful grant writers, they have been able to obtain much higher professional stature based almost entirely on their ability to write logically and coherently (politics plays a crucial role in establishing success, but that requires another serious tome to cover adequately).

PACKAGING GRANTS AND JUMP-STARTING CAREERS

It is fitting that this chapter begins with a quote from Albert Einstein regarding science. I truly believe that the underlying premise of this chapter is about "refinement" of ideas, writing style, and presentation. Refinement and polishing existing ideas is not a new concept to me. I have spent a large portion of my professional training riding on the coattails of some giants in the field of psychology. In one case, I worked in a laboratory renowned for its synthesis of two prominent models or theories of human behavior: self-efficacy[1-3] and problem behavior theories.[4] The melding together of these two models of human action (for lack of a better descriptive term) resulted in one of the most highly acclaimed, evidence-based, school-based drug abuse prevention programs, Life Skills Training. (A wealth of scientific information and commercial product availability on this program can be found at www.lifeskillstraining.com, www.med .cornell.edu/public.health/prevention.html, and www.med.cornell.edu/ipr/.)

During the years I worked with Dr. Gilbert J. Botvin, Professor of Public Health and Psychiatry at Weill Medical College of Cornell University, we had countless late-night conversations about research productivity, grant writing, politics, and family. I treasure these conversations because he was my mentor, collaborator, and friend. I also treasure them because he laid out before me a plan describing how to become a successful grant writer. He answered questions truthfully and honestly. Possessing a young, capacious, and eager mind, I would ask him about his daily schedule, how much time he spent writing, how he formulated his grant ideas, and what strides I needed to make professionally and personally to obtain an equal level of success (or at least be equally prolific). Like a dart board in an Irish pub, he fielded every question and answered them methodically, thoughtfully, and with an earnest eye toward my professional education. Over time, and after several of these thought-provoking late-night meetings, I came to understand that much of what we do for a living concerns "refinement" of existing ideas and theories.

From these and related conversations, one additional item I was able to glean is that the days of the influential psychologists, including Clark Hull, William James, Gordon Allport, Albert Bandura, Edward Tolman, B. F. Skinner, J. P. Guilford, and Kurt Lewin, are over.[5] I also learned that we should not make our careers endless struggles to push the event horizon but rather focus on elaboration and application. In fact, the laboratory at Cornell University Medical College (Institute for Prevention Research) was able to create a successful bridge between basic science (drug abuse etiology) and application (developing and testing school-based drug abuse and violence prevention programs) by focusing on making a difference in the lives of youth through the introduction of cognitive-behavior programs. Our laboratory focused on prevention in action, where causes and consequences, scientific method, and theories of behavior forged a confluence. In this respect, perhaps the most important comment ever given to me by any mentor, professor, or colleague, was a statement by Dr. Botvin to the effect that "the best grant writers are hard-working individuals, some brilliant, others less fortunate in this regard, but all very focused."

When push comes to shove, most grants suffer from largesse, that is, too much information, too many disparate ideas, and too much ambition. As another mentor, himself a highly acclaimed and well-funded drug prevention researcher, once said, "A lot goes into learning how to focus, benefiting from this focus, and then focusing your career." It is thus imperative that we follow this advice, acquire the requisite skills so that our grants address specific and well-delineated ideas, and comport with the rigors of science and peer review. In the words of Einstein, we should continually strive toward refinement.

A BRIEF SYNOPSIS OF THE NIH REVIEW AND SCORING CRITERIA

The NIH scoring template for independent research grants (e.g., R01, R21, and R03) consists of five individual sections required for most reviews: significance, approach, innovation, investigators, and environment. There are some noted exceptions to this review template, and these are handled in the individual chapters that follow. Specifically, readers will find more extensive review criteria elaborated in chapter 9 detailing center grants (P), which require an initial review procedure to determine "centeredness"; chapter 6 on fellowships (F), which evaluate grades and scholastic performance for pre- and postdoctoral candidates; chapter 12 on training awards (T), which include standards for educational components and productivity with regard to mentoring; chapter 11 on independent mid-career and senior scientist awards (K), which contain extensive review criteria based on the candidate's accomplishments, their career plans, and training goals; and chapter 13 on other grant mechanisms (SBIR or STTR) that contain specific review criteria regarding plans for commercialization and distribution of products and how different production and marketing phases are linked.

It is generally understood that the five evaluative components serve as guidelines for the written reviews (summary statements) received by applicants. In many review cycles, these five basic components go as far as to help frame the reviewers' comments during the oral presentation of a review and further help structure any formal discussion among reviewers. When a reviewer starts to dissect an application during peer review, the usual point of departure is a brief discussion covering a summary of the goals of the application. This conversation then advances to a more detailed discussion regarding the significance of the study. Reviewers must always keep in mind that not all members of the internal review group or special emphasis review panel have read the application (or read the application in its entirety). Therefore, in order for the study section members to follow the specific critique that will follow, it is imperative for them to be cognizant of what the study proposes to examine and whether the application is perceived as a significant piece of research that will advance science overall.

The review criteria also serve another distinct function during peer review. Sometimes, and as is often the case when there are discordant scores from different reviewers, a chairperson will go down the list of review criteria, asking for summarization of the key points. In other words, the study section chair will ask, "Did you feel the study was significant, was the approach consistent with current methods, was there an element of innovation, was the investigator appropriately trained, and was their environment supportive?" This point-by-point analysis helps other reviewers in the room prepare themselves to cast a score and find some middle ground in light of the discrepant scores provided by the primary and secondary reviewers. In many respects, the evaluative scoring criteria are critical to successful grant writing because they form an objective means to gauge each application's scientific merit.

In order to obtain consensus during a review, there must be a consistent set of guidelines on which to conduct any review, and to a large degree, the five evaluative criteria used for research grants provide this much needed framework. From my own experience (and my colleagues contributing to this book agree with me in principle), in the days leading up to the grant review and especially as reviewers gear up for their visit to Washington and pore over the application materials, reviewers begin to rely more strongly on a cognitive template or mental framework that helps guide them toward their eventual score (cognitive psychologists would call this template a "schema"). The template consists of certain essential requirements articulated as part of each select funding mechanism and also more general requirements that touch on editorial and presentation concerns (we deal with these issues separately at the end of the chapter). Without question, some reviewers get bent out of shape when grants are not grammatically correct, missing documentation, or simply sloppy. However, most reviewers try to absorb the science first. What will hurt any application is weakness in the science (i.e., the application contains some probing questions but uncertainty about the approach) that is further exacerbated by shoddy writing and a poorly constructed grant (I touch on scholarship and grammar later).

Once reviewers are selected by the various NIH institutes for a particular review (or if they are members of a standing committee), they receive a packet from the institute that arrives about four to five weeks prior to the scheduled review. Along with the individual applications, each reviewer receives a summary scoring sheet (these materials are confidential and must be destroyed immediately following completion of the review). A separate form includes a synopsis of the five basic review criteria (guidelines). If the grant mechanism is unique or if there have been changes in the review criteria, the packet also will include a brief description of the PA or RFA and descriptive information. While most seasoned reviewers have developed institutional memory for the five scoring criteria, they do change from time to time (grants1.nih.gov/grants/peer/peer.htm), and therefore NIH includes a one-page synopsis with each review packet. The review guidelines help steer reviewers toward making concise written comments tethered to the five evaluative criteria. The five criteria also help reviewers remain streamlined during their roundtable conversation.

SCORING

A brief digression into scoring is necessary at this point, particularly because the review criteria help formulate a score. Prior to conducting a review, the institute or center provides reviewers with reams of paperwork. One important piece of paper graphically portrays the priority scoring anchors and is reproduced for readers in figure 3.1. The guide is intended to help reviewers score the scientific merit of an application and is meant for illustrative purposes, not as a complete guide. Reviewers can use their own discretion in applying a score and may not follow the illustrative guide. For instance, an application may contain serious problems in one or more aims that help drag the overall score down. However, a reviewer may point out that these aims are peripheral and not central to the application, thus bolstering a higher score. Naturally, this issue would surface during discussion of the application, but reviewers may disagree as to how germane these aims are and whether the poorly constructed or problematic aims should influence the overall priority score. An application also may suffer from problems in the approach (methods) but reviewers note the application is considerably innovative and would make a significant contribution to the field regardless of the problems in design or methodology. Thus, while it is hard to arrive at a single score, and the process is not foolproof, the final score is reflective of each reviewers scoring based on the priority score range.

With this information in mind, a goal of the present chapter is to provide insight into the cognitive framework used by reviewers as they read over a grant (sometimes, to an applicant's chagrin, grants are read hastily the night before a review). Each of the five review criteria is discussed in detail, with comments enumerated regarding potential pitfalls and remedies. For your benefit, appendix 1 shows how to access various NIH Web sites and obtain detailed definitions of these particular five criteria and other important review guidelines.

Figure 3.1. Scoring Ranges for NIH Grant Reviews

Priority Score Range	Balance of Strengths and Weaknesses
1.0–1.9	1.0 Many substantial strengths; few, if any minor weaknesses Many strengths and some remediable weaknesses 1.9
2.0–2.9	2.0 Several strengths, some problems Limited or few strengths and/or many problems 2.9
3.0–5.0	Limited or few strengths and/or serious problems

Again, the five guidelines or review criteria are significance, approach, innovation, investigator, and
environment.

Significance

Sadly, many a reviewer has read over
an application and, despite finding
outstanding scholarship, has not been
able to find a single sentence outlining

> ### Significance Criteria
> Does the study address an important prob-
> lem? If the aims of the application are
> achieved, how will scientific knowledge or
> clinical practice be advanced? What will be
> the effect of these studies on the concepts,
> methods, technologies, treatments, services,
> or preventive interventions that drive this
> field?

the application's significance. In order to understand how crucial this portion is
to the overall scoring of an application, it is essential that to outline what is meant
by "significance." Significance taps the overall scientific questions and problems
addressed by the application. Significance relates to the pressing questions faced
by NIH addressing the general public health agenda and also the portfolio of
concerns specified for the various institutes and centers. An application sent to
NIMH examining synaptic transmission under the influence of cocaine in rhesus
monkeys may not fit with the current zeitgeist at NIMH (this application would
propose an animal model for testing behavioral drug effects). However, the same
application couched to include examination of the effects of an illicit drug on
synaptic transmission in schizophrenics may dovetail nicely with the current
NIMH portfolio of research activities. This example is used only for illustrative
concerns. Readers interested in learning more about current foci at the various
institutes or centers should consult their respective Web sites as well as carefully
scrutinizing the CRISP database at the eRA Commons to determine the current
funding pattern (crisp.cit.nih.gov/).

Second, and somewhat related to this first point, it is imperative that applicants realize that, by themselves, statistics do not make an application compelling. Most of us have heard the infamous quote attributed to Mark Twain
(1924), "There are three kinds of lies—lies, damned lies, and statistics."[6] This
humorous line contains some truth, and there is little point in providing a litany
of statistics as the sole means to outline a problem. In fact, many an applicant
makes this mistake by usurping almost the entirety of Section B (sometimes
termed "Background" or "Background and Significance") to present the "statistical problem" and not elaborate the "real problem." The argument proffered
by the applicant is that, if enough people have the problem (use of some drug or
some medical disorder), then all efforts under the public health agenda should
focus on remediation of the problem.

Let me expand on this issue for one minute. Consider an application focusing on prevention of cigarette smoking in youth. Pretend for a minute that
you are a reviewer assigned to an internal review group dealing with an RFA for
cigarette smoking interventions targeted to youth. First, we need to establish

some facts regarding prevalence of smoking among youth. You read an application, which contains recent national epidemiological survey data and reports that 13% of American youth (ages 12–17) reported using a tobacco product in the past month.[7] Moreover, the application goes on to state, although the rate of past month cigarette smoking is actually declining (from 13% to 10.8% over a three-year period), the fact remains that 1 in 10 youth smokes regularly. The application provides additional detail indicating that among older youth (14–15 years of age), 9.2% are current smokers, and this figure gets even higher, reaching 20.6%, among youth between the ages of 16 and 17.

Unfortunately, there is little public health significance associated with these data, particularly given the observation that prevalence rates for adolescent cigarette use have been fairly steady over the past 10 years (although this observation may be the focal topic of a separate grant to examine why cigarette use has not declined in light of the large infusion of prevention money to reduce tobacco use among our nation's youth).

To summarize, statistical arguments stripped of any theoretical connections or practical meaning do not excite reviewers or wet their appetites. What is required is a stronger case made for these data in the context of the public health agenda, with regard to focal prevention efforts, and in terms of theories central to explain human behavior (i.e., social learning, social influence, or theory of planned behavior, to illustrate a few). It is possible to extend this argument to include other focal topics that are important with regard to the public health agenda. For instance, it is well known that a significant proportion of the population do not restrict their dietary intake of fatty high-risk food, and likewise, recent data show that a growing number of children can be considered obese using reliable measures of body mass index.

Added to this, transportation and traffic safety data show that many youth drive without using their seatbelts. Stating the obvious does not render an application significant unless it can be somehow linked either with a study of associated risks (etiology) or with efforts focusing on preventing these behaviors. In the case of cigarette use, it is clear that if we do not stop youth from experimenting with cigarettes, a substantial portion will go on to become adult smokers and increase their volume of smoking. An applicant would make a much stronger case underlying significance by examining prevention of medical diseases related to cigarette use. For instance, there are ample data showing that lung cancers, chronic obstructive pulmonary disease, respiratory problems, kidney disease, heart disease, and other medical maladies are related to cigarette use (or any tobacco use, including smokeless tobacco). Tying together the medical argument with the theoretical models that argue cigarettes are a stepping stone to other forms of drug use makes a much stronger case for the significance of the proposed slate of research.

To summarize, what makes an application of this scope and focus significant is joining together the consequences of these behaviors in terms of morbidity and mortality with the fact that many of these behaviors are preventable. Stopping youth from smoking their first cigarette with an evidence-based smoking prevention program that can be readily delivered in the schools can have a significant impact on later coronary heart and respiratory disease and lower mortality rates. In this respect, what needs to be highlighted in these few sample cases are the risks we run if we do nothing with regard to the behaviors in question. For instance, what would happen if we avoid developing prevention trials to stop youth from smoking, or fail to recognize the importance of dietary control for obese youth attending schools (where we can control to some degree their nutritional intake), or do not create stringent guidelines for seatbelt usage among new drivers, and so forth. The public health significance should be the focus of this section of the application, and not a rehashing of statistics showing that some particular problem remains fixed on the radar screen.

While these few examples are meant only to illustrate a potential "trap" applicants face when constructing the significance section of an application, it represents a dangerous trap if they do not take care to correctly position the significance of their grant application. Significance bears directly on three essential concerns: (1) does the study address an important problem, (2) will the proposed research help advance scientific knowledge and inform public policy, and (3) in the event the study gets implemented, will it stimulate changes in the concepts, methods, technologies, treatments, services, or preventive interventions that drive the field? In addition to these concerns, less salient but equally important concerns include (4) whether federal (or state) expenditures will solve the problem articulated in the grant (fiscally prudent?), and (5) whether the proposed research identifies or recognizes a new but as of yet undetected problem (i.e., violence in the schools) that may quickly logjam our national public health agenda. Attention to these issues is of paramount importance if we are to be prepared, as a society, for the next generation of social and health problems.

There are two places where an applicant can both easily highlight the significance of an application and seamlessly connect this statement with the general content of the grant. First, applicants can place a statement regarding significance in the opening paragraph of the grant as part of Section A preceding the detailed listing of Specific Aims (please make this only one paragraph at most!). The statement should articulate the significance of the application in its entirety with a synopsis of the research program. The example provided in box 3.1 comes from a revised R21 grant (funded), and the text appears before the Specific Aims (the different pagination in this book makes the text look longer!).

Whether an applicant chooses to use the R03, R21, or R01 mechanism, all three require a statement of significance. Many other mechanisms do, as well, and

Box **3.1**   Sample Significance Presented Before Specific Aims

This revised R21 proposal addresses the concepts and research imperatives put forth by the NIH Office of Behavioral and Social Sciences Research in their report "Progress and Promise in Research on Social and Cultural Dimensions of Health: A Research Agenda" and more recently included in PA-02-043. Both the NIH report and program announcement outline a compelling research agenda that focuses on examining social and cultural dimensions of health. The report includes suggestions to improve the measurement and clarify the meaning of basic constructs used in health research including race, ethnicity, and culture. In response to these and related concerns, the present study articulates a research agenda that examines the personal meaning of ethnic identity using novel experimental, memory-based strategies. These strategies will be applied using middle ($N=300$) and high school students ($N=300$) as a means of determining whether maturational factors influence ethnic identity formation. As part of a second integrated research component, a one-year prospective study will examine the stability and predictive utility of ethnic identity (using both age cohorts: $N=2000$ combined). The need to amplify our understanding of how social and cultural factors influence health behaviors is particularly noteworthy in the field of adolescent drug prevention where there exists little scientific explanation for noted racial differences in prevalence rates and psychosocial vulnerability. The absence of key information on drug etiology can hinder the development of effective prevention efforts and limit the applicability of existing intervention strategies. At present, there exists no uniformity with regard to research emphasizing measurement of social and cultural influences (i.e., ethnicity and ethnic identity) and there exists little consensus on the precise mechanisms through which identity factors influence the early stages of drug use. Therefore, the proposed study is both innovative in its reliance on novel experimental approaches to learn more about memory accessibility of social and cultural constructs, and in its application of multivariate statistical approaches to develop a more refined understanding of how ethnicity and identity influence drug use. The proposed research is divided into a 12-month developmental and pilot phase, a 12-month prospective study phase, and a 12-month data analysis/scientific dissemination phase.

the chapters on P50 grants, SBIR grants, and K-series grants mentioned above all describe requirements for sections outlining significance of the research. Given that a portion of the application will highlight significance, it is imperative then that each applicant choose where to best locate this information. There is nothing wrong, for instance, in combining the section on significance with the section detailing background. In fact, the overall significance of the proposed research can be stated succinctly in one or two paragraphs, the remaining portion of the background section can be used to detail the problem and provide epidemiological data to support any arguments or research goals, and the remaining text can be used to create a "story" outlining why this particular body of research addresses a "significant public health problem."

The example given in box 3.2 provides an alternative way to state the study's significance. Both methods can be combined (as they were in the R21 example in box 3.1). The materials contained in box 3.2 summarize the strengths of the study and were presented right before the section containing preliminary findings (Section C). Both methods continually highlight the strengths of the study design, the novelty or innovation associated with using implicit cognition memory associative techniques, and the need to find alternative ways to study "identity" as it relates to drug use.

A second place to concisely state a study's significance takes shape as a summary paragraph embedded at the end of Section D (Experimental Design). This is as good a place for applicants to summarize their research agenda as any other place in the application and should be inserted as the last paragraph before introducing Section E (Human Subjects). Box 3.3 provides a sample summarization paragraph from a funded R01 grant. The summarization paragraph should not only highlight the overall significance of this research in the event the study achieves it goals, but also highlight significant features associated with the application, including but not limited to special features of the sample, data collection methods, assessment strategies, special strengths and expertise of the investigative team, enhancements provided through consultants and collaborations (multisite investigations), and extension of current theory or applications of new statistical innovations not tested explicitly.

> **Approach**
>
> Are the conceptual or clinical framework, design, methods, and analyses adequately developed, well integrated, well reasoned, and appropriate to the aims of the project? Does the applicant acknowledge potential problem areas and consider alternative tactics?

Approach

"Approach" concerns the experimental design, statistical analyses, and methodology (i.e., sampling) used to conduct the study. It is critical that investigators take a long hard look at the words that describe "approach" (e.g., well integrated, reasoned, and appropriate). Failure to attend to these "connections" in the body of the grant could represent a fatal flaw. This is particularly true if the reviewer possesses methodological skills and is looking to see beyond the substantive arguments whether the grant pulls together the loose ends of theory, hypotheses, and analysis. This issue was of paramount importance in my earliest grant applications (R29 and R01) and became a raison d'être for my focus on linking theory with appropriate methods and statistics.

Box 3.2 Summary of Concerns

To summarize, there have been numerous recent attempts to develop psychometrically sound and theoretically driven measures of racial/ethnic identity. Despite these efforts, certain methodological and conceptual problems remain unresolved. In some cases, scales are far too abbreviated (less than 20 items to tap multiple dimensions or in some cases 5 items to assess a single dimension), homogeneous with regard both to scale content (one-dimensional scales tapping solely participation in cultural activities) and the respective focal population. In fact, there are only a handful of scales that purport to be able to assess ethnic identity in multiple groups (black and Hispanic), whereas a majority of scales were designed specifically to assess ethnic identity in black or Hispanic youth only. Additionally, in many cases assessment of ethnic identity has been confused with acculturation or scale development has been markedly lacking in theory. Only a handful of researchers have investigated whether racial identity is a core part of an individual's overall identity (i.e., self-concept). This may represent an important conceptual oversight leading to a diminished view of ethnic identity as a type of "racial preference" tapping acceptance of race-specific physical features. In fact, there may be a hierarchical ranking of identities, where ethnic or racial identity represents one component tier formatively linked with other tiers culminating in an integrated "personal identity." The need to employ a multidimensional conceptualization of ethnic identity highlights additional methodological concerns. For instance, many researchers have relied solely on exploratory factor analysis methods to derive dimensional structures for assessing ethnic identity. As a result there exists some uncertainty with regard to the psychometric soundness of many existing measures. Rotational and extraction methods may vary considerably from one study to another contributing to disparate psychometric findings. An even more compelling issue pertains to what Cross (1991) labeled "experimenter-ascribed identity," which refers to experimenter's assumptions regarding racial or ethnic identity based on physical characteristics without attending to the wealth of psychological experience that underlies identity formation[B1]. The strategy of downscaling items written for adult samples to fit ethnic youth coupled with a strict reliance on close-ended, fixed-choice formats for assessing identity formation, may lead to affirmation of a researchers' conceptualization of identity and yet be far removed from *personally affirmed identities*. One remedy offered in the current proposal involves use of experimental protocols to obtain self-generated, open-ended responses regarding ethnic identity. Subsequent analyses can determine accessibility of "cognitions" from memory regarding ethnic, racial, and personal identity. Another level of analysis (i.e., validity network) can then link these responses with known (and psychometrically refined) measures of ethnic identity to paint a more complete social constructivist picture of identity in adolescence.

| Box 3.3 | Sample Summary Statement Regarding Significance |

In summary the proposed study is significant because it: (1) examines empirically several hypothesized intervening mechanisms associated with a multi-component drug abuse intervention and determine the ability of these mechanisms to account for behavioral change; (2) utilizes data from three large-scale school-based randomized prevention trials that share a core assessment battery and that permits extensive testing of construct and external validity; (3) extends current prevention theory by examining the ability of several culture-specific measures to account for variability in hypothesized mediating mechanisms and drug criterion; (4) provides a unique opportunity to test the ability of each hypothesized intervening mechanism to disrupt the developmental progression of drug use; (5) accounts for clustering (i.e., school-level) effects through hierarchical linear model analyses; and (6) enables a research team that is highly regarded in the prevention community and that has obtained a thorough familiarity with the data from each prevention trial to examine further mediation applying state-of-the-art statistical procedures.

Let me illustrate this situation more carefully to better describe how the approach section helps reviewers formulate a score. Take, for instance, a group-randomized trial where schools are assigned to either receive an experimental treatment or be the minimal or no-contact control condition (or they could be wait-listed and receive the treatment immediately following completion of the study). There must be a systematic means of assigning schools to experimental conditions (i.e., using the "urn" method) or based on some prestratification scheme using demographic features to create a balance (in our school-based drug prevention programs, we stratify based on prebaseline cigarette smoking levels and minority enrollment figures).

Given that the design for school-based drug prevention programs calls for schools as the unit of assignment and student as the unit of observation (we anticipate behavioral change in student norms and skills, not school norms and skills), the statistical analysis plan suggests a need to control for any clustering or intraclass correlation that may occur. Schools may contain intact social groups, or clusters of students that share common social norms, thus raising the possibility that a "social climate" is creating dependence among the students' behavioral responses. From a design point of view, this relatedness among students violates the assumption of independence among error terms and may weaken the internal validity of the study (i.e., increase the type I error rate and bias test results by inflating standard errors of parameter estimates). The intraclass correlation coefficient (ICC) provides an estimate of the magnitude of clustering and can be used to statistically correct for intragroup dependence. The ICC can be computed using a one-way ANOVA procedure with school as the single grouping variable.

Standard errors for the variance estimates are computed using a formula for the variance inflation factor provided by Donner:[8]

$$\text{Var}(\rho) = 2(1-\rho)^2 [1+(n-1)\rho]^2 / n(n-1)m,$$

where n = the average (harmonic mean) number of students within each school, m is the number of schools, and ρ is the predicted level of clustering for the outcome variable (i.e., drug use).

The fact is, students within a school are more like each other than like students from different schools, and the occurrence of these "intact social groups" has caused some consternation to methodologists conducting school-based drug abuse prevention trials. Failure to control for the magnitude of behavioral similarity (again, using the ICC as a measure of the magnitude of clustering) will lead to biased estimates of the intervention effect.[9-11]

The real point here is not an exegesis on statistics but rather that a researcher proposing to use group randomization has to be concerned with several issues that fall under the rubric of "approach." First, assignment procedures have to be neatly laid out to comport with current methods of randomization (computers can do this quite deftly). Second, and particularly with the example given above, efforts have to be made to prevent contamination (students will cross barriers between schools), limit compensatory rivalry (parents will scream and raise bloody havoc about why their children are not receiving a beneficial program), and implement appropriate statistical analyses in order to control for clustering. There are many other factors that can influence the internal validity of a study, but for now, they are less intrusive in our brief example.[9]

A researcher proposing to use group randomization at any level will have to make sure to incorporate these issues at every level of their research grant. From the very outset when the aims include a statement such as "Assess the effect of a cognitive-behavioral intervention using a group-randomized trial...," the remaining portions of the grant need to reinforce that the investigator has considered the effect of this particular design on the hypotheses, statistical analyses, conductance of data collection, and a host of related research issues.

This is why the section of the grant dealing with approach requires so much thought and why design concerns are so pervasive in constructing grants. It is not uncommon during peer review to hear a reviewer lament the fact that the applicant did not appear to consider design issues prior to construction of the grant. In other words, the "approach" of the grant is muddled with inconsistency that flourishes and surfaces at numerous places in the grant writing. It also should be mentioned at this point that there are probably many different ways to handle the approach section in a grant. For instance, using the example of computing power for a school-based study where schools were randomized to either receive an experimental treatment or serve as controls, many investigators compute a single power statistic and use this number throughout to support their study design.

The problem is that power is dependent on so many factors, and all of them need to be considered in the computation. Alteration of any one of these factors would unduly influence power calculations and change the investigator's ability to detect significant findings given the current sample size and study design. Power in a group-randomized trial, for instance, will vary according to the magnitude of clustering. Accordingly, some estimates of clustering should be provided based on baseline data collection or obtained from published reports.[11] Power is also dependent on the reliability of the study measures, and the correlation between measures across time in a longitudinal study also influences power estimation. Thus, it may be more prudent to portray the power of a study in tabular form with a wide range of estimates provided based on varying parameters of interest (i.e., sensitivity analysis). This way, using the example of a randomized, school-based, drug prevention trial, the investigator can show how power changes with concomitant changes in sample size (both number of groups and number of subjects within the assigned groups), clustering influences (ICCs will change dramatically based on race, gender, or school geographical location), and other factors that influence power calculations (e.g., reliability of measures).

There is also another side to the approach section that often gets investigators into trouble. This has to do with the explication of statistical analyses appropriate for the design and the nature of relations between variables. It is incumbent on the investigator to defend their choice of statistical analysis in the section labeled Experimental Design (Section D). The nature of statistical relations between measures is clearly part of the "approach" or design of a study and helps reviewers determine whether the investigator has a definitive handle on how to extract meaningful information from the data. But applicants also need to recognize there may be no certain, definitive, and unassailable method to analyze the data. Rather a host of different approaches can tell the "story" about statistical relations. It all depends on which points will help address the specific aims (the analysis section must tie together the aims and the research hypotheses), what particular data are under scrutiny, and the course of action chosen to examine the data.

Applicants need to consider, especially in today's world, with the proliferation of very innovative and technically sophisticated computerized statistical modeling programs, that there are multiple ways to examine the data. In some cases, different analysis choices will lead to common findings, or they can produce disparate pieces of knowledge. Historically, this issue surfaced in the field of psychology with the introduction of a classic piece by Baron and Kenny.[12] In their article, Baron and Kenny raised the issue that in some cases a variable might moderate the relations between two measures (attenuate or exacerbate its influence), whereas in other cases a variable could mediate effects between two variables. In the case of moderation, a variable will augment (make stronger) or attenuate (weaken) the effect of one variable on another. This third variable "moderates" effects at various levels of activity, and the maximal effect zones can be plotted to show the shape or form of moderation (i.e., fanlike or intersecting lines).

Traditional conceptual models of moderation specify the moderator activity in terms of "high" or "low" (e.g., high and low social support) that produce different effects. The significance of a moderator effect is tested using interaction or multiplicative terms (A*B) in an additive linear regression model.[13] The equation depicting moderation would take the form $Y = \mu + A + B + A^{*}B + \varepsilon$, where μ is the group or grand mean stipulating no effect of the predictors on the outcome, A represents one predictor, B another predictor (conceived as a moderator), and the A*B is the interaction term (ε represents an error term or net residual effects after prediction). A significant interaction term (A*B), controlling for the independent predictor terms (A and B), indicates that the effects of A and B are dependent on each other at different levels (e.g., high values of A produce one effect on Y at high values of B and a different effect at low values of B). Either way (A could moderate the effects of variable B on the outcome Y), the nature of these relations is conditioned by the different values or levels of predictors A and B.

In contrast to moderation, mediation captures "generative mechanisms" where an independent variable influences a dependent variable through the influence of a third "intervening" variable. Baron and Kenny made it quite clear that moderator and mediating influences were both conceptually and statistically different and would argue for different statistical tests. In fact, their seminal article offered several methods to test both moderation and mediation using conventions available in linear regression, structural modeling, and other multivariate statistical approaches. In a very simplified version of mediation, the direct effect of variable A on dependent measure Y is mediated by another predictor B. When the mediated effect is not included in the equation, the size or magnitude of A's direct effect on Y is large. However, when B, the intervening variable, is included in the model as a predictor of Y (and A predicts B), the magnitude of A's direct effect on Y diminishes or approaches zero. Thus, B mediates the direct effect of variable A on the outcome Y.

To illustrate mediation, consider a middle school drug abuse prevention trial where several prevention modalities are implemented to change behavior. One hypothesized mechanism of change involves improving refusal assertiveness skills (e.g., taking defective merchandise back to the store, asking a friend to return something borrowed, and telling someone who cut in line to step back). Increased application of these "social skills" is hypothesized to reduce drug use by creating a barrier against negative peer social influences.[14] Armed with better (age-appropriate) social skills and, more specifically, equipped with refusal assertiveness, youth will be more inclined to refuse offers to use drugs and select healthy alternatives. In other words, as this simplified example shows, changes in skills mediate the program effects on the target outcomes. In general, tests of mediation have become a staple practice in prevention science as a means to examine program effects. The methods proposed by Baron and Kenny allow for specific statistical tests of whether, for instance, social skills mediate significantly the effect of program intervention modalities (activities) on the focal behavioral outcomes (i.e., drug use).

The moderator–mediator distinction is important because it raises the issue that variables can have different types of effects on each other. Submitting an application that lacks any specification of the types of relations between variables or that fails to address theoretically guided "cause and effect" relations would diminish enthusiasm for the approach of a study. In other words, it is not acceptable to "fish" around or "trawl" with live bait for shark in the hope you "catch something big." On the other hand, the need to buttress the approach of a grant application with specific statistical tests tied to explicit theoretical models can easily be rectified with the inclusion of a priori hypotheses. These hypotheses would be stated broadly in the specific aims emphasizing moderation (e.g., "Build a more detailed knowledge of factors that affect program effectiveness by examining moderators that may influence skill development") or mediation (e.g., "Evaluate program effects on hypothesized mediators using fixed-effect structural equation modeling and test both general and specific [nonstandard] effects using empirical specification searches"). At a later point in the application, you can insert a set of more refined research hypotheses in either Section D or in Section B where you explore the theoretical tenets of drug abuse prevention (you can even insert hypotheses in Section C, Preliminary Findings). The best way to formally state any relations between measures would be to specify direct influences, indirect influences (moderation or mediation), and third-variable alternatives that are spurious and undetected.

The moderator–mediator distinction opens the door for other considerations about which statistical analysis is best for the question at hand. The "question at hand" becomes the driving force in an application and should be deeply intertwined with the aims (i.e., clearly articulating what will be examined using tests of moderation as opposed to mediation), research hypotheses (i.e., differentiating effects associated with moderation from those anticipated with mediation), experimental design (i.e., are the anticipated effects lagged or delayed?), statistical methods (i.e., testing mediation using mixed-model approaches), and measures (reliability influences power and also effect sizes), to name a few grant components. Readers should note that mediation and moderation can be graphically portrayed to help clarify for reviewers which models are the focus of a particular study. Figure 3.2 graphically shows a simplified three-variable framework for testing mediation. Again, this is for illustrative purposes, and more complex models can be tested; the figure merely alerts the reviewer to the basic format used to test mediation.

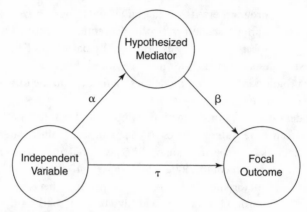

Figure 3.2. A Basic Framework for Testing Mediation

At a more complex level of analysis, when a goal of the study is to ascertain if phenotypes exist (e.g., alcohol abuse vs. dependence), latent class analysis may be appropriate. On the other hand, if determining the efficacy of an intervention is intended, and the intervention was tested in a group-randomized trial, then mixed model, mixture modeling, structural equation modeling, generalized estimating equations, mixed-model analyses, hierarchical or general linear models, or any of the myriad modeling efforts that decompose variance estimates and control for the nested structure of the data may be appropriate. Here again, the investigator has to examine carefully the different estimation methods, how they are influenced by the type of variables used (nominal, continuous, ordinal), and what pieces of information will help address the stated aims. A quick read of the current literature will reveal trademark or signature types of analyses for particular research questions, but there is no fault in proposing alternative modeling efforts, if they can be reasonably applied and are valid to the question at hand. Keep in mind that much of the work done by our predecessors who discovered "psychology" was conducted using very basic analytic designs including Student's t-tests, chi-square proportional tests of independence, ANOVA, or exploratory factor analysis. We should never stray too far from our roots, but be appreciative of the nuances of computer modeling and what they can do with large data sets.

Innovation

No matter what anyone says, it is hard to put a finger on the pulse of innovation. In fact, it can be extremely

---

Innovation

Is the project original and innovative? For example, does the project challenge existing paradigms or clinical practice? Does it address an innovative hypothesis or critical barrier to progress in the field? Does the project develop or employ novel concepts, approaches, methodologies, tools, or technologies for this area?

difficult at times to discern innovation from happenstance. There are so many examples throughout history of luck playing a huge role in scientific discovery, though this should not diminish in any way the enormous time commitment and energy invested by many scientists. In 1921, Menne Minniberg was mixing a batch of bran gruel for some patients. Inadvertently, some of the gruel spilled on a hot stove and sizzled into flakes, leading to the discovery of Wheaties cereal. In 1895, German physicist Wilhelm Röntgen was experimenting with electron beams. When he placed his hand in front of the beam, an image of the bones inside his hand was projected across the room, leading to the discovery of the X-ray machine. Endless stories exist of other inventions that have significantly advanced science, rendering significant changes in our daily lives. A substantial portion of these "discoveries" or innovations were based in part on luck, some minor tinkering with the status quo, or fiddling with existing machinery. In 1948, Swiss mountaineer George de Mestral was out for a stroll and noticed small plant burrs sticking to his trouser leg. Struck by the simplicity of this action, he begins to tinker with "velours crochet," which we now call Velcro. Would it be unfair to suggest all of these examples provide prima facie evidence of innovation, or is it sheer luck that brought about these different advances?

A very successful colleague of mine once told me that some of your "best" scientific ideas may not get funded. In fact, he noted, "great ideas that push the scientific envelope often don't get funded—they are too shocking to review committees." He went on to remark that this happens at times when there are few or no data to support research aims or hypotheses, "but the ideas stated in the grant represent natural (i.e., logical) connections that extend current theory or will be more readily apparent when a new technology becomes available or more ubiquitous." At a grant review for NIAAA, another well-respected colleague who was chairing the meeting engaged the review committee in a lively debate examining the proposed (NIH) definitions for the review criteria "innovative." He argued, quite convincingly to me at least, that science should rarely consider itself innovative because of the slow, almost tortoiselike pace that characterizes development of theory and new revolutionary ideas. My colleague then argued that we yield our desire to be innovative and focus rather on being "accepted" as part of an "old boy's club." Grants that are innovative, he went on "are often rejected because they extend our thinking in 'giant' steps, testing the review committee's resolve and how strongly reviewers are wedded to existing ideas and theory." He also commented that reviewers can be myopic at times, tending to look back at previous work more than they look forward toward new horizons. His views are supported in principle by historians examining trends in thinking. Noted author and chronicler Thomas S. Kuhn[15] argued that paradigm shifts take a long time to foment and can be imperceptible, based on the smaller historical and logical connections required for us to appreciate the growth of knowledge and the sociocontextual changes that grip our lives.

As I began to establish my own career, I took the advice of one of colleagues who suggested I retain the desire to be innovative but also learn how to "package" my grant ideas so they were not regarded by the review committee as too forward thinking or unsubstantiated. In fact, I started to bite off smaller pieces of science in my respective field, weaving together a stronger (and more logically coherent) fabric of understanding. This took shape as my first grant, an NIDA First Award (R29), which provided me the necessary jump-start to iron out some of my own thinking in the context of my predecessors and mentors. Although not offered currently by many of the NIH institutes, first awards are limited in financial scope and, in comparison to R01 awards, maintain a scaled down focus. They do, however, offer a sweet chance for investigators to get started in the financial and administrative management of grants as well as help young investigators learn the ropes of scientific enterprise.

There is another approach to tackle the issue of innovation. It may beg the question of whether your science departs from existing conventions, but you can always extend new thinking by building on the work of historical giants. In fact, extending existing theory to fit new applications has been a staple part of the past 20 odd years of psychology research. For instance, many grant writers cite the Health Belief Model[16] and subsequent refinements[17,18] or self-efficacy theory[1-3] as the cornerstone theories used to guide development of a behavior change intervention. To wit, models of persuasive communication provide a theoretical foundation to the National Youth Anti-Drug Media Campaign, a mass media, public health, social marketing campaign to prevent onset to and reduce existing drug use among youth (www.mediacampaign.org/publications/index.html). Most of the publications examining the efficacy of this campaign cite the Health Belief Model as the central argument for why youth will not consider using drugs following exposure to campaign messages.[19]

Here again, a large, well-funded campaign (the White House Office of National Drug Control Policy and the National Institute on Drug Abuse have provided funds for the campaign and provided financial support for secondary analysis of the campaign using the National Survey of Parents and Youth as an evaluation tool) builds on some very "strong" theoretical evidence attending to behavior change (other examples of innovation using existing theoretical lines could be provided for community-based drunk driving programs, AIDS risk reduction strategies, and mental health education programs). The NIH has extended grants or contracts through third parties to various research groups that combined existing theory with evaluation skills (LARS Research Institute, Inc. has received one such contract). Therefore, innovation in these instances relies more on combining a defined set of analytic skills with existing theory to make the case for extending scientific knowledge.

As another example, one avenue that forms an intersection between innovation and existing theory might include developing a new statistical technique that may have been ironed out mathematically but never applied in principle as a software program. The individuals responsible for developing a new user-friendly version of latent transition analysis and latent class analysis (WinLTA) brought the software to market under the rubric of a NIDA-funded P50 Center (the Center for Prevention Methodology at Pennsylvania State University, method-ology.psu.edu). In addition to this route of securing funds for developing soft-ware, chapter 13 on SBIR grants should prove fruitful in this respect because software development involves establishing avenues for commercialization and product utility in a business plan.

Countless examples exist within psychology of people who did not embark on making a revolutionary discovery but rather sought to fill a notable gap in a particular field. As a case in hand, Robert Sternberg edited a special centennial issue of *Psychological Bulletin*[20] where he researched which 10 articles in this prestigious journal were the most cited. The most cited piece was "Convergent and Discriminant Validation by the Multitrait-Multimethod Matrix," by Donald T. Campbell and Donald W. Fiske.[21] Four of the top 10 articles were written by Lee J. Cronbach and colleagues for their seminal work in quantitative method-ology and the measurement of change. Dr. Sternberg asked all the authors (who were alive) to respond in a short essay to three relevant questions: (1) what makes a good *Psychological Bulletin* article (likely to be widely read and cited), (2) what is the particular contribution of their own article, and (3) what kind of advice should be given to other scholars to help them maximize their influence on the field. All three questions readily form the foundation of what we mean by "in-novative," and whether you answer these questions for an article or a grant, the same formative ideas and basic strategy apply.

It is also worth mentioning that the synopsis provided by Dr. Sternberg addressed what made these top 10 citations reach this pinnacle of recognition. Paraphrasing Sternberg's editorial, what makes a good article, a good theory, a good contribution consists of (1) a timeless message, (2) a broad topic and audience, (3) being well written, (4) comprehensible and interesting, (5) pro-viding fundamental and concrete examples, (6) being persuasive and explicit, (7) being personal and not bland in writing style, and (8) being lucky. With the exception of item 8, if you carefully pick apart the contents of this chapter, you will find that I also have included these same points as staple ingredients in successful grant writing.

One of the top "10" in the classic citation list struck a personal chord with me, given that the author, Dr. Peter M. Bentler, was my postgraduate mentor and that we had co-authored an article.[22] Dr. Bentler, who published a number of seminal pieces on covariance structure analysis and model fit, is author of a structural equation modeling program known as EQS (www.mvsoft.com). In his essay responding to the three questions posed by Dr. Sternberg, Dr. Bentler re-iterated that he felt lucky to have made his contribution in research methodology.

In fact, he went on to comment that he did not start out to write a "citation classic" but rather sought to fill a void in the field with a useful and needed statistic. As Dr. Bentler wrote, the Bentler-Bonett Normed Fit Index[23] "provided a solution to a technical problem, the evaluation of model fit, which most likely accounts for its

Investigators

Are the investigator(s) appropriately trained and well suited to carry out this work? Is the work proposed appropriate to the experience level of the principal investigator and other researchers? Does the investigative team bring complementary and integrated expertise to the project (if applicable)?

more enduring contribution and may be the primary basis for citations."[24] Filling voids is highly regarded and consistent with the process of being innovative.

Investigators

Probably the biggest mistake made by junior investigators is the desire to bite off a big piece of the apple before they are ready to chew. In other words, very junior investigators write R01 grants that fall way short of the mark when it might have been more prudent to tackle an R03 or an R21 funding mechanism (see chapter 5 for more on this topic). Getting started on the road to funded grants may take longer than anticipated, and it is worth the time to invest in learning how to construct and structure grants from more senior investigators. As reviewers, we also see this happen when more junior investigators take on the burden of writing fellowship or independent investigator awards without consulting with more senior investigators who could provide conceptual and editorial oversight. In fact, it is quite common to hear reviewers state, "This application does not appear to have been reviewed by the more senior investigators prior to submission." This comment heralds that reviewers found too many holes and weaknesses to believe the application underwent serious review internally before submission.

One way to appreciate the need for a concerted plan in developing grants requires that we take a look at the number of grants funded in certain categories. Table 3.1 shows the FY 2005 award base and success rate for the different grant mechanisms at NIH. The R01 independent research category rates in table 3.1 indicate that 37% of continuation grants (already awarded and then renewed for a subsequent award year) were refunded. However, only 18% of the 21,745 R01 grants received for the first time were funded. R03 or small grants had a slightly better rate, with 723 of the 3,307 submitted, or 22%, being funded as new grants. R21 grants had the same 18% funding rate as R01 grants based on the 1,495 that were funded out of 8,483 submitted.

Table 3.2 provides more detail by breaking down groups of grants into their constituent parts. For instance, F-series grants have eight different types ranging from F05 to F38, including the pre- and postdoctoral fellowship grants (F31 and F32) covered in this book (chapter 6). Rates of funding are considerably higher for the F series grants: 31% for F31 and 30% for F32, respectively. The number of

TABLE 3.1 Success Rates for Various NIH Grant Mechanisms, Fiscal Year 2005

Activity Code	Award Title	Award Type	Number of Applications	Number of Awards	Award Rate (%)
DP1	NIH Director's Pioneer Award	New	283	13	5
P01	Program Project	Continuation	199	91	46
		New	252	73	29
		Supplements	27	12	44
R01	Traditional	Continuation	6,362	2,347	37
		New	21,745	3,894	18
		Supplements	122	34	28
R03	Small Grant	Continuation	14	2	14
		New	3,307	723	22
R15	AREA	Continuation	66	39	59
		New	595	158	27
R21	Exploratory Developmental Research Grant	Continuation	1	0	0
		New	8,483	1,495	18
R33	Exploratory/Developmental Grants—Phase II	Continuation	1	0	0
		New	97	17	18
R34	Clinical Trial Planning Grant	New	322	74	23

(continued)

TABLE 3.1 Success Rates for Various NIH Grant Mechanisms, Fiscal Year 2005 (*continued*)

Activity Code	Award Title	Award Type	Number of Applications	Number of Awards	Award Rate (%)
R36	Dissertation Support	New	22	8	36
R37	Merit	Continuation	184	178	97
		New	8	8	100
		Supplements	2	2	100
R55	James H. Shannon Director's Awards	Continuation	1	1	100
		New	8	8	100
R56	High-Priority Short-Term Project Awards	Continuation	60	60	100
		New	47	47	100
U01	Research Project— Cooperative Agreement	Continuation	115	80	70
		New	521	175	34
		Supplements	18	3	17
U19	Research Program— Cooperative Agreement	Continuation	22	11	50
		New	96	30	31
		Supplements	1	0	0
UC1	NIH Challenge Grants & Partnerships Program Phase II Cooperative Agreement	New	88	16	18

applications is noticeably smaller for the other types of F-series awards because some of these grants have unique eligibility requirements. For instance, the F05 grant is set up for international fellowships and therefore has a smaller pool of applicants (5 out of 11 were funded, a 45% success rate). Of the remaining F-series grants (all of which have higher funding rates), many are earmarked for international fellows (F06 and F07), scholars in residence (F15), foreign funded fellows (F20), senior fellows (F33), faculty fellowships (F34), and visiting scientist fellowships (F36, not included in table 3.2).

Regardless, a careful inspection of table 3.2 shows a higher funding level associated with many of the more "junior" or early awards that have been established to help individuals transition to research from a medical or clinical background. The K grant mechanisms, in particular, have much higher success rates of funding. For instance, the K01 (NCI Howard Temin Award), which has a 31% success rate, is set up as a Research Scientist Development Award that helps individuals

> bridge the transition from a mentored research environment to an independent basic cancer research career for scientists who have demonstrated unusually high potential during their initial stages of training and development. This special award is aimed at fostering the research careers of outstanding junior scientists in basic research who are committed to developing research programs directly relevant to the understanding of human biology and human disease as it relates to the etiology, pathogenesis, prevention, diagnosis, and treatment of human cancer. (grants1.nih.gov/grants/guide/pa-files/PAR-03–104.html)

Likewise, most of the other K-series grant mechanisms (only some are shown in table 3.2) are specifically established to encourage physicians (K11) or medical programs (K12, 28% success rate), minority school faculty (K14), dentists (K15 and K16), clinicians (K20), and clinical scientists seeking retraining (K21) to advance their careers in a calculated and staged manner. The message here is that investigators need to make sure the mechanism they have chosen is correct for their ability and skill level, fits their career model, and has a relatively high success rate of funding.

Investigators that have completed at most one or two years of postdoctoral studies are cautioned to consider submitting scaled down applications that are not burdened with huge administrative requirements (budget). Likewise, even more senior investigators with established track records compile P50 (research) or P60 (dissemination) center grants based on the premise they are seasoned R01 investigators and should be awarded a center. However, their lack of administrative expertise and absence of true evidence of collaboration beyond their own laboratory weakens their position for a center. Having been a reviewer for NIH on several P50 centers as well as having sat through site visits for our own P50 center, I realize now the importance of "centeredness" and the critical pieces that

TABLE 3.2 Breakdown of NIH Funding Success Rates for Different Grant Mechanisms

Activity Code	Mechanism	Success Rate Base	Number Awarded	Total Cost Awarded*	Success Rate (%)
C06	Research Facilities Construction Grant	152	17	$55,149,836	11
D43	International Training Grants in Epidemiology	36	23	$5,055,325	64
D71	International Training Program Planning Grant	4	2	$162,000	50
DP1	NIH Director's Pioneer Award	284	14	$9,969,924	5
F05	International Research Fellowships	11	5	$286,940	45
F30	Individual Predoctoral NRSA for M.D./Ph.D. Fellowships	105	46	$1,555,098	44
F31	Predoctoral Individual NRSA	1,425	446	$14,620,092	31
F32	Postdoctoral Individual NRSA	2,390	716	$33,239,293	30
F33	NRSA for Senior Fellows	39	14	$665,228	36
F34	MARC (NRSA) Faculty Fellowships	1	0	$0	0
F37	Medical Informatics Fellowship	18	7	$387,720	39
F38	Applied Medical Informatics Fellowship	11	3	$331,793	27
G07	Resources Improvement Grant	37	4	$321,947	11
G08	Resources Project Grant	62	6	$829,673	10
G11	Extramural Associate Research Development Award	18	9	$365,503	50
G12	Research Centers in Minority Institutions Award	4	3	$5,328,398	75

Code	Title				
G13	Health Science Publication Support Awards	50	9	$635,925	18
G20	Grants for Repair, Renovation and Modernization of Existing Research Facilities	100	21	$12,890,078	21
K01	Research Scientist Development Award—Research & Training	645	198	$24,323,695	31
K02	Research Scientist Development Award—Research	112	42	$5,092,989	38
K05	Research Scientist Award	30	19	$2,398,933	63
K07	Academic/Teacher Award	169	37	$5,223,279	22
K08	Clinical Investigator Award	676	266	$35,641,759	39
K12	Physician Scientist Award	126	35	$22,398,472	28
K14	Minority School Faculty Development Award	2	0	$0	0
K18	Career Enhancement Award	9	2	$278,074	22
K22	Career Transition Award	171	50	$7,409,689	29
K23	Mentored Patient-Oriented Research Career Development Award	679	232	$32,796,232	34
K24	Midcareer Investigator Award in Patient-Oriented Research	149	76	$10,762,585	51
K25	Mentored Quantitative Research Career Development Award	113	37	$4,952,585	33
K26	Midcareer Investigator Award in Biomedical and Behavioral Research	1	1	$110,492	100

(continued)

Table 3.2	Breakdown of NIH Funding Success Rates for Different Grant Mechanisms (continued)				
Activity Code	Mechanism	Success Rate Base	Number Awarded	Total Cost Awarded*	Success Rate (%)
K30	Clinical Research Curriculum Award	80	51	$15,137,629	64
M01	General Clinical Research Centers	27	16	$59,772,057	59
P01	Research Program Projects	478	176	$271,525,302	37
P20	Exploratory Grants	167	59	$73,552,770	35
P30	Center Core Grants	174	83	$127,454,156	48
P40	Animal Model and Animal Biological Material Resources Grant	13	6	$3,952,377	46
P41	Biotechnology Resource Grant Program	70	27	$26,909,407	39
P42	Hazardous Substances Basic Research Grants Program	14	0	$0	0
P50	Specialized Center	183	50	$95,497,986	27
P51	Primate Research Center Grants	1	1	$9,440,483	100
P60	Comprehensive Center	1	0	$0	0
PN2		20	4	$5,832,999	20
R01	Research Project	28,346	6,301	$2,277,701,056	22
R03	Small Research Grants	3,361	732	$56,349,623	22
R10	Cooperative Clinical Research	1	0	$0	0

R13	Conferences	599	435	$10,087,577	73
R15	Academic Research Enhancement Awards (AREA)	662	197	$39,740,776	30
R18	Research Demonstration and Dissemination Projects	43	6	$3,482,091	14
R21	Exploratory/Developmental Grants	8,543	1,507	$296,514,631	18
R24	Resource-Related Research Projects	187	73	$30,836,861	39
R25	Education Projects	472	156	$37,089,068	33
R33	Exploratory/Developmental Grants Phase II	98	17	$6,966,902	17
R34	Clinical Trial Planning Grant	322	74	$15,196,502	23
R36	Dissertation Award	22	8	$274,068	36
R37	Method to Extend Research in Time (MERIT) Award	194	188	$83,800,755	97
R41	Small Business Technology Transfer (STTR) Grants—Phase I	649	146	$22,771,532	22
R42	Small Business Technology Transfer (STTR) Grants—Phase II	110	43	$16,607,011	39
R43	Small Business Innovation Research Grants (SBIR)—Phase I	4,320	777	$121,510,132	18
R44	Small Business Innovation Research Grants (SBIR)—Phase II	1,059	340	$168,261,846	32
R55	James A. Shannon Director's Award	9	9	$900,000	100

(continued)

TABLE 3.2   Breakdown of NIH Funding Success Rates for Different Grant Mechanisms (*continued*)

Activity Code	Mechanism	Success Rate Base	Number Awarded	Total Cost Awarded*	Success Rate (%)
R56	High-Priority, Short-Term Project Award	108	108	$26,081,070	100
S06	Minority Biomedical Research Support	66	31	$14,709,130	47
S10	Biomedical Research Support Shared Instrumentation Grants	455	156	$69,674,892	34
S11	Minority Biomedical Research Support Thematic Project Grants	9	1	$1,025,385	11
S21	Research and Institutional Resources Health Disparities Endowment Grants—Capacity Building	5	4	$15,937,500	80
S22	Research and Student Resources Health Disparities Endowment Grants—Educational Programs	1	0	$0	0
T15	Continuing Education Training Program	18	5	$542,819	28
T32	Institutional National Research Service Award	933	389	$126,103,196	42
T34	MARC Undergraduate NRSA Institutional Grants	36	13	$5,512,121	36
T35	NRSA Short-Term Research Training	54	32	$2,778,336	59
T36	MARC Ancillary Training Activities	9	6	$2,936,354	67
T37	Minority International Research Training Grants	46	24	$5,363,559	52
U01	Research Project (Cooperative Agreements)	853	307	$269,576,760	36

U10	Cooperative Clinical Research (Cooperative Agreements)	134	66	$44,966,198	49
U13	Conference (Cooperative Agreements)	32	14	$788,884	44
U18	Research Demonstration (Cooperative Agreements)	32	9	$2,347,678	28
U19	Research Program (Cooperative Agreements)	120	42	$46,302,038	35
U24	Resource-Related Research Project (Cooperative Agreements)	27	21	$21,699,699	78
U2R	International Training Cooperative Agreement	12	4	$1,150,723	33
U41	Biotechnology Resource (Cooperative Agreement)	1	1	$3,325,000	100
U42	Animal Model and Animal Biological Material Resource (Cooperative Agreement)	11	4	$5,465,392	36
U43	SBIR (Cooperative Agreement)	1	1	$139,911	100
U45	Hazardous Waste Worker Health and Safety Training Cooperative Agreements	37	26	$35,997,636	70
U54	Specialized Center (Cooperative Agreement)	157	62	$186,386,920	39
U56	Exploratory Grants (Cooperative Agreements)	2	2	$811,773	100
UC1	NIH Challenge Grants & Partnerships Program Phase II Cooperative Agreement	88	16	$62,629,901	18
UC6	Construction Cooperative Agreement	10	4	$87,541,256	40

*The total cost is the sum of the direct and indirect costs for each fiscal year, and not for the life of the project.

must be put into place in order to "center" research activities logistically and administratively. A great deal of information is presented on the NIH centers in chapters 9 and 10. The price paid by many investigators, junior or otherwise, is a lack of salesmanship in their specific grant and the absence of unequivocal supporting voice in the review room.

There are other factors that need to be considered with regard to investigative strength. For instance, just as politicians work arduously at gaining face recognition in the months preceding an election, so too must junior or new investigators work carefully at building rapport and recognition with leaders in the field (this probably holds true even for more senior investigators). There are many ways to go about this task, including aggressive networking, contacting highly published and well-respected colleagues (it is sometimes helpful to send published articles with a short note to colleagues who can become prospective reviewers), increased visibility at conferences (e.g., chairing symposia), and accepting invitations to review manuscripts for various scientific journals (this exposes you to works in progress before they are published). When I was more junior, I found that inviting very senior members of the field to moderate or chair conference symposia was critical in helping elevate my own exposure and increase face recognition (plus you get to see how experts handle questions from the audience).

Environment

Does the scientific environment in which the work will be done contribute to the probability of success? Do the proposed studies benefit from unique features of the scientific environment, or subject populations, or employ useful collaborative arrangements? Is there evidence of institutional support?

Environment

It is almost fitting that a review of the applicant's environment comes right after any statements made about the investigator. The two components should go hand in hand, particularly if an investigator has been associated with a research group for a long period of time and is building a career in a particular academic center or research think tank. The investigator is essentially "investing" in the productivity of the research group and hopes this affiliation will translate into a productive research career. There are a number of places in an application where you can highlight the strengths of the environment. Individual fellowship and K-series grants have designated places for showcasing the strengths of the environment. It is less clear for R-series grants, where one should specifically highlight the resources available to conduct the science.

One place I found quite useful to showcase environment is the "Resource" page either prior to or immediately following the budget (and budget justification). The resource page is not counted in the 25-page limitation for NIH PHS 398 (or SF424) grant applications, and thus you can expand (within reason) on the strengths provided by your environment. Environment means physical space, resources (equipment, library, supplies, and special materials), and supporting cast. In my current position as president of LARS Research Institute (LRI), Inc., a Nevada-based 501(c)(3) nonprofit company, we pride ourselves on the library and collection of scientific resources we have amassed, the highly trained personnel we involve in our projects, and the physical accoutrements we use to execute our grants (local area network, materials, publishing capabilities). We use the Resources page from LRI to showcase these strengths, but we also highlight resources from collaborators and consortium arrangements to strengthen our "look."

Since we decided that it would not be in the best interest of a small albeit burgeoning company to engage in the labor-intensive activity of data collection (we had enough of that party!), we decided to subcontract out data collection to outside vendors. In one case, for an R21 grant, we used a highly professional group at the University of Southern California that was part of an NIDA-funded P50 Transdisciplinary Prevention Research Center under the leadership of Dr. Alan W. Stacy. Dr. Stacy had in place a very highly trained group of seasoned data collectors that were used to collect survey data from students in the Los Angeles schools (and other surrounding counties). Dr. Stacy is one of the leading thinkers in the area of memory and drug use using associative and implicit cognition techniques, and his laboratory uses computers to collect implicit cognition and neuropsychological data.[25] His ability to engage data collection and gain access to public schools dovetailed nicely with our grant objectives that also required data collection using both laptop computers and paper-and-pencil survey questionnaires. Therefore, we developed a consortium agreement and used the strengths of the USC group in describing our environment. Naturally, we spent an enormous amount of time building and reinforcing the linkages between our respective groups, and we made this collaboration obvious in the grant application. We handled all of the institutional review board and institutional issues that crop up when you utilize the services of outside vendors, met our HIPAA compliance requirements at USC, and developed in-roads between LRI and USC to connect our business office with the USC Office of Contracts and Grants.

Environment also includes library and professional resources (clinics, laboratories, special centers, campus facilities [e.g., student health centers]), staff available for administrative assistance, and various university professional services that can lend their expertise to a particular grant (clinics can be used for testing). Environment also includes the computer system linking work stations at your think tank (including Internet and email access), community resources that may be a part of your grant, the advisory board that will assist you in meeting your professional and community obligations as you execute a grant, and all of the possible resources that bring to bear on a grant. Showcasing these strengths exemplifies for reviewers that an investigator has given thought in advance to all of the components that are required to execute a grant. This thoughtfulness and anticipation is usually a good sign that the business model is operating in an investigator's mind.

Above I mentioned several places to showcase the significance of your study. The same opportunities exist for extolling the virtues of your environment. There are several different places where you can alert the reviewer to the special features of your environment, highlight important community collaborations, outline various means available to collect data with special populations, and note the special strengths of your research team (e.g., noting that you have been collecting school-based data for 10 years). If your environment is unique, and you have access to special populations, or you have developed strong ties to the community (i.e., schools or after school programs), this can be highlighted in the section detailing preliminary findings where you wrap up the discussion of findings by mentioning how you were able to collect such opportune data because of your special relationships with community service groups. Likewise, you can highlight the special nature of your laboratory in the section where you detail the experimental methods and articulate the unique equipment available to test drug effects on synaptic transmission. If you store your laboratory rats in a mental health facility or a Veterans Administration hospital but you work out of a university office, make sure to connect these environments in the budget justification (and resources page), and later when you describe your preliminary findings, make mention of the rat storage facility. Likewise, if you gather data from methadone clinics located throughout an urban locale, but you work in a research think tank, make mention of the connections you have with the different facilities or whether they form a health care network.

If you utilize the services of a consortium, you will be able to provide a budget for the consortium agreement and include a budget justification (see chapter 15 for more on the budgeting of consortiums). This will allow you to take up some space describing the special features of the consortium, its physical facilities, and unique qualities of their staff (which is generally why you chose the consortium services anyway). Don't miss this opportunity to provide a detailed explanation of why the consortium provides a unique service and how you will utilize its services. The consortium is considered part of your environment at the time your grant undergoes review. Use every available space to continually reinforce the opportunities created by your collaborations, shared facilities, and your ability to execute the grant because of unique environmental features.

This brings to a close the portion of this chapter attending to the five review criteria. All five areas come under equal scrutiny during review, even though the criteria do not evenly share the text portions of the application. At this point, I turn to a more protracted discussion of the Specific Aims section, which provides the backbone or structural support to your grant.

SPECIFIC AIMS

Specific Aims are like a constant thorn in your side. They stick with you throughout the construction phase of an application and likewise during the review process. In fact, it is not uncommon for reviewers to flip back and forth between the Specific Aims and other sections of a grant searching for connections and ensuring the applicant has prepared a specific plan (research hypotheses and statistical approaches) that addresses each and every aim. When aims are not delineated clearly, are written loosely, or are not embedded or tracked carefully throughout the grant document, it is not surprising to receive a summary statement that includes a comment such as "Aim #5 was never addressed in the research hypotheses and there was little evidence in the statistical analysis section this aim would even be examined."

One way to appreciate the importance of the Specific Aims section is to consider that aims truly represent a "beacon" presaging and illuminating the organization of a grant with respect to study design, research hypotheses, methods, and statistical approaches. In their entirety, aims provide reviewers with a taste of what will come, represent a framework on which to determine the overall significance of the application, and help tether the more abstract or theoretical parts of an application to the methodology, core statistical analyses, and experimental procedures.

Well-worded applications with carefully specified aims and logically coherent scientific goals are usually reviewed favorably and can easily be distinguished from applications containing feebly developed aims. For example, if the aims are poorly specified, overly ambitious, errantly framed, inconsistent, or not written clearly, this will not bode well during review. There is no hard and fast rule about how many aims should be included in a grant application. Some applications contain only a few, and others exceed 10. What is important is that the applicant use the aims as a framework for discussion and planning as the grant unfolds. Applicants that construct ambitious aims that are never subsequently addressed in the body of the grant will suffer scoring letdowns, missing essential detail to shore up the application. Conversely, applications that contain specifically worded and detailed aims that deftly form a backbone to the grant fare better during review because of their conceptual clarity and organization. Keep in mind, however, the aims must be scientifically meritorious and not just worded correctly. Again, using the analogy of a "beacon," the aims point out the direction of the grant, provide a rationale for conducting the science, and showcase the applicant's various strengths (brief descriptions of analyses that will help test aims should be embedded in the aims and highlight statistical or experimental skills).

Notwithstanding, an important part of constructing well-written Specific Aims section involves the use of "power words," words that clearly delineate

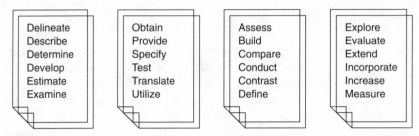

Figure 3.3. Sample Power Words for the Specific Aims.

intent, purpose, direction, and organization. Figure 3.3 provides some examples of power words that can be used to construct aims.

A second issue concerning aims regards precision. Aims need to detail precisely what will happen when the grant is funded (we say "when" rather than "if" in this business!). In the business world, we often use the term "deliverables" to connote the product that will arise from a contract. Deliverables can refer to scientific papers, products, inventions, software programming, and physical things (i.e., inventions) that will be turned over following conclusion of the contract. Another term, often used by lawyers when they construct service contracts, is "works," which is quite similar to "deliverables" but usually refers to written/textual creations, such as software code, manuals, papers, and products of an intellectual nature.[26] To go even one step further, sometimes you can define intellectual property rights as part of the deliverables, but more often since intellectual property rights are "intangibles," you obligate the party involved on the production end (grantee institution) to provide all deliverables, including "works," and have the party agree that they are transferring therewith all rights therein, including rights in inventions, copyrights, and so forth. Universities are known to want control over intellectual property when the rights are part of a grant, housed at the university; however, many scientists work this out contractually if they intend to develop intervention materials as their focus.

From a legal standpoint, "works" are considered products in the same vein that an edited book is a collected "work." This very same legal framework can be used to understand that execution of a grant will also result in deliverables and works (e.g., interventions) are the "product." SBIR grants, for example, are notorious for resulting in the creation and testing of training programs and intervention materials with potential market commercialization.

The long and short of this brief digression into legal vernacular is that the aims are a good place to detail precisely the products, works, or deliverables of a grant. In other words, the aims outline what will take place once the grant is funded. The aims detail what product will be delivered, in what time period, and how the product will take shape (manual, software code, book, intervention materials, and evaluation tools, to name a few examples). Good examples of precisely worded aims include ones that detail how the study will be conducted (i.e., experimental design and, if necessary, laboratory procedures), what sample will be used, what intervention will be delivered and in what sequence, data collection methods (e.g., surveys, assays, interviews), timelines, and data analysis strategies (techniques and purpose). Since there are some noted differences between aims for various funding mechanisms, these are covered separately in the chapters examining SBIR grants (chapter 13), R01 mechanisms (chapter 8), and center grants (chapter 9).

To help summarize this section on Specific Aims, boxes 3.4 and 3.5 show two different examples of aims (with slightly different composition styles) taken from a funded NIDA P50 Center grant and an R01 grant submission.

THE ESSENTIALS OF SCHOLARSHIP

Undoubtedly, scholarship plays an important part in grant writing. Stripped to its bare essentials, scholarship consists of careful and logical writing, historical accuracy, and attention to detail. Careful writing is perhaps the strongest element of any grant. Sloppy and poorly constructed grants replete with widows, orphans, grammatical errors, missing text, typographical errors, and erroneous statements can really piss off a reviewer, leading to a climate of "death."

Box 3.4

One of the central aims of the proposed studies is to test several new integrations of research paradigms (assessments and theory) developed from previous research independently conducted in the United States and in the Netherlands (NL). More specifically, the joint studies proposed will:

A. Directly compare the different ways to assess implicit drug cognitions developed in the US and in the NL, with respect to their relative predictive power to explain later drug use and abuse.

B. Investigate potential interaction effects between the implicit associations assessed in the reaction time (RT) paradigms developed by the NL team and the implicit memory association tests used by the US team. These different paradigms may tap different aspects of implicit cognition that may act in concert to influence drug use.

C. Investigate whether a brief but novel intervention is feasible as a prevention tool, and whether it moderates (decreases) the influence of implicit cognition on drug use in high-risk youth.

D. Compare the new integrations across parallel studies in the NL and US in high-risk adolescents.

Box 3.5   Aim 1

What is the benefit of the workplace-based parenting program compared to a dosage equivalent contact intervention including an online parenting education program and a nutrition and exercise class for this population in improving five latent cluster outcome variables (worker job satisfaction and supervisor performance ratings, substance use, depression, family relations, social skills, and healthy behaviors (improved nutrition, exercise and reduced health care claims, workman's compensation)?

To address this question, a repeated measures, experimental design (2 groups by 5 times) will be employed to randomly assign 360 "families" (828 participants) in 10 cohorts of 36 families to the family intervention (n=180 families) or a placebo online parent education and control weight management class (n=180 families).

At the very outset, I suspect that most readers of this book, and hence this chapter, came through a similar educational training as I did, obtaining either an advanced doctoral degree in some discipline of behavioral science or advanced training in medicine. As a result, we can all acknowledge that very little of our education focused on the principles of teaching. Other than teaching a laboratory class or an introductory graduate school course, we had limited exposure to the fundamentals of teaching. After exiting graduate school, those of us who chose careers in academia were put to task acquiring the requisite teaching skills and scholarship. The only problem is that during our graduate school experiences we had minimal training in both of these areas. We were ill prepared to face the demands and vicissitudes of teaching and left prey to the whim and caprice of students and end-of-year student evaluations.

With respect to scholarship, the bulk of our work in graduate school concerned coursework, papers, theses, and dissertations. Once in a while a precociously bright and energetic student would squirrel themselves away in a laboratory and, when shepherded under the wings of an appropriate mentor, publish a few scientifically relevant articles prior to graduation (but those are few and far between). More and more, however, many of us realize that a lacuna exists with respect to our own professional training. While this may be a long-winded way of informing readers their skills need honing, it is imperative that graduate schools change their approach to teaching and learning. Of utmost importance is that graduate training programs incorporate more of the skills required in the professional arena. Just as medical students undertake clinical rounds in their third and fourth years of medical school (and some even engage rounds earlier, depending on their curriculum), graduate schools need to take heed that we are not preparing our students with the requisite skills essential for scholarship in general and grant writing specifically. By hiding graduate students from the very skills required to be successful in the "real" world, we do considerable damage to them and to the field. Most important for readers of this book, we create a vacuum with respect to producing successful grant writers. Succinctly stated, we simply don't impart enough grant writing skills to eager young graduate students until it is far too late and the crunch hits them full force.

As an example, I was at least four to five years post-Ph.D. and following two postdoctoral fellowships before I was asked to even consider writing a grant (this scenario was not uncommon among my junior colleagues, as well). After receiving a much sought after and heralded offer to write a grant, I did what I believe was the best thing I could at the time, which was to examine carefully the style and format of my mentor's grants (those were R01 grants) and map my own writing style to that very successful template. The material in this chapter is therefore, on balance, a rehashing of what I learned in those early years and since that time have preened and refined into my own style of grant writing. In essence, there is a template on which to construct grants—the government makes clear this template through a scoring and evaluation system—and applicants should pay close attention to the format and style of this system to better position their grant applications and increase their funding success rates.

Another crucial and important concept to consider is that explanation is the keystone that holds a grant together. It is not uncommon for reviewers to note that an application seems rife with haste. In other words, applicants sometimes put too much content inside the 25 pages of an NIH application and yet still fail to address essential concepts. In their effort to defend, rather than explain, a proposed study, in their effort to reinforce, buttress, and justify their position with citations, examples, and more data, many applicants omit the careful explanation of science that helps the reviewer journey into the applicant's line of reasoning. Well-written applications, whether in their first submission or second revision, will "explain" scientific concepts, account for statistical relations, and combine or cross-fertilize ideas generated from different disciplines. In effect, an application will elevate reviewers to a new level of understanding, showcasing innovative thinking encased in the traditional scientific language we artfully use.

There is no hard and fast rule about what should be inside the 25 pages of a grant, though the NIH application suggests page limitations for standard grants (communication with colleagues and your project officer should help clarify page limitations for sections). In one case, one of the NIH institutes permitted 15 pages for an R03 small grant award (including revised applications), whereas another institute recommended no more than 10 pages for a revised R03 application. Regardless of the different institute rules for PHS applications, use your space judiciously!

THINGS THAT YOU CAN DO TO LEARN SCHOLARSHIP

There are a few tried and true methods that will help you learn scholarship along the way. People working at think tanks or nonprofit groups can hire outside consultants with extensive grant-writing expertise, using this as an avenue to model writing skills. Individuals residing at academic centers can seek consultation from faculty with well-funded laboratories regardless of their substantive focus (good writing is good writing whether in chemistry or in anthropology). Something else to consider is making oneself available as a reviewer. In other words, let your parent institute become aware that you are willing to review grants or serve on committees in any capacity. This will enable you to learn first hand and gain precious insight into the machinations of how committees review grants and what criteria help applications get over the hurdle or, conversely, potentially hurt grant applicants. Importantly, this experience should help shape future submission because it should lead you to incorporate a more refined picture detailing how committees make their respective decisions regarding the suitability of a grant in addressing the prevailing science.

One positive experience that helped me to see the incredible importance of editing grants prior to submission came from a consulting relationship I had with a beltway bandit group (i.e., consulting firms located around the Washington, DC area that respond to government contracts). This company had in place a remedy to help them meet the press of submitting large volumes of grants in short spans of time. This solution consisted of using the services of an in-house "red team" consisting of writers or individuals with advanced graduate degrees in English, composition, or scientific writing that help improve the readability of a grant prior to submission. The "red team" reviews all grants emanating from the research and investigative teams at least a week prior to the submission deadline (this may not work for investigators who are up writing the night before the submission deadline!). Grammar, typos, and problems with basic sentence structure were chief targets that red team members examined. These individuals also read the grant carefully to determine if the basic appeal of the grant was driven by thematic integration. If the grant doesn't make sense to a lay person, it won't make sense to a reviewer, even with their stated professional expertise. Grants that have dangling participles, widows, orphans, typos, and poorly constructed grammar are headed for the rejection bin, regardless of the powerful science that may be embedded in the text.

If you don't have the financial resources to obtain professional red team services, put one together from existing staff, including use of a thesaurus and dictionary. Further, obtain a writing style manual, such as the *Publication Manual of the American Psychological Association*,[27] which helps dress up grants nicely, and proofread your grant until you are sick and tired of seeing it! As a starter, you can go to Amazon.com and type in APA Publication Manual—a host of resources, DVD and CD-ROM guides, and books come up that will give you the inside professional scoop on how to write research papers, format grants, and learn a particular publication style. There are many other styles to consider (several manuals and books by Kate L. Turabian, including the Chicago style and the Vancouver biomedical style established by the International Committee of Medical Journal Editors (1978), to name a few, are also available by typing in "Turabian" in the search box at Amazon.com)—simply pick one and utilize this style consistently.

In this regard, the following two items are critical to consider as you engage in grant writing, whether it is for the first or fifteenth time:

1. Don't submit a grant application containing typographical errors. This is perhaps the biggest mistake even seasoned investigators make. Typographical errors are one of the foremost painful mistakes made by novice grant writers. In their haste to present a polished grant idea, investigators often fail to thoroughly check their own writing. There is no more egregious error than submitting a grant that is marred with problems, marked by grammatical errors, and replete with missing documentation and is characteristically plumb sloppy.

   Take my word for it (or, for that matter, the word of any of the contributors to this book), grant reviewers are careful readers. Also note that the level of compensation for grant reviews is not what brings us to Washington, DC to engage in peer review. Rather, our concern for science, the opportunity to sit in a room with 20 or more of the leading scientists in the field, the chance to serve the institute or center that may eventually fund our own research, and the valued friendships we build are all reasons cited by our colleagues for participating in the NIH grant reviews. But the common thread that binds us all is a level of scholarship and attention to detail, which always surfaces during grant reviews.

   I can think back to one review when we decided that missing sentences, poor documentation, and lack of effort in providing essential detail dropped a grant from the "outstanding" (1.0–1.5) category to "unscored." As you may recall, unscored applications are in the lower half of the applicant pool, do not receive a score, but receive summary statements containing critiques. How damaging this must be to know, upon receiving your summary statements, that your overall scientific ideas were considered novel and appropriate but the manner in which you presented them considered so sloppy that this adversely affected your overall priority score. In essence, even though reviewers don't make funding decisions, the grant plummeted in appeal from the higher scoring pile that is considered meritorious to the lower end of the scoring continuum, which in all likelihood meant the death knell for this grant.

2. Don't violate the PHS 398 rules regarding font selection (a number of different font types are accepted, including Arial and Helvetica), type size (11 pt is recommended), appendix materials, and which materials belong in which section of a grant. Perhaps the most important document we suggest reading is the guidelines section for PHS 398 forms and applications (the new guidelines can be downloaded from www .grants.nih.gov/grants/guide/notice-files/NOT-OD-05-006.html and the actual forms can be accessed at www.nih.gov/forms/PHS398). For example, if you intend to submit a T32 training grant, which requires a statement of mentoring experience, don't embed this highly important material in an appendix if reviewers are told up front to consider this material germane to reading a training fellowship application. Oftentimes, applicants are uncertain about how important a particular table or figure will be to reading the grant. This is always the case when the background, significance, preliminary studies, and research plan must conform to the 25-page limit. The rule of thumb is that if you have concisely stated the material in the text and the figure or table reinforces the text, delegating it to an appendix will not make a big difference to the reviewer. However, if you have not addressed an important point that you believe is germane to reading the application (and this material is critical toward understanding the logical content of the grant), then embed the figure, chart, or table in the 25 allowed pages of the grant (sections A through E).

The following points should also be very helpful as you craft your grant application:

- Don't miss on the opportunity to build essential collaborations that will help launch your own career. Make friends with colleagues who can help you during all the various stages of grant construction. Colleagues can be used to proofread your grant, submit the grant for preview scrutiny, provide necessary expertise during execution, and give you the "once over" in case the grant does not muster a high evaluation and needs revisions.
- Don't diminish the importance of the "lesser" sections of a grant. These might include the environment, resources page, and supplemental materials that help your grant transition from one review evaluation pile to another. All sections of the grant are treated equally during review!
- Be fastidious in the way you put your grant together, allowing yourself time for preparation, writing, routing, and obtaining necessary approvals, institutional review board certification, and eventual permission to submit from the various departmental chairs, division chiefs, and supervisors.

Make ready for this feedback throughout your career, be earnest, compliant, and dutiful, engage in due diligence—it pays off.

SUREFIRE TIPS AND POINTERS

Here are some editorial pointers you may want to implement the next time you submit your grant application:

- Connect the different sections of your grant. One means of doing this deftly is to write a summary of specific aims at the very end of the grant (last paragraph before Human Subjects). Use this space to help summarize the research goals, unique features of your scientific approach, and strengths of the investigative team.
- Read through the grant repeatedly and make sure the different sections are tethered together by some common thread. For instance, are the aims justified in the experimental design? Does the analytic section leave the reader (reviewer) with a reassuring feeling that the proper statistical methods are used to address the specific research hypotheses?
- Have other people review your grant prior to submission, especially if you are a new investigator. It is one thing to "love" your own ideas and feel proud of your accomplishment when you put the final brushstroke on a 25-page grant. However, it is essential that you make sure your ideas are consistent with the existing fund of knowledge in your respective field (don't be an iconoclast when you are young!).
- Keep in mind that your job when you write a grant is not to convince your own mind that you are onto something special, but rather to convince the reviewer that you are capable of conducting a scientific project with all its logistical trimmings. Make your grant a story that has a fabric of understanding running pervasively throughout.
- With respect to using available resources, seek out and find consultants who embellish your project. The best piece of advice here is to bring on consultants who are going to help you shape your ideas and at the same time are capable of fine-tuning your career progress. It is not uncommon for consultants to return the favor, using your strengths to support their grant initiatives, which can lead to long-term collaboration, co-authored books, joint attendance at symposium and conferences, and other professional opportunities that help you bridge the gap between your own knowledge and strengths and the larger body of scientific inquiry.
- Make sure there is an element of positive thinking and "realism" running rampant through your grant. Positive thinking includes the absence of derogatory materials aimed at other researcher's work. Realism underscores the special abilities and characteristics of your team, laboratory,

and thinking. Science is about the obvious, or as Thomas Henry Huxley said, "Science is nothing but trained and organized common sense."[28] Make sure the grant is feasible and represents state-of-the-art thinking and techniques but is written in a way that anyone can understand the grant's basic tenor.

SUMMARY AND CONCLUSIONS

If I have not already said enough on the subject of writing grants, there are 18 other formidable chapters in this book to read, digest, and contemplate their contents. The focus of my energy and effort in this chapter has been to highlight the scholarly nature of grant writing. With a modicum of attention to detail, and a penchant for writing consecutive and iteratively refined drafts, you should be able to eventually construct a meaningful grant application that should merit high regard in the peer review system. There is enough ammunition in this book, and sufficient instruction on how to load the writing gun; nevertheless, you must be prepared to pull the trigger.

4 | Sample Size, Detectable Difference, and Power

A power analysis is only as good as the formulae and estimates that are used and the analyst who uses them.

—DAVID MURRAY, *Design and Analysis of Group-Randomized Trials*

THE ESSENTIAL NATURE OF A POWER ANALYSIS IN ANY NIH GRANT APPLICATION

Many factors influence the level of enthusiasm that a reviewer will have for a grant application. These include the significance and innovation of the proposed work, the quality of the proposed methods, the strength of the research team, and the environment. Even though power is not listed explicitly among these evaluation criteria, it is an essential part of the experimental design section (section D for an R01 grant). Unless the reviewers are satisfied that the investigators have provided an appropriate power analysis and shown that the power is adequate, their enthusiasm will be reduced, with a consequent reduction in the likelihood that the project will receive a good priority score (and eventually get funded).

The power of a study is the probability that the investigator will find an effect of a specific form and magnitude given the design, analysis, sample size, and type I error rate chosen for the study. The

89

effect of interest can take many different forms, depending on the nature of the proposed study. In a randomized controlled trial or group-randomized trial, the effect of interest will be the effect of the intervention, often measured as a difference between the intervention and control conditions in their mean or rate for the primary endpoint. In a longitudinal study, the effect of interest will be a measure of association between an exposure and an outcome, often expressed as an odds ratio, regression coefficient, or mean difference. This chapter summarizes the factors that influence power and offers a generic approach to estimating the appropriate sample size, detectable difference, and power with examples for several types of studies.

It is important to note that a power analysis is only as good as the formulas and parameter estimates that are used and the analyst who uses them. Power analysis should be done by someone who understands the formulas and why they are structured as they are. This type of knowledge allows the analyst to tailor the formulas to the particular needs of the study. In addition, investigators should take care that the parameter estimates accurately reflect the expected state of affairs in the population to be studied. Without good estimates, power analysis is at best only guesswork.

FACTORS THAT DETERMINE POWER

Many factors influence the power of a statistical test. These include the form and magnitude of the effect of interest, the type I and II error rates, the choice of a one- or two-tailed test, the number of primary analyses or endpoints, the structure of the variables, and the structure of the analysis. Below I briefly review each of these factors in terms of how they can influence power.

The Form and Magnitude of the Effect

An investigator must determine in advance what form and magnitude of effect are worth detecting in terms of its clinical or public health significance. If the investigator anticipates an effect that is well described as a difference between two means or a difference between two slopes, then the test statistic should be constructed to evaluate such a difference. If the investigator anticipates an effect that changes in magnitude over time, then the test statistic should be constructed to evaluate such a pattern. The pattern expected for the effect is cast as the alternative hypothesis, and the pattern expected in the absence of the effect is cast as the null hypothesis. The test statistic should be chosen to be sensitive to the form and magnitude of the departures from the null hypothesis that define the effect.

Typically, an investigator may ask a biometrician or statistical analyst, "If I conduct an experiment in a certain manner, what kind of effect can I get?" The reply from the analyst should be, "What form and magnitude of effect is important to detect from a clinical or public health perspective?" If the investigator only stares back blank-faced, the analyst might then further ask, "What form and magnitude of effect would be viewed as important by experts in the field?"

The original question from the investigator is an example of approaching the problem from the wrong direction. The form and magnitude of the desired effect should lead the way in planning the study; they should not emerge only at the end, as a finishing touch in the planning process. For example, if an investigator wants to examine change, observations must be taken over time and the design must be structured to include multiple observations. If an investigator expects the intervention effect to follow a particular pattern, the design must be structured to include enough observations scheduled at the proper times to be able to detect the designated pattern. If an investigator expects the effect to take some time to develop, sufficient time must be provided so that the effect can mature and be captured in full force.

Type I and II Error Rates

The type I error rate is the rate at which the effect will be reported as significant due to chance alone. In general, investigators try to minimize that rate. The type II error rate is the rate at which the effect will be reported as nonsignificant when it occurs. In general, investigators try to minimize that rate, as well. Unfortunately, the forces that govern the type I and II error rates often act in opposition, such that reducing one error rate serves to increase the other. The desired type I and II error rates define the critical values in the distribution against which the observed value of the test statistic is assessed. The actual values depend both on the type I and II error rates and on the expected distribution of the test statistic under the null hypothesis. The research community has come to look at 5% as an acceptable type I error rate. Many view 10%, 15%, or 20% as an acceptable type II error rate. In fact, the type I and II error rates should be matched to the study at hand, in consideration of the relative danger of making a type I or type II error. If a type I error would be serious, that rate should be set quite low. If a type II error would be serious, as well, that rate should also be set quite low. On the other hand, if one or both errors would be troublesome but not ruinous, their rates might be set somewhat higher. Setting the rates should be done in full recognition that they have a substantial effect on the size of the study.

One- or Two-Tailed Tests

If the investigator expects that the effect will be in a particular direction and does not care if the direction is reversed, then a one-tailed test is appropriate. If the investigator is not sure of the direction of the effect, or if the investigator cares if the effect is reversed, a two-tailed test should be used. Often investigators remember only the first part of each of those two rules. Many scientists believe that as long as they have a clear a priori expectation that the effect will be in a particular direction, they should use a one-tailed test. In fact, that represents only half of the requirement.

There is also a risk in reporting a one-tailed test, particularly when the result is only barely significant. Some members of the scientific community will wonder whether the investigators reported a one-tailed test because a two-tailed test would not have provided a significant result. The best way to avoid this problem is to publish a design paper in which the primary analysis is laid out in detail, as a one-tailed test. By having the plan on record in advance, there is no reason to speculate later about the motivations of the investigator.

The Number of Primary Analyses or Endpoints

If there is but one primary analysis for one primary endpoint, then the type I error rate for that analysis can be set at the nominal level, usually 0.05. If there is more than one primary analysis or primary endpoint, the type I error rate for each test should be reduced so as to safeguard the type I error rate for the study. Otherwise, the type I error rate for the study may be inflated well beyond the nominal level. For example, given $k = 5$ primary endpoints or analyses, the true type I error rate is $1 - (1 - \alpha)^k$, or $1 - (1 - 0.05)^5 = 0.226$ rather than 0.05. This is a considerable difference going from an expected error or chance occurrence in 5% of the cases to 22.6% of the time.

The best way to avoid this problem is to identify a single primary endpoint and a single primary analysis for that endpoint. Other variables may be identified as secondary endpoints, and other analyses as secondary analyses. If there must be multiple primary endpoints, then the investigator should consider an omnibus test both to avoid an inflated type I error rate and to improve power over any of the individual tests.[1,2]

The Structure of the Variables

In general, an analysis of Gaussian data is more powerful than an analysis of non-Gaussian data, other factors constant. Here, power depends entirely on the variance because the mean and variance are independent. For non-Gaussian variables, power often depends on both the mean and the variance, because the two are often related. In both cases, power increases as the variance decreases, through better measurement, adoption of a more precise endpoint, or more exacting analytic strategies.

The Structure of the Analysis

Any action that reduces the standard error of the effect will improve power, other factors constant. The size and form of the standard error of the effect are influenced by the design, the analysis and the nature of the dependent variable. Analytic tools such as regression adjustment for covariates, stratification, matching, and repeat observations can be used to reduce the standard error of the effect, depending on the nature of the effect of interest and the analysis used to evaluate that effect.

FUNDAMENTALS OF POWER ANALYSIS

Several excellent treatments of power analysis are available. Cohen's text[3] provides a good background discussion of power analysis, many useful formulas, and, for the computationally reticent, extensive tables of power and sample size for a variety of metrics and analyses. Fleiss and colleagues[4] provide a good discussion of power analysis for rates and proportions and also provides tables of sample size as a function of the magnitude of the expected effects and the desired type I and II error rates. Other familiar texts on clinical trials and observational studies also include material on power analysis.[5–8]

Even for a single research question, a well-defined endpoint, an appropriate design and statistical analysis, there are many different approaches to power analysis. Some analysts focus on computing power. Others focus on computing detectable differences. Yet others focus on computing the number of participants required to detect an effect of a given magnitude. Even if two analysts intend to compute the same quantity, they may use different formulas. Add the rich variety in research questions, endpoints, designs, and analyses, and power analysis can seem very complex or, at the very least, confusing.

One of the reasons for the apparent complexity and confusion is that there are so many factors that influence power. Any equation that has many parameters can be written in many different ways, with each formulation solving for a different parameter. At first glance, these formulas may appear to be quite different, when in fact most of the basic formulas can be manipulated into a common form. Unfortunately, the algebra can get complicated, and for the inexperienced, it is easier to believe that all those formulas are doing different things. But that simply is not the case. These formulas use estimates for many different parameters to compute detectable differences, power, sample size, or some other single parameter that is temporarily treated as the dependent variable in a complex expression.

Another reason for the apparent complexity is that there is no standard notation for power analysis. An inexperienced investigator can look at two formulas that are in fact equivalent and believe they are different simply because they use different notation. Adding to this confusion, not all writers include the same set of parameters in their equations. This is particularly true for such parameters as the expected rate of attrition, noncompliance, and others. Formulas that ignore such parameters are effectively assuming that their value is zero. On the other hand, the author may simply plan to deal with those factors at a later time.

Yet another reason for the apparent complexity is that discussions of power analysis are often cast in the context of a particular scale of measurement or a particular analysis plan. Certainly the scale of measurement and analytic plan affect the power analysis, but it also is possible to structure the formulas so that they can accommodate a wide variety of measurement scales and analysis plans. No single presentation can resolve all of these relevant issues. Even so, we can consider the steps that all power analyses have in common and examine a few examples. This information should be helpful and stimulate even the most reluctant investigator to include a stronger and more clearly defined power section in their grant application.

Steps in a Power Analysis

Seven steps are involved in a power analysis:[5]

1. Specify the form and magnitude of the effect of interest.
2. Select a test statistic for that effect.
3. Determine the distribution of that test statistic under the null hypothesis.
4. Select the critical values in that distribution that determine whether or not the investigator will reject the null hypothesis.
5. Develop an expression for the standard error of the effect under the null hypothesis in terms of parameters that are easily estimated.
6. Gather estimates of those parameters.
7. Estimate power given the results of the first six steps.

The seventh step should include a sensitivity analysis that varies the estimates of the most important parameters. The investigator should select the design and analysis that optimizes power and cost for the effect of interest under assumptions that are easily defended.

Reporting the Results of the Power Analysis

Many investigators insert power analyses early in the methods section, often right after the description of the study design and hypotheses. This necessarily means that the power analysis is presented before the data analysis plan, and this can be awkward. The power analysis should be based on the analysis plan, and it can be difficult for reviewers to evaluate the power analysis without first reading the analysis plan. For this reason, it is better to report the results of the power analysis after the presentation of the analysis plan.

The presentation should provide enough information for the reviewer to evaluate the power analysis. It is simply not adequate to report that "the study has 80% power." Instead, the presentation should include the formulas used, the parameter estimates used, and a justification both for the formulas and for the parameter estimates. Importantly, there should be sufficient detail that a good analyst can replicate the power analysis. Reviewers who are good analysts will want to do that, and if they try but cannot replicate the power analysis, they will report that to the study section, with adverse consequences for scoring the application.

METHODS FOR SPECIFIC STUDY DESIGNS

Power in a Simple Randomized Clinical Trial

The simplest randomized clinical trial is a posttest-only control group design with n participants allocated to each of two conditions. If the primary endpoint satisfies the normality assumption, the simplest analysis is a t-test or, equivalently, a one-way analysis of variance (ANOVA). If regression adjustment for covariates is included, then the analysis becomes a one-way analysis of covariance (ANCOVA). The model for the unadjusted analysis is

$$Y_{i:l} = \mu + C_l + \varepsilon_{i:l} \tag{4.1}$$

The observed value for the ith participant in the lth condition is a function of the grand mean and the effect of the lth condition; any difference between the observed value and the predicted value is allocated to the residual error ($\varepsilon_{i:l}$).

Assume that the investigator determines that the intervention effect is well described by a difference between the two conditions in their posttest means. Let $\hat{\Delta} = \hat{\bar{y}}_1 - \hat{\bar{y}}_C$ estimate that difference. Let $\hat{\sigma}_\Delta^2 = \hat{\sigma}_{\bar{y}_1 - \bar{y}_C}^2$ estimate the variance of that difference under the null hypothesis. Assuming the residual error is distributed Gaussian, the intervention effect is evaluated using a t-statistic in combination with the appropriate df. The general form of that t-statistic is

$$\hat{t} = \frac{\hat{\Delta}}{\hat{\sigma}_\Delta} \tag{4.2}$$

In this case, the t-statistic is estimated as:

$$\hat{t} = \frac{\hat{\bar{y}}_1 - \hat{\bar{y}}_C}{\hat{\sigma}_{\bar{y}_1 - \bar{y}_C}} \tag{4.3}$$

The expected distribution of this t-statistic is determined by its df, here $2(n-1)$, where there are n participants in each of the two conditions.

Assume further that the investigator has determined that the desired type I and II error rates are 5% and 20%, respectively. Assume as well that the investigator expects a positive intervention effect but would be concerned about a negative effect; as a result, the investigator chooses a two-tailed test. These decisions define the critical values that are used to determine whether or not to reject the null hypothesis.

At this point, the investigator is ready to develop an expression for the variance of the intervention effect under the null hypothesis in terms of parameters that are easily estimated. In the current case that variance is the variance of a difference between two condition means, given above as $\hat{\sigma}_\Delta^2 = \hat{\sigma}_{\bar{y}_I - \bar{y}_C}^2$. That form is not given in terms of parameters that are easily estimated, and some elaboration is required.

Given the random assignment of members to conditions, it is reasonable to assume that the two study conditions are independent. The variance of the difference between two independent conditions means is

$$\hat{\sigma}_{\bar{y}_I - \bar{y}_C}^2 = \hat{\sigma}_{\bar{y}_I}^2 + \hat{\sigma}_{\bar{y}_C}^2 \tag{4.4}$$

The estimated variance of a single condition mean is the estimated variance of the dependent variable, $\hat{\sigma}_y^2$, divided by the number of observations contributing to that mean, n:

$$\hat{\sigma}_{\bar{y}_C}^2 = \frac{\hat{\sigma}_y^2}{n_c}$$

The variances for the two condition means are then estimated as

$$\hat{\sigma}_{\bar{y}_I}^2 = \frac{\hat{\sigma}_{y_I}^2}{n_I} \quad \text{and} \quad \hat{\sigma}_{\bar{y}_C}^2 = \frac{\hat{\sigma}_{y_C}^2}{n_C}$$

If the number of participants observed in each condition is assumed equal, $n_I = n_c = n$, and the variances in the two conditions are assumed equal, $\hat{\sigma}_{y_I}^2 = \hat{\sigma}_{y_C}^2 = \hat{\sigma}_y^2$, then

$$\frac{\hat{\sigma}_{y_I}^2}{n_I} = \frac{\hat{\sigma}_{y_C}^2}{n_C} = \frac{\hat{\sigma}_y^2}{n}$$

The estimate of the variance of the difference becomes

$$\hat{\sigma}_\Delta^2 = \frac{2\hat{\sigma}_y^2}{n} \tag{4.5}$$

As a result, the t-statistic is estimated as

$$\hat{t} = \frac{\hat{\Delta}}{\sqrt{\dfrac{2\hat{\sigma}_y^2}{n}}} \tag{4.6}$$

The advantage of this formulation is that it is written in terms of three simple parameters: the usual population variance, estimated as $\hat{\sigma}_y^2$, the number of participants per condition, n, and the difference between the two sample means, estimated as $\hat{\Delta} = \hat{\bar{y}}_I - \hat{\bar{y}}_C$. These parameters are relatively easy to estimate, drawing on data from published reports, from analyses of existing data, or from preliminary studies.

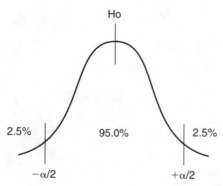

Figure 4.1. Selecting Cut Points for the t-Distribution to be $\pm\alpha/2$ Ensures That the Type I Error Rate Will Be α

To ensure that the two-tailed type I error rate is α, $\hat{t}$ is considered statistically significant only if $|\hat{t}| > t_{\text{critical}:\alpha/2}$, where $t_{\text{critical}:\alpha/2}$ defines the $\alpha/2$ percentile of the t-distribution for the available df. Figure 4.1 illustrates the division of the t-distribution into two tails, each containing 2.5% of the distribution. The probability that $|\hat{t}| > t_{\text{critical}:\alpha/2}$ will be the sum of the probabilities in the tails, or 5%. Thus under the null hypothesis (H_o), the probability that $|\hat{t}| > t_{\text{critical}:\alpha/2}$ will be α.

The observed $\hat{t}$ also is but one possible value from the sampling distribution under the alternative hypothesis (H_a) that the point estimate has some specified nonzero value. If the alternative hypothesis is true, we want to reject the null hypothesis as often as possible. If we fail to reject the null, we are making a type II error. In order to ensure that the type II error rate is β, the probability that $|\hat{t}| > t_{\text{critical}:\alpha/2}$ must be $1 - \beta$ for the expected value of the point estimate under the alternative hypothesis. This happens only when $\hat{t} > t_{\text{critical}:\alpha/2} + t_{\text{critical}:\beta}$, or equivalently, when $\hat{t} > t_{\text{critical}:\alpha/2} - t_{\text{critical}:1-\beta}$. Here $t_{\text{critical}:\beta}$ and $t_{\text{critical}:1-\beta}$ define the β and $1 - \beta$ percentiles, respectively, of the sampling distribution under the alternative hypothesis that the point estimate has some specified nonzero value, given the available df. Figure 4.2 illustrates the relationship between the distribution of $\hat{t}$ under both the null and alternative hypotheses.

Written quite generally, the power for a single df contrast of size $\hat{\Delta}$ and evaluated via the t-test given in equation 4.2 is

$$\text{power} = \text{prob}(\hat{t} \le \hat{t}_\beta), \quad \text{where } \hat{t}_\beta = \frac{\hat{\Delta}}{\hat{\sigma}_\Delta} - t_{\text{critical}:\alpha/2} \qquad (4.7)$$

or, equivalently,

$$\text{power} = \text{prob}(\hat{t} \ge \hat{t}_{1-\beta}), \quad \text{where } \hat{t}_{1-\beta} = t_{\text{critical}:\alpha/2} - \frac{\hat{\Delta}}{\hat{\sigma}_\Delta} \qquad (4.8)$$

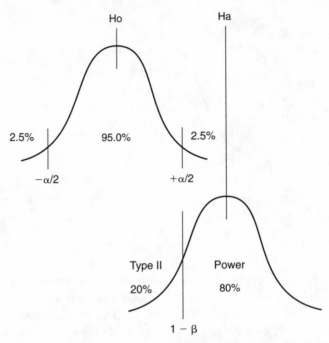

Figure 4.2. The Relationship Between the Distribution of $\hat{t}$ Under Both the Null and Alternative Hypotheses

Written in terms of n, $\hat{\sigma}_y^2$, and $t_{critical:\alpha/2}$, the structure of $\hat{\sigma}_\Delta^2$ is made explicit, and the power to detect a difference as large as or larger than $\hat{\Delta}$ is estimated as

$$\text{power} = \text{prob}(\hat{t} \le \hat{t}_\beta), \quad \text{where } \hat{t}_\beta = \frac{\hat{\Delta}}{\sqrt{\frac{2\hat{\sigma}_y^2}{n}}} - t_{critical:\alpha/2} \qquad (4.9)$$

or, equivalently, as

$$\text{power} = \text{prob}(\hat{t} \ge \hat{t}_{1-\beta}), \quad \text{where } \hat{t}_{1-\beta} = t_{critical:\alpha/2} - \frac{\hat{\Delta}}{\sqrt{\frac{2\hat{\sigma}_y^2}{n}}} \qquad (4.10)$$

To illustrate, consider the example provided in table 4.1. The values for the observed $\hat{t}$ and the a priori $t_{critical:\alpha/2}$ are arbitrary. The values for $\hat{t}_{1-\beta}$ and $\hat{t}_\beta$ are calculated using equations 4.7 and 4.8. The probabilities are determined for the computed values of $\hat{t}_{1-\beta}$ and $\hat{t}_\beta$ assuming many df. When the effect is large enough to generate a value of $\hat{t} = 2.80$, the probability prob $(\hat{t} \ge \hat{t}_{1-\beta})$ is 80%, as is the probability prob $(\hat{t} \le \hat{t}_\beta)$. That indicates that the power of the test is 80% to find an effect that large or larger to be statistically significant. This result is achieved whether power is calculated based on $\hat{t}_{1-\beta}$ or $\hat{t}_\beta$ as long as the proper

TABLE 4.1	The Relationship Between $\hat{t}$, $\hat{t}_{1-\beta}$, $\hat{t}_\beta$, and Power When the Type I Error Rate Is Fixed and df Are Many

$\hat{t} = \frac{\hat{\Delta}}{\hat{\sigma}_\Delta}$	$t_{critical:\alpha/2}$	$\hat{t}_{1-\beta}$	prob $(\hat{t} \geq \hat{t}_{1-\beta})$%	$\hat{t}_\beta$	prob $(\hat{t} \leq \hat{t}_\beta)$%
0	1.96	1.96	2.5	−1.96	2.5
1.96	1.96	0	50	0	50
2.8	1.96	−0.84	80	0.84	80

expression is used. When the effect is large enough to generate a value of $\hat{t} = 1.96$, the test is still large enough to be reported as statistically significant, but the power to detect an effect that large or larger is reduced to only 50%. When the intervention effect is zero, such that $\hat{t} = 0$, the probabilities prob $(\hat{t} \geq \hat{t}_{1-\beta})$ and prob $(\hat{t} \leq \hat{t}_\beta)$ each represent one tail of the two-tailed type I error rate.

There are several different ways to characterize the power of a randomized controlled trial. Investigators may report power for a given $\hat{\Delta}$, or for a range of $\hat{\Delta}$, where the range reflects variations in the assumptions made for the parameters that are used in the calculations. Another way is to report the sample size required for the study; here, too, a range of sample sizes may be reported. Yet another way is to report the detectable intervention effect, often called the detectable difference when the intervention effect is estimated as a difference. Here, too, a range of detectable differences may be reported. These three approaches (detectable difference, sample size, and power) are simply three different ways of arranging the terms that help the investigator determine the size of the study.

Written in terms of $\hat{\sigma}_\Delta^2$, the detectable difference between two independent condition means is estimated as

$$\hat{\Delta} = \sqrt{\hat{\sigma}_\Delta^2 (t_{critical:\alpha/2} + t_{critical:\beta})^2} \qquad (4.11)$$

Written in terms of m, $\hat{\sigma}_y^2$, and $t_{critical:\alpha/2}$, the structure of $\hat{\sigma}_\Delta^2$ is made explicit, and the same detectable difference is estimated as

$$\hat{\Delta} = \sqrt{\frac{2\hat{\sigma}_y^2 (t_{critical:\alpha/2} + t_{critical:\beta})^2}{n}} \qquad (4.12)$$

In either form of expression, the values for $t_{critical:\alpha/2}$ and $t_{critical:\beta}$ depend on the df for the t-test.

Written in terms of $\hat{\sigma}_\Delta^2$, the sample size per condition required for a specified value of $\hat{\Delta}$ is estimated as

$$n = \frac{n\hat{\sigma}_\Delta^2 (t_{critical:\alpha/2} + t_{critical:\beta})^2}{\hat{\Delta}^2} \qquad (4.13)$$

Written in terms of $\hat{\sigma}_y^2$, $t_{critical:\alpha/2}$, and $t_{critical:\beta}$, the structure of $\hat{\sigma}_\Delta^2$ is made explicit and the same sample size is estimated as

$$n = \frac{2\hat{\sigma}_y^2(t_{critical:\alpha/2} + t_{critical:\beta})^2}{\hat{\Delta}^2} \qquad (4.14)$$

The solution of either expression may require two or three iterations. The initial values of $t_{critical:\alpha/2}$ and of $t_{critical:\beta}$ often have to be changed given the preliminary result and its effect on the df.

If we anticipate including regression adjustment for covariates to improve power, we can make a small modification in equation 4.14:

$$n = \frac{2\hat{\sigma}_y^2(1-R_{y\cdot x}^2)(t_{critical:\alpha/2} + t_{critical:\beta})^2}{\hat{\Delta}^2} \qquad (4.15)$$

Here, $R_{y\cdot x}^2$ is the proportion of variance explained by the covariates. To the extent that $R_{y\cdot x}^2$ is greater than zero, the sample size required based on equation 4.15 will be smaller than required by equation 4.14. The df available for the analysis will be reduced by the df required for the covariates, such that $df = 2(n-1) - x$, where x and df are required for the covariates.

If we anticipate matching or stratification prior to randomization, followed by a matched or stratified analysis, we can make a different modification in equation 4.14:

$$n = \frac{2\hat{\sigma}_y^2(1-r_{y\cdot s})(t_{critical:\alpha/2} + t_{critical:\beta})^2}{\hat{\Delta}^2} \qquad (4.16)$$

Here, $r_{y\cdot s}$ is the correlation between the matching or stratification factor and the primary outcome. To the extent that r_{ys} is greater than zero, the sample size required based on equation 4.16 will be smaller than required by equation 4.14. The df available for the analysis will be reduced; in a matched analysis, the df are reduced by half ($df = n - 1$), and in a stratified analysis, the df are reduced by the df used for the stratification factor ($df = 2(n-1) - (s-1)$), where there are s levels of the stratification factor.

If the dependent variable is dichotomous, the analysis will proceed in parallel to the ANOVA/ANCOVA described above but using logistic regression analysis. As a result, two modifications are required. First, the variance of the dependent variable is calculated as pq, where p is the average proportion and $q = 1 - p$, so that $\hat{\sigma}_y^2 = pq$. Once the preliminary result for n is calculated, it must be adjusted to reflect the fact that the dependent variable has a binomial distribution, not a normal distribution. There are a number of corrections for continuity, but with a moderately sized study, this expression from Fleiss et al.[4] is appropriate:

$$n_{corrected} = \frac{n}{4}\left(1 + \sqrt{\left(1 + \left(\frac{4}{n|p_l - p_c|}\right)\right)}\right)$$

Power in a Simple Group-Randomized Trial

The methods for a clinical trial must be adapted for group-randomized trials wherein identifiable groups rather than individuals are allocated to each condition. The simplest group-randomized trial is a posttest-only control group design, with g groups randomized to conditions and m members within those groups observed at posttest to determine if there is an intervention effect. Because both groups and members must be modeled as nested random effects, the appropriate analysis is a mixed-model ANOVA or ANCOVA.[5] In the unadjusted analysis of posttest data, the model is

$$Y_{i:k:l} = \mu + C_l + G_{k:l} + \varepsilon_{i:k:l}$$

Here $G_{k:l}$ represents the effect of the group, estimated as the deviation between the group mean and the condition mean. The variation among the condition means is assessed against the variation of the average within-condition group means with $2(g-1)$ df.

Assume that the investigator has determined that the intervention effect is well-described by a difference between two posttest condition means. Let $\hat{\Delta}$ estimate that difference. Let $\hat{\sigma}_\Delta^2$ estimate the variance of that difference. Then the t-statistic given in equation 4.2 is used to assess that effect. The distribution of $\hat{t}$ is determined by the available df. The critical values in that distribution in turn are determined by decisions on the type I and II error rates and on whether to conduct a one- or two-tailed test.

The investigator still must develop an expression for the standard error of the difference between two condition means under the null hypothesis. Consider first the variance of the group mean. If that mean were based on m independent observations, the variance of that mean would be estimated as shown in equation 4.1:

$$\hat{\sigma}_{\bar{y}_g}^2 = \frac{\hat{\sigma}_y^2}{m}$$

However, because the members within an identifiable group almost always show positive intraclass correlation coefficient, $ICC_{m:g:c}$, those observations cannot be assumed independent. This intraclass correlation reflects an extra component of variance attributable to the groups nested within conditions, expressed as $\sigma_{g:c}^2$. As a result, the variance of the group mean in the group-randomized trial is estimated as

$$\hat{\sigma}_{\bar{y}_g}^2 = \frac{\hat{\sigma}_e^2}{m} + \hat{\sigma}_{g:c}^2 = \frac{\hat{\sigma}_y^2}{m}\left[1 + (m-1)\hat{ICC}_{m:g:c}\right] \tag{4.17}$$

The condition mean is estimated as the average of g group-specific means. Assuming equality across conditions for the components of variance, the number of members per group, the number of groups per condition, and the intraclass correlation among the members within a group, the estimated variance of the condition mean under the null hypothesis is

$$\hat{\sigma}_{\bar{y}_c}^2 = \frac{\hat{\sigma}_{\bar{y}_g}^2}{g} = \frac{\hat{\sigma}_y^2(1 + (m-1)I\hat{C}C_{m:g:c})}{mg} \qquad (4.18)$$

The estimate of the variance of the difference between two independent condition means is then

$$\hat{\sigma}_\Delta^2 = \frac{2\hat{\sigma}_y^2(1 + (m-1)I\hat{C}C_{m:g:c})}{mg} \qquad (4.19)$$

Given a moderate number of members per group and groups per condition, the t-statistic to assess the difference between the two such means is estimated as

$$\hat{t} = \frac{\hat{\Delta}}{\sqrt{\dfrac{2\hat{\sigma}_y^2(1 + (m-1)I\hat{C}C_{m:g:c})}{mg}}} \qquad (4.20)$$

As noted above, the value of df for this t-statistic is $df = 2(g-1)$.

In a group-randomized trial, the variance of the condition mean is based not on the variance of the member-level data, which may have a decidedly non-Gaussian error distribution, but on the variance of the group mean. Under the Central Limit Theorem, the group means have errors that are distributed approximately Gaussian, even if the member-level errors are non-Gaussian, as long as there are moderate numbers of members within each group and groups within each condition. A recent simulation study confirmed that the Central Limit Theorem provides good protection for a dichotomous endpoint in a group-randomized trial with only four groups per condition and 30 members per group.[9]

The formulas presented for power, detectable difference, and sample size from the clinical trial are easily adapted to accommodate the variance of the condition mean in the group-randomized trial. Written quite generally, power is estimated as shown in equation 4.7:

$$\text{power} = \text{prob}(\hat{t} \le \hat{t}_\beta), \quad \text{where } \hat{t}_\beta = \frac{\hat{\Delta}}{\hat{\sigma}_\Delta} - t_{\text{critical}:\alpha/2}$$

or, equivalently, in the manner shown in equation 4.8:

$$\text{power} = \text{prob}(\hat{t} \ge \hat{t}_{1-\beta}), \quad \text{where } \hat{t}_{1-\beta} = t_{\text{critical}:\alpha/2} - \frac{\hat{\Delta}}{\hat{\sigma}_\Delta}$$

In this form, the only difference between the clinical trial and the group-randomized trial is in the structure of $\hat{\sigma}_\Delta^2$.

Written in terms of m, g, $\hat{\sigma}_y^2$, $\hat{\text{ICC}}_{\text{m:g:c}}$, and $t_{\text{critical}:\alpha/2}$, the structure of $\hat{\sigma}_\Delta^2$ is made explicit, and the power to detect a difference as large as or larger than $\hat{\Delta}$ is estimated as

$$\text{power} = \text{prob}(\hat{t} \le \hat{t}_\beta)$$

$$\text{where } \hat{t}_\beta = \frac{\hat{\Delta}}{\sqrt{\dfrac{2\hat{\sigma}_y^2\left[1 + (m-1)\hat{\text{ICC}}_{\text{m:g:c}}\right]}{mg}}} - t_{\text{critical}:\alpha/2} \qquad (4.21)$$

or as

$$\text{power} = \text{prob}(\hat{t} \ge \hat{t}_{1-\beta})$$

$$\text{where } \hat{t}_{1-\beta} = t_{\text{critical}:\alpha/2} - \frac{\hat{\Delta}}{\sqrt{\dfrac{2\hat{\sigma}_y^2\left[1 + (m-1)\hat{\text{ICC}}_{\text{m:g:c}}\right]}{mg}}} \qquad (4.22)$$

Written in terms of $\hat{\sigma}_\Delta^2$, the detectable difference is estimated as shown in equation 4.11:

$$\hat{\Delta} = \sqrt{\hat{\sigma}_\Delta^2 (t_{\text{critical}:\alpha/2} + t_{\text{critical}:\beta})^2}$$

Written in terms of m, g, $\hat{\sigma}_y^2$, $\hat{\text{ICC}}_{\text{m:g:c}}$, $t_{\text{critical}:\alpha/2}$, and $t_{\text{critical}:\beta}$, the structure of $\hat{\sigma}_\Delta^2$ is made explicit and the same detectable difference is estimated as

$$\hat{\Delta} = \sqrt{\frac{2\hat{\sigma}_y^2\left[1 + (m-1)\hat{\text{ICC}}_{\text{m:g:c}}\right](t_{\text{critical}:\alpha/2} + t_{\text{critical}:\beta})^2}{mg}} \qquad (4.23)$$

In either form, the values selected for $t_{\text{critical}:\alpha/2}$ and $t_{\text{critical}:\beta}$ depend on the df for the t-test, df $= 2(g-1)$.

Written in terms of $\hat{\sigma}_\Delta^2$, the sample size of groups per condition required for a specified value of $\hat{\Delta}$ is computed using a modification of equation 4.13:

$$g = \frac{g\hat{\sigma}_\Delta^2 (t_{\text{critical}:\alpha/2} + t_{\text{critical}:\beta})^2}{\hat{\Delta}^2} \qquad (4.24)$$

Written in terms of m, $\hat{\sigma}_y^2$, $\hat{\text{ICC}}_{\text{m:g:c}}$, $t_{\text{critical}:\alpha/2}$, and $t_{\text{critical}:\beta}$, the structure of $\hat{\sigma}_\Delta^2$ is made explicit, and the same sample size is computed as

$$g = \frac{2\hat{\sigma}_y^2\left[1 + (m-1)\hat{\text{ICC}}_{\text{m:g:c}}\right](t_{\text{critical}:\alpha/2} + t_{\text{critical}:\beta})^2}{m\hat{\Delta}^2} \qquad (4.25)$$

Either form may require two or more iterations. The initial values of $t_{\text{critical}:\alpha/2}$ and of $t_{\text{critical}:\beta}$ often have to be changed given the preliminary result for g.

Written in terms of $\hat{\sigma}_\Delta^2$, the sample size of members per group required for a specified value of $\hat{\Delta}$ is computed using a modification of equation 4.13:

$$m = \frac{m\hat{\sigma}_{\Delta}^2(t_{critical:\alpha/2} + t_{critical:\beta})^2}{\hat{\Delta}^2}$$

Written in terms of g, $\hat{\sigma}_y^2$, $\hat{ICC}_{m:g:c}$, $t_{critical:\alpha/2}$, and $t_{critical:\beta}$, the structure of $\hat{\sigma}_{\Delta}^2$ is made explicit and the same sample size is computed as

$$m = \frac{2\hat{\sigma}_y^2\left[1+(m-1)\hat{ICC}_{m:g:c}\right](t_{critical:\alpha/2} + t_{critical:\beta})^2}{g\hat{\Delta}^2} \tag{4.26}$$

Either form may require two or more iterations, because the value of $\hat{\sigma}_{\Delta}^2$ will change with the value of m.

Modifications are required if the analyst plans to employ regression adjustment for covariates, repeated observations on members or groups, or matching or stratification in the analysis. Details on those modifications are beyond the scope of this chapter (for details, see chapter 9 in my text on group-randomized trials).[5]

Power in a Simple Cohort Study

In a cohort study, participants who differ in their level of the exposure of interest are followed over time to determine whether the exposure is associated with the outcome of interest. One analysis that may be of interest is to compare the time trends in the outcome of interest for groups that differ in their level of the exposure of interest. If the outcome is continuous, linear regression methods are appropriate, and this expression (adapted from Diggle and colleagues)[10] can be used to estimate sample size:

$$N_s = \frac{2}{\Delta}\left(\frac{\sigma_y^2(1-\rho)(t_{critical:\alpha/2} + t_{critical:\beta})^2}{ns_x^2}\right)$$

Here, N_s refers to the number of persons contributing to each slope, ρ is the over-time correlation in the outcome of interest, and ns_x^2 are the corrected sums of squares for time at the person level.

We can estimate ns_x^2 based on the survey schedule and the expected participation rates using equation 4.25:

$$ns_x^2 = \sum_{u=1}^{s}\left(p_u\sum_{j=1}^{n_u}(t_j - \bar{t}_u)^2\right) \tag{4.27}$$

Here there are $u = 1 \ldots s$ schedules, p_u is the proportion of participants providing information on schedule u, there are $j = 1 \ldots n_u$ observations for each participant on schedule u, t_j are the values of time on schedule u, and $\bar{t}_u$ is the mean value of time on schedule u.

EXAMPLE: A SIMPLE RANDOMIZED CLINICAL TRIAL

Consider a placebo controlled trial to evaluate a new blood pressure medication. The investigators plan a pretest–posttest design and will use ANCOVA to analyze posttest diastolic blood pressure, adjusting for pretest diastolic blood pressure. With this plan, we can use equation 4.15 to estimate the sample size required for analysis. The variance of diastolic blood pressure for the target population is 110, and the over-time correlation for the one-year follow-up period proposed is 0.7. The investigators plan a two-tailed test with a type I error rate of 5% and 80% power. Assuming large df, we can use 1.96 and 0.84 as the initial values for $t_{critical:\alpha/2}$ and $t_{critical:\beta}$. If the investigators want to detect an effect of 3 mm Hg, they will need 98 participants per condition with data available for analysis:

$$n = \frac{2(110)(1 - 0.7^2)(1.96 + 0.84)^2}{3^2} = 97.7$$

This would provide $2(98 - 1) = 194\,df$, so the t-values should be revised slightly to 1.97 and 0.843. With these adjustments, the sample size required is

$$n = \frac{2(110)(1 - 0.7^2)(1.97 + 0.843)^2}{3^2} = 98.6$$

This would provide $2(99 - 1) = 196\,df$, so these t-values are appropriate.

Because there will be some loss to follow-up over the one-year follow-up period, a few additional calculations are required. If we are to allow for 15% loss to follow-up, and if we are to use multiple imputation procedures to replace the lost data under an assumption of no intervention effect, then we would re-calculate the average expected intervention effect as

$$\Delta = (0.85 \times 3 + 0.15 \times 0) = 2.55$$

Substituting this revised effect into the sample size equation, we see that this attrition rate will increase the size required of the study to 136 per arm:

$$n = \frac{2(110)(1 - 0.7^2)(1.97 + 0.843)^2}{2.55^2} = 136.5$$

This estimation procedure shows that the sample size per condition will increase to 137 to allow for 15% attrition and imputation of missing data under a conservative approach. The df will be $2(137 - 1) = 272$ with this sample size, and the appropriate t-values are still 1.97 and 0.843.

EXTENSION TO OTHER DESIGN AND ANALYSIS PLANS

As outlined toward the beginning of this chapter, the first step in any power analysis is the specification of the form and magnitude of the effect. The research question should define both the design and the analysis, which in turn define the structure of the effect. If the question is whether two randomized conditions differ in the average level of y, after adjustment for baseline levels, the study is a randomized clinical trial with pretest and posttest measures, and the analysis is built around a comparison of two means after regression adjustment for baseline values. Other questions may lead to other designs and analyses and to other definitions for Δ.

To simplify the power analysis, the investigator should simplify the structure of the effect as much as possible. For example, if several contrasts among means, slopes, mean slopes, or their differences are of interest, the investigator should pick one as primary and focus the power analysis on that contrast. Similarly, if there are more than two conditions, the investigators should pick the two that define the primary contrast of interest and focus the power analysis on that contrast. All the methods presented in this chapter presume that the effect is defined as a single df contrast.

The second step is to select a test for that effect. As long as the intervention effect is defined as a single df contrast, and the data are normally distributed, the familiar t-test in equation 4.2 is appropriate. The third step is to determine the distribution of that test under the null hypothesis. With the t-test, the distribution is known as soon as the number of df is known.

The fourth step is to select the critical values in that distribution that determine whether or not the investigator will reject the null hypothesis. The critical values are tied to the investigator's decisions on the type I and II error rates and the use of a one- or two-tailed test.

The fifth step is to develop an expression for the variance of the effect under the null hypothesis in terms of parameters that are easily estimated from the literature, from available data, or from new data. This is the reason that the formulas presented above are written in terms of such parameters as σ_y^2. Those parameters are far easier to estimate than parameters such as $\sigma_{\bar{y}_I - \bar{y}_C}^2$.

The sixth step is to gather estimates of those parameters. This is a critical step, because the quality of the power analysis will depend substantially on the quality of the estimates of the parameters. Investigators should seek to estimate the parameters from data that are similar to the data likely to be collected in the study. For example, if the study will involve school children from a predominantly Hispanic neighborhood, estimates drawn from children of a different age or ethnic group may not be valid. It would be far better to gather limited data from the target population and develop the estimates from those data.

Once the estimates are available, the seventh step is the mechanical generation of the detectable differences, sample sizes, or power estimates, usually across a range of levels for several of the parameters. Here computer spreadsheets can be very helpful, because they often have built-in statistical functions and can perform repetitive calculations more accurately than can be done by hand. Of course, care must be taken to ensure that the spreadsheet is created and used properly.

5 Exploratory/Developmental and Small Grant Award Mechanisms

KENNETH W. GRIFFIN

The creative process takes its own course. If it did otherwise,
it would not be creative.

—P. W. MARTIN, *Experiment in Depth: A Study of the Work of Jung,*
Eliot and Toynbee

THIS CHAPTER DESCRIBES two NIH grant mechanisms, the R03 Small Grant Program and the R21 Exploratory/Developmental Research Grant Program. These mechanisms can be found in the research portfolios of most of the NIH institutes that fund behavioral sciences research. The R03 Small Grant and R21 Exploratory/ Developmental Research Grant programs were introduced by the NIH in order to provide the institutes with more flexibility for funding research projects that vary in scope and degree of risk: R03 grants for projects of limited scope or duration and R21 grants for projects that explore highly innovative topics. These mechanisms can be attractive alternatives to the R01 for a number of reasons. They can help newly independent investigators obtain funding and establish track records as principal investigators before applying for an R01. Pilot data obtained from projects executed using these mechanisms can strengthen subsequent R01 applications for junior investigators, as well as more senior investigators exploring research areas that are relatively new to them. In many cases, R03 and R21 applications have higher funding success rates compared to R01 applications. Thus, R03 and R21 projects often serve as useful stepping stones to larger R01 applications that are broader in scope, duration, and funding.

The R03 and R21 funding mechanisms are used differently across the NIH institutes. Investigator-initiated (or "unsolicited") small grant or exploratory/developmental grant submissions are accepted by most institutes. However, some institutes accept grants using these mechanisms only in response to specific program announcements (PAs) or requests for applications. The NIH institutes change their policies regarding R03 or R21 submissions from time to time (as seen during the recent transition from paper to electronic applications). Therefore, potential applicants must obtain recent information from institute staff and the NIH Web site to ensure that their application follows the most recent institute submission requirements and funding opportunity announcements.

In order to introduce readers to these funding mechanisms, the first section of this chapter describes the goals and objectives of the NIH Small Grant Program according to the NIH-wide guidelines, and the second section describes the NIH Exploratory/Developmental Research Grant Program according to the NIH-wide guidelines. Each mechanism is described in a trans-NIH PA referred to as the "parent R03" and "parent R21" PAs, respectively. These PAs standardize the application characteristics, requirements, preparation, and review procedures for all investigator-initiated submissions using these mechanisms, unless otherwise specified in a separate announcement. In the third section, information is provided regarding how several of the NIH institutes approach these funding mechanisms for behavioral research and where they differ from the NIH-wide guidelines. The institutes included here are the National Institute on Drug Abuse (NIDA), National Institute on Alcoholism and Alcohol Abuse (NIAAA), National Cancer Institute (NCI), National Institute of Mental Health (NIMH), and National Institute on Child Health and Human Development (NICHD). Some of these institutes adhere closely to the parent R03 and parent R21 announcements (e.g., NIAAA, NIMH, NICHD), whereas others have their own grant programs that differ in important ways from the parent announcements (e.g., NCI's Small Grants for Behavioral Research in Cancer Control, and NIDA's B/START Program). The chapter also examines recent trends in the funding success rates for R03 and R21 applications across these five institutes, relative to R01 applications. Examples of recently funded R03 and R21 proposals with a behavioral sciences focus are reviewed for each NIH institute to frame a discussion on the how R03 and R21 grants differ from the R01 funding mechanism in scope, content, and size.

R03 SMALL GRANT PROGRAM: THE NIH GENERAL GUIDELINES

The NIH Small Grant Program provides support for research projects that are typically limited in time, amount of funding, and scope of research aims. These submissions can include pilot projects and feasibility studies to determine the whether a proposed plan of research is worthwhile, practical, scientifically meritorious, and consistent with an institute's research portfolio. The R03 mechanism is also appropriate for secondary analyses of existing data sets that address new research questions, as well as research projects that develop and test new research methods or innovative technologies. Given the relatively short period of time and limited financial support provided with R03 grants, it is expected that researchers will use R03 funding to conduct small projects that may provide a basis for more extended research that fits more closely with R01 initiatives.

The NIH-wide R03 funding mechanism is described in detail in PA-06-180, called "NIH Small Research Grant Program (Parent R03)." This document lists general guidelines for submitting an investigator-initiated R03 application. Most of the institutes reviewed in this chapter participate in the parent R03 program (NIDA, NIAAA, NICHD, and NIMH), with the exception of NCI, which does not accept investigator-initiated R03 applications. According to the parent R03 guidelines, applicants using the R03 mechanism may request project funds for a period lasting no more than two years and a budget with direct costs up to $50,000 per year. The fine print of the NIH PA emphasizes that R03 small grant support is for new projects only, and that competing continuation applications and grants to support dissertation research are not accepted. Other mechanisms covered in this book address these specific forms of funding.

There have been a number of recent changes in the NIH guidelines for R03 funding. In 2006, R03 applications switched to electronic submission, and paper versions are no longer accepted (chapter 17 covers this issue more closely). All R03 applications must now include an appropriate PA number and title. If an R03 application is assigned to an institute or center that does not participate in the parent R03 program, it may be returned without review. According to the parent R03 PA, the research plan of an R03 application (i.e., the Specific Aims, Background and Significance, Preliminary Studies, and Research Design/Methods sections) may not exceed a total of 10 pages. Furthermore, an investigator may submit up to two revisions of a previously reviewed R03 small grant application (this follows a general rule for applications upheld throughout NIH). Applications submitted under the parent R03 announcement currently have the standard postmark/submission deadlines for competing applications (February 5, June 5, and October 5, effective January 2007). Many of the recent guideline changes summarized above reflect broader NIH-wide regulations that affect other types of funding mechanisms as well, including the R21.

R21 EXPLORATORY/DEVELOPMENTAL RESEARCH GRANT AWARD: THE NIH GENERAL GUIDELINES

NIH uses the R21 mechanism to encourage new research initiatives that involve an especially high degree of innovation, novelty, and risk. This would include support for pilot testing potentially groundbreaking ideas and research methods that would have a major impact on biomedical or behavioral research. R21 applications do not require the inclusion of preliminary or pilot data regarding feasibility or efficacy, a fact that can facilitate the exploration of novel and highly innovative research ideas for which no data are available. Notwithstanding, if available, pilot data can be included.

Similar to the directives regarding R03 grants, not all of the NIH institutes accept R21 applications. Most of the institutes discussed in the present chapter participate in the parent R21 PA, again with the exception of NCI (as described in a later section). According to the parent R21 PA, an applicant may request a project period of up to two years with direct costs for the two-year period up to $275,000. For example, investigators may request $100,000 in the first year and $175,000 in the second year to meet the needs of their projects. Normally, no more than $200,000 may be requested in any single year, and all budgets should be in modular format (i.e., in $25,000 increments). Furthermore, the R21 research plan may not exceed a total of 15 pages. Applications submitted under the parent R21 PA currently have the standard postmark/submission deadlines for competing applications (February 5, June 5, and October 5). In the following sections, specific information is provided for several of the NIH institutes that fund behavioral research with the R03 and R21 grant mechanisms, including if and how they differ in emphasis from the general NIH-wide parent PA guidelines.

NIH INSTITUTES THAT FUND BEHAVIORAL SCIENCE RESEARCH USING THE R03 AND R21 GRANT MECHANISMS

National Institute on Drug Abuse (NIDA)

NIDA participates in both parent PAs for the R03 and R21. Consistent with R03 grant mechanisms in general, NIDA's small grants program is designed for less experienced new investigators, researchers at institutions without well-developed research histories and resources, experienced investigators who are interested in pursuing a research direction that is new for them, and investigators that would like to test new research methods or techniques. NIDA small grants submissions must adhere to the parent R03 requirements. Accordingly, NIDA R03 grants provide research support of a maximum of $50,000 per year in direct costs for up to two years. Similarly, for R21 applications, NIDA follows the NIH-wide parent R21, which provides research support of a maximum of $275,000 per year in direct costs for up to three years. The mechanism an investigator chooses would reflect the proposal's scope in size, anticipated expense, required time for execution, and level of innovation.

NIDA uses a special R03 grant award mechanism for early career investigators, the Behavioral Science Track Award for Rapid Transition (B/START), which is meant to facilitate the entry of new investigators into behavioral research related to drug abuse. NIDA's B/START (described in PAR-05-541) provides funding for a period of one year with a maximum of $50,000 in direct costs. Because the B/START mechanism is for new independent investigators, a goal of the program is to provide awards rapidly, within about six months from the date the application is received at NIH. The NIDA B/START funds small-scale or pilot research projects that focus on a variety of topics that NIDA is particularly interested in funding, including determinants, correlates, and consequences of drug use, abuse, and addiction; the epidemiology and risk/protective factors for drug abuse; research related to drug abuse services in treatment and prevention; and behavioral research on drug abuse and HIV/AIDS. Eligibility requirements for the NIDA B/START are that an applicant must be five or fewer years beyond training status and must not have been a principal investigator on an NIH research project (including mentored K-awards) or received similar support from another federal agency. Investigators who previously received a dissertation research grant or a National Research Service Award (institutional or individual) are eligible for the NIDA B/START program.

How do R03 and R21 applications submitted to NIDA fare in funding decisions compared to R01 success rates? Figure 5.1 shows the number of new grant applications submitted to NIDA from the 2003–2005 fiscal years using the R03 and R21 funding mechanisms, along with the success rates for funding and average award amounts in dollars. For comparative purposes, data for R01 applications are provided alongside. Juxtaposition of this information helps paint a picture of the highly competitive nature of R01 grants versus R03 and R21 mechanisms. At NIDA, for instance, there has been an increase in the number of applications submitted each year using the R03, R21, and R01 funding mechanisms. Compared to R01 grant applications, the R03 and R21 mechanisms were fewer in number and smaller in dollar amount, as would be expected. This is also true for each of the other four institutes examined in this chapter. However, in general, a higher percentage of R03 and R21 applications submitted to NIDA were funded relative to the R01 success rate. Another trend clearly shown in figure 5.1 is that the application success rate has decreased for all three funding mechanisms from FY 2003 to FY 2005. About one in three R21 applications submitted to NIDA were funded in FY 2003, whereas fewer than one in five applications were funded in FY 2005. Thus, although funding for all three mechanisms has decreased in recent years, R03 and R21 applications submitted to NIDA are slightly more likely to obtain funding relative to R01 submissions, all other things being equal.

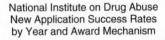

National Institute on Drug Abuse
New Application Success Rates
by Year and Award Mechanism

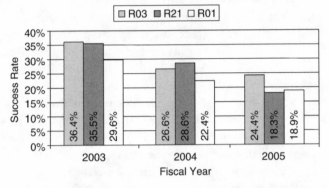

	Submitted	Awarded	Success Rate	Average Award
R03 Small Grant Program				
2005	176	43	24.4%	$88,690
2004	139	37	26.6%	$76,602
2003	132	48	36.4%	$85,441
R21 Exploratory/Developmental Research Grant Program				
2005	378	69	18.3%	$178,427
2004	213	61	28.6%	$176,670
2003	172	61	35.5%	$157,104
R01 Research Project Grant Program				
2005	935	177	18.9%	$407,244
2004	892	200	22.4%	$387,906
2003	713	211	29.6%	$395,760

Figure 5.1. New Application Success Rates by Funding Mechanism for NIDA

National Institute of Alcohol Abuse and Alcoholism (NIAAA)

NIAAA participates in both parent PAs for the R03 and R21. Similar to the other institutes, NIAAA has several PAs that accept applications through multiple mechanisms including the R21 and R03. At NIAAA and throughout NIH, one of the many recent changes is a trend to divide PAs into separate funding opportunity announcements for different funding mechanisms. For example, the previous PA for "Secondary Analysis of Existing Alcohol Epidemiology Data" (PA-05-088) stated that submissions could be made via the R03, R21, or R01 mechanisms. Recently, this PA was reissued as two separate announcements: PA-06-558 for R03 submissions and PA-06-557 for R21 submissions. This strategy may be helpful to applicants because more detail is provided regarding the expected scope of research projects according to each funding mechanism. It may also help reviewers keep the specific criteria for each funding mechanism in mind during the review process. Again, the mechanism an investigator chooses would reflect factors such as the work scope, the time and budget needs, and degree of novelty.

For small grants and exploratory/developmental grants, NIAAA funds projects that explore the feasibility of innovative or creative research questions within the research interests of the institute. These topics may include applied research on behavioral mechanisms leading to pathological drinking behavior, and behavioral approaches to more effective diagnosis, prevention, and treatment of alcoholism, alcohol abuse, and alcohol-related problems, to name a few. To expedite the review and award process for new investigators applying for R21 grants, NIAAA allows new applicants receiving scores within five percentile points of the pay-line to write a letter to NIAAA program officials, responding to the critiques raised in the summary statement, and program staff then have the option of making a recommendation for award to the institute director.

What about NIAAA's track record for funding R03 and R21 applications relative to R01 grants? Figure 5.2 shows the number of new grant applications submitted to NIAAA from the 2003–2005 fiscal years using the R03, R21, and R01 funding mechanisms, success rates for funding, and average award in dollars. Interestingly, these data show that at NIAAA the number of applications submitted using the R03, R21, and R01 funding mechanisms has not fluctuated tremendously over the past few years. A careful inspection of these data show no clear trends in funding success rates for the different mechanisms. For example, in FY 2004 there was a 40.3% success rates for R03 applications, while 21.7% of R01 applications were funded; however, in FY 2005 the success rate for R03 grants was 17.5% while 27.5% of R01 applications were funded. Thus, it is not clear given recent trend data or funding priorities that—everything else being equal—an investigator would be better off applying to NIAAA for an R03 or R21 as opposed to an R01, except perhaps for a new investigator applying for an R21.

National Cancer Institute (NCI)

Out of the five NIH institutes reviewed in this chapter, NCI is the only one that does not currently participate in the parent R03 or parent R21 programs. Thus, NCI does not accept investigator-initiated R03 submissions. However, NCI does have an ongoing program for R03 applicants in the behavioral sciences called "Small Grants for Behavioral Research in Cancer Control (R03)" (PAR-06-458). This NCI small grants program is designed to facilitate the growth of a nationwide cohort of scientists with a high level of expertise in behavioral research related to cancer control. This program differs in important ways from the general parent R03 announcement: Applicants may request funding for up to three years with a budget for direct costs that does not exceed $100,000 for the entire project

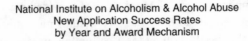

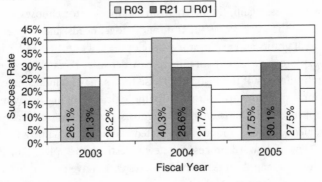

	Submitted	Awarded	Success Rate	Average Award
R03 Small Grant Program				
2005	40	7	17.5%	$80,970
2004	67	27	40.3%	$52,137
2003	46	12	26.1%	$73,825
R21 Exploratory/Developmental Research Grant Program				
2005	183	55	30.1%	$189,586
2004	168	48	28.6%	$182,821
2003	178	38	21.3%	$156,327
R01 Research Project Grant Program				
2005	313	86	27.5%	$369,063
2004	337	73	21.7%	$353,989
2003	298	78	26.2%	$395,415

Figure 5.2. New Application Success Rates by Funding Mechanism for NIAAA

period. Unlike the parent R03, small grant support obtained from this announcement may be used for dissertation research; however, investigators who
have been awarded an NCI-funded cancer control research grant (R03, R21, R01
U01, or P01) are not eligible. Applicants who have received these awards from
other institutes are eligible to apply for the NCI R03 small grant award for
behavioral research in cancer control. In addition to those differences already
mentioned for the NCI R03, applicants must identify a mentor, and foreign
applicants are not eligible for this program. Applications submitted under this
NCI small grant award have three postmark/submission deadlines (currently
April, August, and December), but these are different than the standard submission dates listed in the parent R03. Submissions are reviewed by an NCI ad hoc

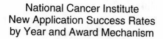

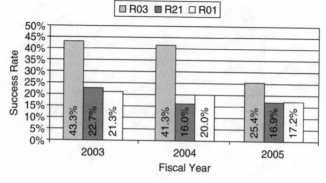

	Submitted	Awarded	Success Rate	Average Award
R03 Small Grant Program				
2005	350	89	25.4%	$75,897
2004	327	135	41.3%	$76,492
2003	247	107	43.3%	$75,443
R21 Exploratory/Developmental Research Grant Program				
2005	1,474	249	16.9%	$173,703
2004	1,509	242	16.0%	$173,840
2003	963	219	22.7%	$195,229
R01 Research Project Grant Program				
2005	3,434	592	17.2%	$328,651
2004	3,246	650	20.0%	$327,918
2003	2,987	636	21.3%	$345,123

Figure 5.3. New Application Success Rates by Funding Mechanism for NCI

review group that selects reviewers with specific expertise to match current batch of applications. NCI also has a similar specific R21 PA titled "Exploratory Grants for Behavioral Research in Cancer Control (R21)" that describes the submission and eligibility requirements in detail (PA-06-351).

What is the recent history of funding success at NCI for the R03, R21, and R01 mechanisms? Figure 5.3 shows the number of new grant applications submitted to NCI for the period from 2003 to 2005 fiscal years using the R03, R21, and R01 funding mechanisms, along with the success rates for funding and average award amounts in dollars. At NCI, there has been an increase in the number of R03 and R01 applications submitted each year during this time period, and a corresponding decrease in funding success rates. Interestingly, the success rate for R03 applications dropped precipitously from 43.3% in FY 2003 to 25.4% in FY 2005.

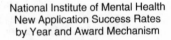

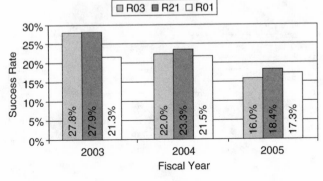

	Submitted	Awarded	Success Rate	Average Award
R03 Small Grant Program				
2005	300	48	16.0%	$73,786
2004	368	81	22.0%	$71,903
2003	299	83	27.8%	$70,339
R21 Exploratory/Developmental Research Grant Program				
2005	326	60	18.4%	$189,831
2004	343	80	23.3%	$170,149
2003	315	88	27.9%	$156,754
R01 Research Project Grant Program				
2005	1,352	234	17.3%	$373,415
2004	1,316	283	21.5%	$366,966
2003	1,229	262	21.3%	$379,989

Figure 5.4. New Application Success Rates by Funding Mechanism for NIMH

The success rates for R21 applications submitted to NCI were even lower, ranging from 16% to 22.7%, which was similar to the success rates for R01 submitted to NCI. So despite the notable drop in success rates for R03 applications submitted to NCI over this time period, success rates for R03s still remained higher than those for the R21 and R01 mechanisms.

National Institute of Mental Health (NIMH)

NIMH participates in both parent PAs for the R03 and R21 as well as several PAs that accept applications through multiple mechanisms. NIMH began the B/START R03 program to facilitate the entry of new investigators into the field of behavioral research in areas consistent with the institute's mission of reducing mental illness and behavioral disorders. While NIDA continues its B/START program, NIMH recently discontinued its B/START program because staff felt the applications were increasingly similar to R03 grants submitted through other funding opportunity announcements.

Figure 5.4 shows the number of new grant applications submitted to NIMH for the fiscal period from 2003 to 2005 using the R03, R21, and R01 funding mechanisms, along with corresponding success rates for funding and average award in dollars. While the number of applications submitted to NIMH using the R03, R21, and R01 funding mechanisms has not fluctuated greatly during this designated time period, there is a clear trend for reduced funding success rates corresponding to each mechanism. The drop in success rates was largest for R03 applications, from 27.8% in FY 2003 down to 16% in FY 2005. In FY 2005, the success rates for the three funding mechanisms were approximately the same, ranging from 16% to 18.4%.

National Institute of Child Health and Human Development (NICHD)

NICHD participates in both parent PAs for the R03 and R21 and does not have institute-specific instructions for submitting R03 and R21 grants. However, NICHD does maintain a higher pay-line for small grant applications as a way of supporting new investigators. NICHD reviews applications submitted by new investigators that received priority scores beyond the funding range, and in some cases NICHD may give special funding consideration for these applications. Program staff may decide to fund a small grant out of sequence or provide partial funding of larger grants to allow preparation and submission of revised applications for review. As far as funding success rates, figure 5.5 shows the number of new grant applications submitted to NICHD from the 2003 to 2005 fiscal years using the R03, R21, and R01 funding mechanisms, along with success rates for funding and average award in dollars. In recent years, there has been an increase in the number of applications submitted to NICHD using all three mechanisms. The success rates for the three mechanisms was highest in FY 2003, lowest in FY 2004, and improved somewhat for FY 2005 despite an increase in applications for each mechanism.

CONCLUSIONS

The R21 and R03 mechanisms were first introduced by NIH for the purposes of funding research projects that might not fare well in a standard R01 review because they are either of limited scope or duration (R03) or explore highly innovative topics (R21). For smaller projects or those that explore research ideas not incorporated into mainstream thinking, these funding mechanisms provide new and established investigators with an attractive alternative to the R01 grant application.

Investigators may choose to submit a research grant proposal using the R03 mechanism if they are planning to conduct a smaller scale study that can be

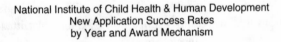

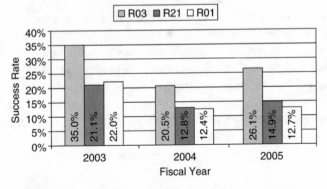

National Institute of Child Health & Human Development
New Application Success Rates
by Year and Award Mechanism

	Submitted	Awarded	Success Rate	Average Award
R03 Small Grant Program				
2005	494	129	26.1%	$74,707
2004	409	84	20.5%	$74,753
2003	354	124	35.0%	$74,547
R21 Exploratory/Developmental Research Grant Program				
2005	450	67	14.9%	$181,363
2004	196	25	12.8%	$162,428
2003	90	19	21.1%	$199,605
R01 Research Project Grant Program				
2005	1,478	188	12.7%	$345,064
2004	1,385	172	12.4%	$352,761
2003	1,084	238	22.0%	$331,020

Figure 5.5. New Application Success Rates by Funding Mechanism for NICHD

completed within two years for less than $50,000 in direct costs per year. Table 5.1 lists the titles of several recently funded R03 grant applications with a behavioral sciences focus, by NIH institute. From this table, one can see that investigators have used the R03 mechanism in recent years for projects that are of limited scope because they test very specific hypotheses (e.g., "The Boomerang Effect of the Anti-drug Media Campaign"), examine unique populations (e.g., "Obesity in Hispanic Children With Leukemia"), conduct research that develops new self-report measures and tests their psychometric properties (e.g., "Development of the Trauma Appraisal Questionnaire"), or conduct secondary analyses of existing data sets in order to answer very focused and previously untested scientific questions (e.g., "Patterns and Transitions in Alcohol Use for Urban Youth").

TABLE 5.1	Examples of Funded R03 Grant Applications With a Behavioral Sciences Focus, by NIH Institute, 2003–2006
Institute	Grant Title
NIDA	Child Maltreatment and Later Drug Use The Boomerang Effect of the Anti-drug Media Campaign HIV Risk Behaviors and Depression Among Drug Users Predictors of Adolescent Ecstasy Use in National Survey Nonmedical Prescription Drug Use Among College Students
NIAAA	Migration, Alcohol Use and HIV Risk in Rural Mexico Patterns and Transitions in Alcohol Use for Urban Youth Alcohol Effects on Smoking Urge and Behavior Runaway Youth: Precursors and Consequences Alcohol-Related Sexual Assault Among Adolescents
NCI	Obesity in Hispanic Children With Leukemia Race-Specific Occupational Risk Factors for Cancer Culture and Cancer Literacy Among Immigrant Women Diet and Cancer in Puerto Rican Men Health Behaviors in Adolescent Cancer Survivors
NIMH	Primary and Mental Health Services for Rural Children Effects of Context on Fear Behaviors in Toddlers Mother–Infant Conflict and Problem Behavior Development Prevention of Depression Among Adolescents in Iceland Development of the Trauma Appraisal Questionnaire
NICHD	Out-of-School Child Care for Children With Disabilities Causality Between Youth Employment and Problem Behavior Marriage, Birth and Divorce After Terrorist Attack Father Involvement and Child Well-being in Poor Families Wealth and Health: Race, Assets and Child Development

Investigators may choose to submit a research grant proposal using the R21 mechanism if they are planning an especially innovative or exploratory study for which pilot data is unavailable and that can be completed within two years for less than $275,000 in direct costs total. Table 5.2 lists the titles of several recently funded R21 grant applications with a behavioral sciences focus, by NIH institute. As shown in this table, investigators have recently used the R21 mechanism for projects that test the feasibility of new research approaches (e.g., "Assessing HIV in Hidden Populations: A Feasibility Study"), explore new ideas (e.g., "Effects of Alcohol on Human Self-aggressive Behavior"), or examine the use of new research methods (e.g., "Handheld Computer Diaries to Enhance Alcohol Assessment").

TABLE 5.2	Examples of Funded R21 Grant Applications With a Behavioral Sciences Focus, by NIH Institute, 2003–2006
Institute	**Grant Title**
NIDA	Does Psychological Wellness Predict Treatment Response?
	Home Based Treatment for Drug Use in Early Adolescents
	Assessing HIV in Hidden Populations: A Feasibility Study
	Deconstructing HIV Interventions for Female Offenders
	Mechanisms of Smoking Reinforcement
NIAAA	Alcohol-Involved Sexual Risk Behavior among HIV+ Persons
	Effects of Alcohol on Human Self-aggressive Behavior
	Handheld Computer Diaries to Enhance Alcohol Assessment
	Alcohol, Mortality and Ethnicity in the US
	Alcohol, Risky Behavior, and HIV / AIDS in Zimbabwe
NCI	Cultural Model of Prevention in African-American Women
	Smoking Cessation in African-American Men: A Pilot Study
	Involving Adolescents in Physical Activity Promotion
	Psychosocial Impact of Cancer-Related Female Infertility
	Computerized Assessment of Cancer Symptoms
NIMH	Indicated Prevention With At-Risk Gamblers
	Developing a Model of Transitive Behavior
	Development of a Tailored Treatment for Angry Mothers
	Preventive Intervention for Children at Risk for ADHD
	Developing Effective Treatments for Child Physical Abuse
NICHD	Tipping the Energy Balance for Latino Children
	Health Patterns: Hispanic and Non-Hispanic Children
	Promoting Condom Use among African American Males
	Home Visiting With High Risk Teen Mothers
	Measuring Developmental Idealism and Family Life

In deciding whether to submit an R03 or R21 application, an investigator should consider several factors. The first would be how innovative and novel a research idea is. If a project idea is very novel and no preliminary data are available, it might be best suited to an R21 application, which does not require pilot data. Another obvious consideration is the time and resources needed to carry out a project. R21s allow for longer project terms and greater funding than do R03s, although they do not have to use the maximum resources allowed, of course, if the research plan does not call for it.

There is some debate within and outside of NIH as to whether the R03 and R21 mechanisms have the advantages over R01s that had been envisioned when these selective funding mechanisms were introduced. Do review committees adequately consider the differences between the R03 and R01 mechanism, for example, or do reviewers sometimes hold R03 grants to the same high standard as R01 grants? Every grant reviewer and NIH study section is different, and it is impossible to know in advance what will happen during the review of a grant application. However, in preparing an R03 or R21 application, it may be worthwhile to remind reviewers of the specific characteristics of the application that make it appropriately aligned with the less stringent requirements for small and exploratory/developmental grant mechanisms.

6 Funding Your Future

What You Need to Know to Develop a Pre- or Postdoctoral Training Application

JENNIFER WEIL, SUSANNA NEMES, & KELLY MUNLY

The danger lies in refusing to face the fear, in not daring to come to grips with it. If you fail anywhere along the line, it will take away your confidence. You must make yourself succeed every time. You must do the thing you think you cannot do.

—ELEANOR ROOSEVELT, *You Learn by Living*

THE MISSION OF NIH is to lead the nation in bringing the power of science to improve people's health. This broad undertaking involves four expressed goals: (1) fostering innovative research methods that advance the nation's ability to protect and improve health, (2) providing and maintaining the physical resources necessary to prevent disease, (3) increasing scientific knowledge and further the nation's public investment in research, and (4) maintaining the highest standards of integrity, accountability, and social responsibility in the conduct of science.[1] An essential component toward achieving the mission of NIH is the nurturing, development, and growth of individual researchers capable of conducting high-quality research in areas that are priorities to the current 27 NIH institutes and centers.

THE HISTORY AND PURPOSE OF CAREER DEVELOPMENT AND TRAINING AWARDS

NIH involvement in training new scientists to conduct biomedical and behavioral research began in the 1930s with the enactment of the Ransdell Act. This congressional act established the agency as a premier training center fostering research activities and maintaining a critical research workforce. As each institute was formed, training support for new investigators was a primary goal highlighted by its mission statement and sustained financially by the federal government budget. By the 1960s, NIH dedicated 15% of its extramural research budget to developing training programs and supporting the training of 16,000 new investigators each year.

Unfortunately, the burden of economic difficulties cropping up in the late 1960s hindered government support and threatened to eliminate research training programs. The Nixon administration contended that supply of research scientists was inordinately high, essentially diminishing any pressing need for training new investigators. As a result, Congress consolidated research-training activities into a single program of training grants and fellowships known as the National Research Service Award (NRSA) program. To date, the NRSA program has provided research training in the biomedical and behavioral sciences to more than 130,000 students and young investigators through a combination of individual fellowship awards and institutional training grants at approximately 750 universities, research institutes, and teaching hospitals.[2]

HOW DOES AN NRSA BENEFIT A STUDENT, MENTOR, AND INSTITUTION?

When one of the many NIH institutes awards an NRSA, numerous parties benefit including the award recipient, recipient's sponsor, and the funding government agency.[2] The award substantially reduces a student's financial concerns and possibly any need for outside employment, allowing students to focus more intensely on their research and learning. Minimizing financial and situational stress for university students enhances their subjective well-being and future scholarly success.[3,4] Moreover, the prestige associated with receiving an award inspires future success in the research world. The university or research institute providing sponsorship also benefits from its receipt of the grant award, not only in terms of prestige, but also financially because the award reduces the necessity of providing student financial support. The government agency providing the funding also benefits from the service research award mechanism by inspiring new research ideas, increasing recognition in a specific field, and developing a critical mass of highly trained scientists needed to sustain future innovation.

GOALS OF THIS CHAPTER

Information on the NIH career training programs is readily available to the public. Graduate and postdoctoral students alike have access to this information. However, it appears that not many individuals take advantage of these grant funding mechanisms. The lack of clear interest in these funding opportunities coupled with the lack of formal education in grant writing results in a diminished number of applications submitted by doctoral candidates and postdoctoral students. According to the National Opinion Research Center, approximately 42,683 doctoral degrees were awarded in the United States during 1998.[5] However, the majority of Ph.D. graduates do not seem to be pursuing F awards; in 1998, there were only a total of 2,839 applicants for this award, approximately 15% of the total number of Ph.D. graduates in the United States. The latest statistics offer evidence of depicting only minimal growth, yielding a total of 3,030 new applicants.[6]

Graduate and postdoctoral students need to excel within a climate where NIH funding is becoming increasingly competitive, peer review of applications is becoming more streamlined and rigorous, and costs associated with preparation and review of applications are escalating. To help offset these apparent obstacles and smooth the transition from graduate school mentality to the professional research arena, this chapter provides tips to both mentors and students on developing an NRSA application. The chapter reviews the different types of awards available to entry level scientists, highlights crucial elements of the application process, and outlines the main components of the scientific review process for the various F awards.

WHAT TYPES OF AWARDS ARE AVAILABLE FOR PRE- AND POSTDOCTORAL STUDENTS?

Three types of NRSA awards are available to students at the pre- or postdoctoral levels. These grant mechanisms, known as F30, F31, and F32, maintain different eligibility requirements and are intended specifically for applicants desiring advanced research or clinical training. The following sections describe in greater detail requirements for each of the fellowship awards. Table 6.1 provides details for the F-series NRSA grant mechanisms.

Predoctoral Awards

F30

Training the nation's medical students to become active biomedical researchers is a primary goal of this F-series award. Because a majority of medical schools do not provide either the requisite training or experience required to develop

TABLE 6.1	Types of F Awards	
Type of Grant or Award	Eligibility Requirements	Comments
Individual Predoctoral National Research Awards for M.D./ Ph.D. Fellows (F30)	Applicants must be enrolled in M.D./ Ph.D. program, Ph.D. program, and supervised by a mentor in that scientific discipline when the application is submitted	• Stipend: $19,968 per year • Institutional Allowance: up to $2,750 per year • Tuition Costs: 100% of tuition costs up to $3,000 plus 60% above $3,000
National Research Service Awards for Individual Predoctoral Students, Minority Students, and Students With Disabilities (F31)	Applicants must be enrolled in a program leading to a doctorate and be supervised by a mentor	• Stipend: $19,968 per year • Institutional Allowance: up to $2,750 per year • Tuition Costs: 100% of tuition costs up to $3,000 plus 60% above $3,000
NIH National Research Service Awards for Individual Postdoctoral Fellows (F32)	Applicants must have received a Ph.D. or M.D. and have identified a mentor	• Stipend: from $34,200 to $50,808 per year • Institutional Allowance: up to $5,500 per year • Tuition Costs: 100% of tuition costs up to $3,000 plus 60% above $3,000

Applicants are encouraged to visit the respective Web sites for each NIH institute or center (see appendix 2) in order to obtain current information about the scientific missions, program priorities, research topics of interest, and policy guidelines. In addition, applicants are advised to visit the NIH Web site to obtain current information about funding. Appendix 1 provides extensive detailed information covering relevant Web sites for F-series awards.

research scientists, it becomes essential to reinforce or supplement training and education of medical health researchers through NRSA awards. Students enrolled in M.D./Ph.D. programs are eligible for this award and are encouraged to develop training projects that will foster their scientific acumen in the areas of clinical, translational, epidemiologic, prevention, and services research. Students from a wide range of disciplines are encouraged to apply, including public health, epidemiology, economics, bioethics, computer science, and pharmacy.[1]

F31

Three different awards fall under the umbrella of the F31 funding mechanism: the NRSA Predoctoral Fellowship, the NRSA Predoctoral Fellowship for Minority Students, and the NRSA Predoctoral Fellowship for Students With Disabilities.

These awards provide up to five years of support for research training leading to the Ph.D. or equivalent graduate research degree in biomedical, behavioral, and health services. The NRSA that targets minority students and the NRSA for students with disabilities were created to enhance the overall diversity of the field.

Postdoctoral Awards: F32

The F32 award is provided in support of postdoctoral training in the areas of biomedical, behavioral, or clinical research. Individuals interested in this grant mechanism strive to enhance their expertise in health-focused sciences. Awardees must dedicate no less than 40 hours per week to a research training program, restricting clinical duties outside of their research training experience. The F32 may not be used to support studies leading to the M.D., D.O., D.D.S., D.V.M., or other similar health-professional degrees. Furthermore, this specific F-award may not be used to support medical or other health professional residency training.

THE APPLICATION PROCESS

This section first highlights special considerations from the perspective of the applicant and then provides useful information appropriate to the mentor's perspective.

The Applicant's Perspective

If you are a graduate student or current postgraduate fellow considering submitting an F-series application, this section may be particularly relevant.

Should You Be a Researcher?

Making the decision to become an independent researcher early in your career may appear quite daunting and challenging. As a graduate student or postdoctoral candidate, you may feel overwhelmed with innumerable professional opportunities and facing a broad range of career choices. When determining whether a research career is in your future, consider the questions listed in box 6.1. If you respond yes to all or most of these questions, you may find a career in research appropriate and an incredibly rewarding experience. In general, researchers gradually become experts in a particular area, and most have dedicated a lion's share of their professional lives to studying specific phenomena. Most researchers are quite methodical, very detail-oriented, and creative individuals who continue to pursue the "truth" that deductive and inductive research investigation can provide. Researchers strive to communicate and disseminate their knowledge for the purpose of improving services and extending science. If you believe or already know this type of work is appealing and can be professional rewarding, then applying for an NRSA may be the right step for you.

Box 6.1 Pop Quiz: Are You Ready to Be a Researcher?

- Are you the type of person who is passionate about learning?
- Do you notice even miniscule details?
- Do you enjoy writing?
- Are you willing to work on a project for multiple years without instant gratification?
- Are you interested in brainstorming alternative explanations to information presented?
- Do you enjoy working in a group environment with a team of individuals?

How Do You Find a Mentor?

Choosing an appropriate mentor represents an important key to developing a successful application and training experience. Typically, your graduate or postdoctoral mentor will serve as your NRSA project mentor. There are numerous reasons to choose your graduate or postdoctoral mentor. First, in most academic institutions, your primary mentor was assigned based on his/her ability to provide research opportunities in your interest areas. These opportunities support your career development by allowing you to obtain specialized training consistent with your career goals. Second, many investigators will develop NRSA projects that represent an extension of their mentor's current area of study. This helps to build on an existing research program, establishes a continuous train of research endeavor, and allows the candidate to draw favorably from the mentor's expertise. Third, there is already an established professional relationship that exists between you and your graduate or postdoctoral mentor. An NRSA will serve only to extend and consolidate this professional relationship, retaining a key ingredient based on an apprenticeship model. Finally, your graduate or postdoctoral mentor will typically have experience in obtaining grant funding as well as mentoring other students to become independent research scientists. This track record and accumulated expertise are vital to your success. A sponsor who has already served as a mentor to other predoctoral or postdoctoral candidates would be ideal. This serves to strengthen your application, demonstrating the mentor's interest in training. However, you should not choose someone who has so many graduate students or fellows that he/she would not have sufficient quality time set aside for you. A major point of review, as discussed further below, is the quality of mentoring with respect to time commitment.

In the case where your NRSA project is not based on your graduate or postdoctoral mentor's current area of study, it may be beneficial to recruit a co-mentor. A co-mentor can provide you with additional expertise and training that will ultimately support your career development. A co-mentor's experience should enhance your NRSA application, exemplifying specific opportunities that will further develop your skills and research acumen. Although it is recommended that co-mentors be easily accessible, it is not mandatory they reside at or near your institution. If you choose to retain a mentor located at another institution or located in another state that is not geographically accessible, be sure to create a realistic plan to access his/her expertise. This plan should detail the number of visits per year and the frequency of email and phone contacts necessary to ensure appropriate mentorship. With the advent of internet access and file transfer protocols, review committees recognize that collaborations can take place over longer distances from institution to institution, even across continents. When this occurs, the supervision plan should outline the necessity of the co-mentor making sure to emphasize the realistic communication that will happen utilizing the mentorship bridge. In addition, the application should carefully articulate the alliance created between co-mentor and usual mentor, making sure to highlight the recognition of each other's expertise, their scientific relationship, and the handshaking that will occur during the supervision period. Both the mentor and co-mentor should recognize each others scientific reputation and affinity toward training in their letters of support. This is no small matter, and on many occasions reviewers have noted that the mentor or co-mentor did not recognize his/her counterpart's contribution to science, as if unaware of this important relationship.

Your mentor's credentials, his/her ability to oversee your research goals, and where he/she has established expertise weigh very heavily in the review process of your application. It is not uncommon for mentors to contribute a significant portion to the construction and writing of the NRSA application. A good piece of advice is to choose a person who adds strength to your application and will assist you in honing your writing and research skills. There is much to be learned during graduate school, focusing on particular theory, methods, history, and technique, to name just a few scholarly foci. Often, however, one of the most overlooked skills is the ability to generate research grants (interestingly, we make a living doing this particular task but receive so little preparatory training) through effective writing. This emphasis on writing effectively and successfully is one of the highlights or main features of this book, and you will find numerous contributors repeatedly emphasizing the importance of communication through writing skills!

Developing a Research Project and Training Plan

The first step in writing any application revolves around preparation. To start, applicants should download the application forms and corresponding instructions from the appropriate NIH institute or center Web site and carefully read this information (see appendix 1). Make sure you meet eligibility requirements and that your background/project topic is appropriate to the NIH institute where you will direct your application. Next, establish a working meeting with your primary mentor and begin brainstorming a research project. There is any number of ways to go about this task, and as some contributors have made clear in their chapters, there is no formal means to specify how these meetings should proceed. One contributor made reference to a discussion that ended up outlined on a Marriot Hotel napkin and eventually turned into this book. Whole dissertations as well as research articles and even grants have been outlined in a similar fashion. The meeting can be more formal, use a chalkboard to outline ideas, or take shape as a formal research presentation to colleagues who then critique your ideas to the point of refinement. Regardless of technique, the end result is the same.

You can ask your mentor for sample proposals from other students who might be willing to share them. Having a chance to review the content and layout of another NRSA application can prove to be invaluable. Also if there are other F-grant awardees in your program or in other graduate or postgraduate programs at the same university or institute, consult with them and seek their advice. Even if the grant comes from someone who applied and did not get funded, reading his/her reviewer comments can be very helpful in strengthening your own proposal. Remember, to the reviewers, evaluation of the project emphasizes the training environment and research plan. The goal of an F award is to focus more on acquiring, developing, and refining skills as a researcher rather than on discovering something new or testing a specific theory. Developing a project that will provide training in new or innovative statistical techniques or allow you to hone additional data collection skills represents an appropriate endeavor.

When considering a research project, think about the amount of time you will have from the moment of award until graduation to complete the project. It is important to be realistic with respect to "deliverables" and "timelines." Although, once awarded, an NRSA consumes a lot of time, there are numerous other activities that require attention. For instance, applicants are involved in classes, may have clinical obligations related to their training, and additional responsibilities teaching laboratories or grading papers or tests for their graduate advisors. It is likely that most reviewers were at one time graduate or postdoctoral students, and as a result, they have a keen understanding regarding what is practical and feasible. Reviewers will not be impressed with applications that are unrealistic and/or do not appear to have developed a reasonable timeline and that may not be completed in a timely manner.

Developing a Project That Makes Sense

The next step involves thinking about what research niche you want to fill throughout your career and then map out the necessary steps required to pursue such a goal. What is the first step? How does this step naturally progress from everything you have already done in graduate school and your experiences outside of graduate school? Think about how your mentor's experience and research support your goals and what additional training you require to become an independent researcher in your field of interest. Sit down with your mentor and discuss career objectives and research ideas and plan a program of study that can contribute to the field and toward your education and provide you with the necessary skills to develop into an independent scientist.

Once you have identified your niche, make sure your understanding of the research question is both current and comprehensive. Bounce your ideas off your mentor, and perhaps gain some feedback from colleagues during a graduate student colloquium or research seminar. Map out the desired steps needed to improve your skills and at the same time address a pressing research question. Determine the appropriate scale of the plan based on similar applications, advice from your mentor, or feedback from program officials at the appropriate NIH institute or center.

Creating a Sound and Executable Training Plan

At the bare minimum, your training plan should include basic coursework in research and your field of interest, as well as statistics and ethics. It is highly essential to draw a connection between your training plan and what you plan to accomplish in your research project. Far too often, applicants lay out an ambitious program of study to supplement graduate coursework but lack essential training involving areas deemed critical to the research plan. For example, if the stated career goal outlines a program of study in the combined areas of juvenile forensic psychology and substance abuse, and your project involves developing a psychometric measure to evaluate substance abuse among juvenile offenders, a course or two in instrument development would be an appropriate component to any training plan. Likewise, additional coursework in ethnographic research or qualitative interview or survey techniques may be instrumental in the component dealing with juvenile offenders. In addition to coursework, you can outline a concerted plan that involves attending regional or national conferences, grand rounds, seminars, and workshops, as well as provide a list of additional readings in your area of study, and other professional experiences that will augment your skills as a researcher. Perhaps the most important piece of advice is to "be creative." Other chapters in this book, most notably chapter 3, focus on the pertinent issues related to "innovation" and how best to showcase creativity within a grant. Added to this, you should get the basics by seeking advice both from your mentor and other faculty members available to you. Table 6.2 provides a sample training plan as an example of the essential requirements.

Preparing the Application

Applicants should keep in mind that writing an NRSA application is not a weekend project. These applications require a lot of thought, preparation time,

TABLE 6.2   Sample Training Plan

Task	Training Objectives	Time Commitment
Year 1 **Reading List**	Articles, chapters, and books focused on adolescents, substance abuse measures, substance abuse treatment, and juvenile justice will be collected and reviewed to assist me in thinking of the optimal set of questions for the substance abuse screening instrument.	10 hours per week
Coursework: Fall: Research Methodology I, Substance Abuse Treatment, Introduction to Ethics, Forensic Assessment I; Spring: Research Methodology II, Introduction to Measurement, Forensic Assessment II, and Psychopharmacology	This coursework will enhance my expertise in research and substance abuse, fostering my abilities to apply theory to and think critically about research related to substance abuse, assessment, and treatment in juvenile justice settings.	3 credits per course=10 hours per week per course—4 classes per semester is a standard courseload for a third year doctoral student at my university
Practicum: Institute of Addiction, Clinician	This practicum will help develop my skills as a clinician and provide me with the extensive clinical background in working with substance abusing populations.	8 hours per week
Practicum: Children's Hospital of Connecticut, Assessor	This practicum will assist me in honing my assessment skills working with youth.	8 hours per week

Activity	Description	Time
Conference: American Psychological Association Annual Conference	Conference presentations will help me learn to communicate research findings, network with other professionals in my substantive area, and prepare for publications.	4 days
Mentor's Research Study: Assessment of Youth Miranda Rights	This research will provide expertise in measurement principles and allow me to further my education in assessment of youthful populations.	8 hours per week
Year 2 **Coursework:** Fall: Special Topics in Statistics—Factor Analysis; Advanced Measurement; Law and Mental Health, Child Psychopathology, and Multicultural Psychology	These classes will build on previous coursework, enhancing my knowledge base in the areas of research, substance abuse, and juvenile justice.	3 credits per course= 10 hours per week per course—3 classes per semester is a standard courseload for a fourth year doctoral student at my university
Practicum: Adolescent Substance Abuse Unit	This practicum will allow me to obtain experience in treating substance-abusing adolescents.	8 hours per week
Practicum: Forensic Assessment Clinic	This practicum will allow me to apply my assessment skills to offender populations.	8 hours per week
Conference College on Problems of Drug Dependence	This annual conference will enable me to further hone my oral presentation skills, reinforce my networking, and gain professional exposure.	3 days
Manuscript Development with Co-mentor	This project will allow me to further my analytical and writing skills. All manuscripts will focus on the area of substance use.	4 hours per week

and much discussion between the applicant and mentor. For applicants who choose a co-mentor, there should be advanced communication and partnerships created between the usual mentor and co-mentor. Geographical stretches between institutes (universities or think tanks) may require conference phone calls that need to be scheduled way in advance of the actual writing time. Additionally, applicants may need to obtain support letters from recruitment sites and testing facilities depending on the type of project proposed. You also will need to obtain letters of recommendation from individuals who can address your skills as a future researcher. These letters are important and serve to ensure that your project is feasible and that you are an appropriate and deserving NRSA candidate.

Applicants also should consider they need to include the appropriate amount of time to both fill out the NRSA forms and allow the application to be approved by the office of contracts and grants as well as receive departmental approval. This may be the first "go-through" for an applicant, and there are many obstacles to receiving the appropriate signatures. NIH requires signatures on every application from the business administrator, contracts and grants office, or dean to submit an application. Depending on each individual applicant's institution, others (e.g., department chair, mentor) may need to sign the application or a face sheet indicating the applicant has the chair or dean's approval prior to being accepted or routed to the contract and grants management office. Thus, before starting this process, it is generally a good idea to create a proposal timeline that incorporates the time required from brainstorming the project idea to submitting the finished proposal.

Again, applicants are advised to be realistic and consider that their application will end up on a pile alongside of other multimillion dollar research grants from established professors also seeking to advance their grants in a similar time frame. We cannot overstate how important it is that the application be error free and have approval at each institutional step. The formative steps taken in building an application will not change from the F-series through the R-series (or even P-series). All investigators face the same submission deadlines, demand for signatures, approval processes, and paperwork trail to monitor the flow of a grant from preparation to submission. Thus, it is important to consider putting aside time as the semester progresses to address these issues, and gathering the appropriate components of the grant (letters, approvals, budgets, and ancillary documents) cannot wait for the last minute. Doing so would jeopardize the application and result in a hastily prepared and sloppy application that is less likely to be funded.

The Mentor Perspective

If you are considering becoming a mentor for an NRSA candidate, this section of the chapter is particularly relevant to you. There are several pertinent questions that need to be addressed prior to establishing whether you are suitable for mentorship.

Should You Be a Mentor?

Mentoring should and can be a rewarding experience. As a mentor, you are responsible for guiding an individual's career path and assisting him/her with achieving his/her goals. A mentor is a teacher who collaborates with students to meet their educational needs. First and foremost, being a mentor requires time and patience.

Prospective mentors should consider their current position and whether mentoring a graduate/postdoctoral student will dovetail with their natural professional duties, time commitments, and administrative, research, or teaching responsibilities. Although it is not a requirement to have prior experience mentoring researchers for the development of an NRSA application, mentors should present their acumen based on their experience in the applicant's substantive area along with their ability to provide a high level of training. It goes without saying the application should reinforce and highlight any supervisory and training experience by the mentor, showcasing strengths in providing research and professional learning experiences.

Helping the Applicant Develop a Research Project

Whether the project represents an extension of the mentor's current work, fills a particular void in the field, tests a novel technique, or extends a current line of thinking, the mentor should guide the applicant toward presenting a feasible, well-managed, and timely project. A critical area in the presentation of the project, and one that should be within the purview of the mentor, is to help the applicant showcase how the project will advance or help refine his/her research skills. Ultimately, the research project should be the first step in a student's pursuit of a career as an independent researcher. The mentor should discuss with applicants with great clarity their goals and how these should be presented and bundled in the NRSA application. It is essential the mentor understand the applicant's research goals may depart somewhat or significantly vary from the mentor's current research platform. It may thus be appropriate for the mentor to advise a suitable co-mentor and form a team approach. The mentor should offer suggestions of individuals that complement the applicant's training and research goals. The nature of the supervisory and training component should be given great thought, particularly in light of the centrality of training underlying an NRSA fellowship. A key component is the "relationship" between the applicant and mentor and the professional horizons provided by this supervisory learning experience. Previous training, collaboration, classroom study, laboratory experience, co-authored papers, and professional alliances should be highlighted. The same applies to collaborative experiences with co-mentors. The goal is to demonstrate that the mentoring relationship will be fruitful and positive.

Developing the Mentor Section of the Application

Inevitably, mentors will be tasked with writing a significant portion of the proposal. This effort will include preparation and development of the training plan, describing relevant experience as a mentor, providing a written description of the applicant's potential as an independent researcher, and carefully outlining materials concerning human subject issues. Mentors are advised to carefully and thoroughly read the application instructions prior to writing their material. An important goal in this effort is to provide an honest and truthful overview of the applicant's strengths, while at the same time indicating areas that will benefit from further study, training, and professional honing. Hand in hand with this discussion should be a listing or accounting of activities needed to improve the applicant's research skills. The mentor should describe whether previous work with the applicant has been successful, even if this work stems from graduate-level coursework, papers, or research assistantships.

It is essential that mentors familiarize themselves with the applicant's past experiences and relate these experiences to how he/she has been successful in a laboratory or research environment. In addition, the application should include specific details with respect to the precise nature of mentoring. Move beyond a mere statement that "meetings will occur" to a level that describes the nature and content of these meetings over time (this information can be presented in tabular form). Reviewers also provide mentorship at various points in their career or have been selected for review based on extensive mentoring. Thus, they want to see, at a minimum, weekly supervision, discussion of how research and human subject protocols are reviewed, the nature of shared decision making, and a high level of accessibility. If either the applicant or mentor resides in a geographically distinct region of the country, describe specifically how you plan to be involved in the project.

Tips for a Successful Mentor

Creating a Positive Climate for Learning

Applicants should feel comfortable in approaching mentors and obtaining constructive feedback that will improve their research skills. A good piece of advice for mentors is to articulate any reasons for decisions that are made and help the applicant student develop managerial and research autonomy. Both of these skills will prove to be useful later on when the applicant undertakes more involved research projects or collaborates on larger program projects. The application process should serve as a critical learning experience in this regard.

Areas that should be covered to help hone the research and administrative skills of the applicant include financing science (see chapter 15 on budgeting grants), developing timelines, paper production, constructing new grants, grant supplements, laboratory administration, presentation and oratory skills, collaboration, and, most critical to the applicant's success, writing at a high level.

Promoting Professional Growth

It goes without saying that mentors need to keep informed of the latest research in their field not only for their own edification and knowledge but also to remain informed during any discussion with the applicant. Remind the applicant that developing grant writing skills at this early point in their career will be critical for him/her to succeed professionally as a researcher.

Being Supportive and Realistic

Another key point is to remind applicants that regardless of how much work they invest in any particular proposal, the reality is that only a certain percentage of NRSA proposal will be funded. The same highly selective and rigorous review criteria applied to independent research awards are also used to evaluate NRSA fellowship applications. Be supportive if the applicant doesn't receive a fundable score and, conversely, celebrate with them if he/she does. The bottom line is that applicants are both receptive and sensitive to their mentor's comments and critiques. If reasonable and there is still sufficient time, work with the applicant to revise and resubmit an unfunded application. The revision and resubmission process (covered in greater detail in chapter 18) can be a good learning experience and will provide a firm base from which applicants can rebound and discover the nature of persistent scholarship required for success as an independent scientist.

REVIEW CRITERIA

A primary goal of the NRSA fellowship program is to support applicants who have the highest potential to develop into productive, independent scientists. Therefore, rather than evaluating these proposals in the traditional "independent research" fashion, these applications are reviewed more with regard to the applicant's potential for a successful career and specifically how the proposed training experience will help develop and realize this potential.

The main areas of review are (1) the applicant, (2) the research training plan, (3) the sponsor, and (4) the institutional environment/commitment. Human subject or vertebrate animal protections and ongoing plans for training in the responsible conduct of research must also be addressed in the proposal (failure to do so will result in an unscored application). The following section highlights areas that reviewers critique when reviewing an NRSA fellowship proposal.

The Applicant

Information about the applicant represents one of the "core" review areas in a fellowship proposal. When we speak of "core" review areas this very feature enables the reviewers to sift through any number of applications and determine which applicants have the most potential as future researchers. The materials below provide clear guidelines that will help applicants meet the core requirements when filing F-series applications.

It is especially important that the applicant describe his/her commitment to doing research and to having a productive scientific career. This is done by assessing past accomplishments and providing solid evidence of commitment to a research career, including supporting reference letters. When reviewing NRSA fellowship applications, reviewers will examine the extent and level of previous education, including any undergraduate or graduate degree(s), field(s) of study, conferment and date of degrees, and academic performance (evidenced by submitted transcripts and GRE scores). Awards, honors, other relevant research experience, professional training, scholarly publications, and presentations are also important. Applicants should include any information about forthcoming publications, their expected publication date (if known) and citations if already published. Presentations at workshops, seminars, and professional conferences (both national and regional) also demonstrate potential for success, particularly among applicants who are in the earlier stages of their careers. It is also essential that the applicant maintain substantive interests in line with those of the selected mentor and that the NIH institute or center is highly supportive of the type of work being proposed. If the mentor and the applicant have a strong preexisting relationship, this should be mentioned and can be demonstrated by work on joint projects, presentations, or publications. Also important is that recommendations are complete and speak highly of the applicant. A recent biographical sketch, formatted for the NIH PHS 398 forms, should be included both for the applicant and the sponsor.

Letters of recommendation provide a point of contention for most reviewers. There are two styles of letters: one very comprehensive and detailed with respect to the candidate, and others that pay short shrift to the applicant. The former boosts the candidate's chances of a favorable review because the letter provides an inkling or litmus test of the mentor's involvement. The latter can be quite damaging because there is a sense of "ennui" pervasive in the application when a letter of recommendation is one or two paragraphs and looks to be "stamped" out with little concern. If the mentor is too busy running a shop and has no time to construct a nice full-page letter (more can be better sometimes), the reviewers will sense this lack of commitment and harangue the mentor endlessly during review. The letter provides a chance for the mentor to describe the talents, skills, and personality of the candidate, showcasing his/her strengths as an independent scientist at this early juncture. Special skills, special experiences, and interesting parts of the candidate's life that surface during conversation with the mentor should find their way into the letter. Box 6.2 showcases a review of two different letters for a fellowship applicant to NIH.

The Research Training Plan

In this section, reviewers evaluate the merit of the research proposal and general design issues (approach). At the same time that reviewers sift through this information, they consider the applicant's background and the respective contributions of the applicant and the sponsor in the development of the research proposal. First and foremost, the research design should be sound and reasonable. A study that is not feasible or realistic for a person early in his/her career will considerably weaken the application. If the study is an extension of the mentor's work, it is essential the application distinguishes between the larger study and the proposed project. The proposal should not in any shape or form represent a "copy and paste" version derived from any parent study that is already funded. Rather, the application should present a project that will independently facilitate the applicant's training in a specific area.

The majority of the applicant's time should be devoted to research during the time of the fellowship award, and this should be specified in detail as part of the proposal. This section of the proposal needs to focus, not only on the research design, but on the steps the applicant will take to achieve his/her training goals. Both before and during the actual review session, reviewers will be instructed by the scientific review administrator and the chair of the review committee to avoid a detailed critique of the technical aspects of the research. Notwithstanding, reviewers will check for serious design flaws inherent in the research plan that might cast doubt on the applicant's or the sponsor's scientific judgment. Any major or even "fatal" flaw will raise questions about the mentor's candor regarding their desired level of involvement and provision of supervision. This type of reviewer concern holds both for the present and future and will lurk in the background on revisions (see chapter 18). This component of the review foreshadows an important item in preparing an NRSA fellowship application: The application should demonstrate a joint effort, led by the applicant, but with sufficient oversight provided by the mentor.

The emphasis of the critique will be on the potential of the training plan to provide the applicant with the individualized supervised experiences that will develop the candidate's knowledge and research skills. The critique will not focus on whether the proposed study will have a formidable impact on the field or rigorously extend our current scientific knowledge. In this regard, reviewers are cognizant that the goals of the fellowship program focus exclusively on helping launch new promising researchers into the field. Coupled with this focus, reviewers also recognize that fellowships pave the way for young "budding"

| Box **6.2** | Sample Reviews of Applicants |

Candidate 1

The candidate received her B.A. in psychology and urban planning from Malpensa College. After finishing her undergraduate work, the candidate simultaneously pursued and received an M.P.H. and M.S.W. degree from the University of Bologna. The candidate's grades are considerably average, ranging from a low of C+ to a high of A+, with a multitude of B's and C's. The candidate showed some improvement in grades during the period commensurate with her graduate studies. The candidate has taken several relevant courses on older adults/aging, the Latino population, ethnic identity, and health education. The candidate's research background is based in public health. She has applied her research findings to develop programs that serve both the older adult and Latino populations nationally and locally. The candidate has successfully disseminated the research findings through presentations at various conferences, namely the American Public Health Association national conference. She has also been invited to lecture at the Padua School of Public Health and has presented at the American Psychological Association Annual Conference. She has also published a research guide for social workers and program for Latino families, which are research-based, and have proven efficacious, although these are not peer-reviewed publications. The candidate received excellent recommendations from several well-known scientists working at prestigious universities. Each recommendation emphasized that the award would assist the candidate in pursuing training, education, and research in a field the candidate exhibits much knowledge of and passion for. It should be noted, however, the letters of recommendation appear incomplete as Dr. Faenza's recommendation is not accompanied by an actual letter and Dr. Pontebba's letter is not accompanied by a reference form. Notwithstanding, the letters of recommendations all underscore very high regard for the applicant. All recommendations address her prior experience in the field, her dedication to the subject matter, as well as her desire and motivation to pursue her academic and career goals.

Candidate 2

Candidate received her B.S. in Psychology and Biology from Texas University in 1999. In 2005, she received her master's in psychology from the University of Oklahoma where she is currently pursuing her doctorate in psychology. She is currently a Research Assistant at the University of Oklahoma. At Texas she received mostly A's and B's, with a few C's in Biology, Chemistry, and Calculus. At the University of Oklahoma she has received all A's and one A minus. The candidate lists four publications—two in preparation, one in press and one under review. She is first author of one of the articles in preparation. She lists eight presentations and was lead author on three of those. The candidate has been given outstanding recommendations from all of her professors. She received only one score of 2 in all of the recommendations. Her GRE scores are excellent. Dr. Sliver referred to her as "one of the top two individuals who I've had the pleasure of working with at the graduate level in my 23 years in academics." Everyone believes her to be extremely intelligent, ambitious, eager, mature, motivated, and an overall pleasant person to work with. She is a very promising applicant.

---

scientists to conduct larger and more rigorous studies that can influence their respective field. In this respect, the applicant's training plan should be detailed, providing specific activities that will be conducted each year, including coursework, research, seminars, conferences, grand rounds, workshops to be attended, plans for presentations and writing journal articles, supervision and mentoring sessions and any other tasks which will help the applicant reach his/her training goals. The plan should be directly tied to the goals of the applicant. A strong proposal will describe exactly how each activity will help the applicant reach the training goals described in the proposal. The activities can be tied to short- and long-term career goals, both of which should be well articulated. The role of the sponsor(s) should be described in detail, as well as the role of any other key figures or consultants that are providing support in other areas of expertise to the applicant.

Box 6.3 showcases excerpts taken from peer reviews for sample research training plans submitted as part of fellowship applications to NIH.

The Sponsor

In assessing the sponsor, reviewers look for evidence of his/her research expertise and success competing for research support. The sponsor should provide details of proposals that have been funded with him/her as principal investigator or co-investigator, including the length of the projects and the funding agencies. The sponsor's background will be carefully reviewed, including his/her academic background, his/her track record of publishing and obtaining funding, and his/her research interests, to see if they match those of the applicant. The sponsor should also demonstrate the understanding of and commitment to fulfilling the role of mentor. A description of any previous mentorship experiences should be included, along with a listing of previous fellows and their current professional employment if they have graduated from the program (this can be presented in tabular form). It is important that mentors carefully outline their success with previous fellows. A track record of mentoring is viewed very positively by reviewers. It is also important the sponsor demonstrates that he/she is able to work collaboratively with others on projects and publications. A sponsor who has multiple publications that reflect single authorship or have published always as first author may inadvertently send mixed messages to the review committee.

| Box **6.3** | Sample Reviews of Research Training Plan |

Research Training Plan 1

In year 1 the candidate plans to devote 20% of her time to research and 80% of her time to completing required courses. In year 2 the candidate plans to devote 30% of her time to research and 70% to completing required and elected course. In year 3 the candidate proposes to devote 40% of her time to research and 60% of her time to completing coursework, as well as preparing and defending her dissertation. The candidate's goals include gaining a better understanding of minority aging from a public health perspective, acquiring skills for independent research in the field, acquiring expertise in the area, and disseminating her research findings. The candidate intends to conduct research on Hispanic older adults in the New York City metropolitan area with chronic health conditions, such as diabetes. The candidate does not articulate how her required and elected coursework will help her pursue her goals, nor does the candidate clearly state how her training, mentorship, and participation in ongoing or independent research will assist her in effectively carrying out her research plan. A number of details are missing from the research training plan, which makes it difficult to assess if the plan will be effective in meeting her goals.

Research Training Plan 2

Training under the award will be focused primarily on applicant's research development. The applicant's specific aims are to: assess motivation to smoke a cigarette as a consequence of threats to body image and cues of smoking by the use of urge assessment and smoking behavior; evaluate level of trait body satisfaction and trait self-objectification as moderating variables in the body image experimental manipulations; and evaluate whether negative affect mediates the relationship between the body image manipulation and the subsequent measures of smoking motivation. She is requesting three years of funding. During years one and two, she will devote 75% of her time to research and 25% of her time to clinical work. During year three, the applicant's designated internship year, she will devote 25% time to research and 75% time to clinical work. Her research training plan is well thought out and focused. She has preliminary data related to her research plan. Her research design is fairly well thought out, although there are some areas that could be strengthened. The main concern regards the smoking manipulation, where it seems that the experimental group will be more likely to smoke because they are almost being encouraged to smoke, since they are told they can smoke and are exposed to their cigarettes, an ashtray and lighter. The research design seems somewhat biased. Another question is what will happen with participants who are found to have smoked in the hour before the study? These research questions could likely be addressed with oversight from the sponsor.

The sponsor should also demonstrate that he/she has the time to commit to this applicant and to the applicant's training program. The sponsor should also demonstrate an understanding of the applicant's research training needs and ability to meet those needs. If the sponsor is not located at the same institution as the applicant, there should be a detailed plan outlining how the communication and mentoring will transpire. There should be a plan in place for how the relationship will be maintained and if a long-distance mentoring relationship has already been established, it should be described. The application will be stronger with a sponsor that is in the same institution or at a nearby institution. However, if the sponsor does not have expertise in all of the areas needed for the training program, it may be necessary to include co-sponsors with other areas of expertise. The relationship and plan for communication with each sponsor should be detailed, as well as the role of each sponsor, to ensure that each sponsor plays a vital role in the candidate's training. Sponsors should not be included if they do not play a specific role and merely because they are highly respected in the field. If several sponsors are listed (e.g., one might have statistical expertise, one with expertise in mental health, and another with expertise in studies of health disparities), it is helpful to include a table or figure defining the role of each sponsor, regularity of communication and meeting plan. Box 6.4 shows excerpts taken from two reviews for fellowship applications.

The Institutional Environment/Commitment

For this section, reviewers will evaluate the training environment, including the institutional commitment to research training and career development. It is important to highlight any programs the institution has in place that support research training or the career development of students or trainees. The applicant should describe how students are advised and whether there is a plan in place for monitoring student progress. The quality of the facilities and related resources, such as equipment, laboratory space, computers, access to subject populations, and the availability of research support, should also be delineated. Research being conducted in the substantive area of the applicant should be described. In addition, the applicant's rationale for choosing this program should be provided. It is important to describe the institution even if it is a well-known institution that is respected for its research portfolio. If there is more than one institution that will play a key role, both should be described, and if there is a history of collaboration between the institutions, this should also be described. In the case of combined M.D./Ph.D. programs, any special features to facilitate the integration of, and transition between, the graduate and medical components should be described. Letters of support from any organizations that will assist in the project, such as community organizations that will provide access to the client populations, should be included. Box 6.5 shows how peer review is conducted for evaluating institutional commitment.

Box 6.4	Sample Reviews of Sponsors

Sponsor 1

Erica Ravenna, Ph.D. is the candidate's chosen mentor and sponsor. Dr. Ravenna received her doctorate in Sociology from Dobaccio University. Dr. Ravenna has published several articles relevant to the candidate's career goals, including articles addressing caregiving for older adults, end-of-life care, and older adult and minority health. In addition, Dr. Ravenna is the PI or Co-PI on several studies focusing on adult and minority health and well-being. Dr. Ravenna is currently the Co-Director of the Health Disparity Research Program and the Co-Director of the Center for Research on Minority Medical Care. Both positions should facilitate the candidate's ability to achieve her research goals. Dr. Ravenna speaks very highly of the candidate's goals and indicates an excellent working relationship. Dr. Ravenna is currently the candidate's advisor.

Sponsor 2

Enrique Spalda, Ph.D., received his A.B. in Psychology from the University of Minnesota in 1981 and his Ph.D. in Clinical Psychology from the University of Vermont, in 1990. He is currently Professor of Psychology at the Ohio State University and the Interim Director of the Clinical Training Program. Dr. Spalda has over 62 peer-reviewed publications, many of which are first authored. Dr. Spalda is currently the PI on two research grants, one from NCI and one from the Cancer Research Foundation of America. Dr. Spalda has supervised nine doctoral students and three previous doctoral fellows. Dr. Spalda has known the applicant since 2001 and believes her to be ambitious, extremely dedicated, and hard-working. He also indicates that she possesses high intelligence, intellectual curiosity, theoretical thinking, work ethic, and social conscious. The applicant has selected a good combination of mentors for the proposed project, although she might benefit from having a female expert as well when dealing with the proposed topic.

Plans for Training in the Responsible Conduct of Research

Plans for the training in the responsible conduct of research need to be described in detail and need to be ongoing. It is not sufficient to indicate that a course was taken or will be taken one semester. This should be an ongoing part of the training plan. Many applications fall short of the mark because they indicate the "applicant will take courses." This does not sit well with reviewers, all of whom are well aware of the need for "ongoing" training in the responsible conduct of research. Reviewers are instructed to consider the program of training, coursework, supervision, meetings, seminars, and instructional materials as part of the

---

| Box 6.5 | Sample Reviews of Institutional Environment/Commitment |

Institutional Environment/Commitment 1

The applicant chose to attend the University of North Carolina at Chapel Hill (UNC-CH) for her doctoral degree because she wanted training from a program that was highly regarded for its quantitative and qualitative methods, for its multidisciplinary training strengths, expertise in intervention and evaluation research, as well as for the opportunity to train with her sponsor, Dr. Ravenna. This is an appropriate and strong environment for the proposed work.

Institutional Environment/Commitment 2

The candidate has selected the Mailman School of Public Health (MSPH) in New York City, where the candidate is currently working toward her doctorate. This is an appropriate environment in which to carry out the research. The MSPH has a demonstrated commitment to supporting research training and its student career development.

---

overall responsible conduct training. This type of ongoing program of study must be carefully delineated in the application. In the sample plans listed below in box 6.6, plan A is not adequate because it does not carefully delineate an ongoing plan of education and training in responsible conduct. Plan B, on the other hand, provides more details on the training and ensures the candidate will participate in ongoing educational training throughout the course of the fellowship or any additional scientific work.

Human Subjects/Animal Welfare

If the application involves human subjects, the application will be evaluated with reference to the following criteria: risk to subjects, adequacy of protection against risks, potential benefits to the subjects and to others, and importance of knowledge to be gained. All of these areas need to be addressed in the application. If a clinical trial is proposed, a data and safety monitoring plan must be included. A table indicating gender and race for targeted enrollment is also required. Women, minorities, and children (up to age 21) should be included in the sample. If they are not, justification needs to be provided outlining sound reasons for their exclusion. For details on documenting human subjects protections and procedures, see chapter 16.

Animal welfare needs to be addressed in a similar fashion if a study involves vertebrate or invertebrate animals rather than humans. Any procedures that are harmful to the animals should be limited to those that are unavoidable in the conduct of scientifically sound research.

Box 6.6	Sample Reviews of Plans for Training in the Responsible Conduct of Research

Plans for Training in the Responsible Conduct of Research A

Candidate has completed NIH's Web-based Human Participants Protections Education for Research Training and has received a certification in HIPAA authorization. Applicant completed a semester long course on Ethics and Professional Problems in 2002.

Plans for Training in the Responsible Conduct of Research B

Appropriate and ongoing. The Department of Health Behavior and Health Education at the University provides all doctoral students with formal and informal training designed to develop a firm understanding of and respect for proper standards for the ethical conduct of science. Faculty advisors, who are responsible for modeling appropriate methods for conducting research, provide formal training. There are frequent opportunities for one-on-one discussions between faculty and students about issues such as conflict of interest, data recording and retention, professional standards and codes of conduct, responsible authorship, and ideals of science. In addition, all HBHE doctoral seminar courses address various aspects of the responsible conduct of research. In accordance with NIH requirements, University policy requires all persons engaged in research involving human subjects to complete the training in the ethical conduct of research and protection of subjects.

Scores and Resubmissions

Unlike most other grant review streamline mechanisms, where the "bottom half" of the applications will be "unscored," all of the "F" applications submitted to NIH receive a score. Scores reflect the reviewers' opinion of the application's merit and range from 1.0 (most meritorious) to 5.0 (least meritorious), with increment of 0.1 unit. The goal is for 3.0 to be the median, for "average" applications. All reviewers who are present during the review will score each application, based on the discussion that takes place, which is led by the primary and secondary, and sometimes even tertiary reviewer. There may be more than 20 reviewers present during a review cycle; however, the primary, secondary, and tertiary reviewers may be the only individuals who have read the complete proposal. The primary and secondary reviewers verbally recount their critiques to the other reviewers. The primary and secondary reviewers alone play a key role in determining the response the proposal will receive by the other reviewers. The remaining reviewers may only read the abstract and listen to the critique of the primary and secondary reviewers. For this reason, it is imperative that the proposal abstract be excellent (this point is reinforced in chapter 3), with no typos or errors, and that it convey all essential information about the proposal.

If a proposal does not receive a favorable score, based on the NIH regulations it can be resubmitted two additional times. It is discouraging to receive a score that is not in the fundable range, but it is important to remember that even the best grant writers will have applications that do not get funded on their first submission. In order to resubmit an application, the first step is for the applicant and the mentor to review the reviewer comments carefully and determine whether the application should be resubmitted. This decision will be based on whether the reviewer comments can be addressed and if there is sufficient time to apply, get funded, and complete the proposed project prior to the applicant's graduation. It is critical to address all of the reviewer comments, even if the applicant or mentor does not agree with the critiques. Often, proposal will go back to the same reviewers, and it is important to acknowledge all of their comments and to make revisions accordingly. In a resubmission, the applicant should also focus on any progress she/he has made in publishing or presenting since the previous submission.

CONCLUSION

The majority of graduate school programs do not include grant writing as an established component. Given the lack of formal training in grant writing, it is surmised that the only venue for students and new researchers to learn the art of grant writing is through experience with mentors, in the workplace, or through self-study. Moreover, the lack of didactic training and minimal experience associated with developing proposals prevents students and new researchers from developing applications. For example, students may believe they lack the experience and knowledge to write a "winning application" and decide not to pursue the NRSA programs. This chapter provides the essential tools to help doctoral candidates and postdoctoral fellows familiarize themselves with the NRSA application process and encourage potential applicants to approach their mentors regarding the opportunity to pursue such awards.

7

Unique Funding Opportunities
for Underrepresented Minorities
and International Researchers

JENNY N. KARP, IDA K. NAMUR, & SUSANNA NEMES

You must be the change you wish to see in the world.

—MAHATMA GANDHI

IN AN EFFORT to increase the involvement and success of under-represented minorities in public health and science, a number of public, private, and federally funded programs have been developed to encourage the participation of both American and international minorities in research. Categorization of minorities includes individuals underrepresented in the field of research based on their race, ethnicity, or gender, and in some instances citizenship. The materials explored in this chapter encompass funding outlets for three primary activities: (1) educational and/or training activities, (2) fellowships, and (3) research.

Public, private, and federal programs are available to fund educational, training, and fellowship activities for minorities and international citizens at various monetary levels. Minorities and international citizens can apply for federal grants or specialized minority research programs ranging in support from $5,000 to $500,000 per year. Monetary support can include (1) full coverage of tuition and expenses, (2) flat stipends, (3) course or training specific assistance for undergraduate, graduate, or postdoctoral studies, or (4) specialized training.

This chapter provides a compendium of sources detailing access to information on funding opportunities for minority and international researchers. This information is by no means meant to be exhaustive, but rather illustrative of the wide range of funding opportunities that have consistently focused on the professional advancement of underrepresented minority and international researchers. In order to simplify the vast database of information earmarking these opportunities, we have divided the chapter into four sections. The first three sections highlight funding opportunities available for each of the primary activities described above: educational and training activities, fellowships, and research. Within each of these three sections, we provide an overview of each funding mechanism, a "notes" section that gives more specific information regarding eligibility, availability of monies, and funding cycles, and the Web address that can be used to obtain additional information specific to each mechanism. Appendix 1 at the end of this book gives a brief description of each Web site and provides any necessary links. The fourth and final section of the chapter addresses specific tactics and helpful tips for identifying, qualifying, and obtaining opportunities for funding in the three core areas. Minority and international researchers may find this information useful as a template upon which to construct new grants. Mentors also can use these tips as an organizational tool and to encourage students in search of funding.

SUPPORT FOR EDUCATIONAL AND/OR TRAINING ACTIVITIES

American Association for University Women's Career Development Fund

Web site: www.aauw.org/fga/fellowships_grants/career_development.cfm

Overview

The Career Development Grants support women who hold a bachelor's degree and are preparing to advance their careers, change careers, or re-enter the workforce. Special consideration is given to American Association for University Women (AAUW) members, women of color, and women pursuing their first advanced degree or credentials in nontraditional fields. Grants provide support for coursework beyond a bachelor's degree, including a master's degree, second bachelor's degree, or specialized training in technical or professional fields. Funds are also available for distance learning. Coursework must be taken at an accredited two- or four-year college or university, or a technical school that is fully licensed or accredited by an agency recognized by the U.S. Department of Education. Funds are not available for doctoral-level work.

Notes

To be eligible for the program, individuals must (1) be a U.S. citizen or permanent resident, (2) currently possess a bachelor's degree, and (3) enroll to take
courses at a regionally accredited two- or four-year institution, technical institution, or distance learning program (all of the intended coursework must be
related to your professional development in a significant way).

American Association for University Women's International Fellowships

Web site: www.aauw.org/fga/fellowships_grants/international.cfm

Overview

International fellowships are awarded for full-time study or research to women
who are not U.S. citizens or permanent residents. Both graduate and postgraduate studies at accredited institutions are supported through this mechanism.
Members of International Federation of University Women affiliate organizations are eligible to apply and a number of international fellowships are set aside
for these women each year. International fellowship recipients may study in any
country other than their own. The AAUW also awards several annual Home
Country Project Grants ($5,000 to $7,000 each) to women. These grants support
community-based projects designed to improve the lives of women and girls in
the fellow's home country.

Notes

To be eligible for an international fellowship, individuals must (1) be a citizen in a
country other than the United States (or hold a nonimmigrant visa if residing
in the United States), (2) have completed an academic degree equivalent to a
bachelor's degree from a U.S. college or university, (3) devote full-time study to
their proposed academic plan during the fellowship year, (4) intend to return to
their home country to pursue a professional career, (5) be proficient in English,
and (6) be a member of an organization affiliated with the International Federation of University Women (IFUW) to be considered for one of the fellowships
awarded for study in any country other than their own country. AAUW members
are not eligible to apply for international fellowships.

Gates Millennium Scholars Program

Web site: www.gmsp.org/(gr23jz55ttigtn55jrw40crn)/default.aspx

Overview

The Gates Millennium Scholars (GMS) program is funded by a generous contribution from the Bill and Melinda Gates Foundation. The scholarship was

established in 1999 to provide academically outstanding African American, American Indian/Alaska Native, Asian Pacific Islander American, and Hispanic American students with an opportunity to complete an undergraduate college education. Students pursuing advanced studies in mathematics, science, engineering, education, or library science also can obtain funding to further their graduate education. The goal of GMS is to promote academic excellence and provide an opportunity for thousands of outstanding students with demonstrated financial need to reach their fullest potential.

Notes

To be eligible for the program, individuals must (1) be of African American, American Indian/Alaska Native, Asian Pacific Islander American, or Hispanic American ethnicity; (2) be a citizen/legal permanent resident or national of the United States; (3) have attained a cumulative GPA of 3.3 on a 4.00 scale (unweighted) at the time of nomination; (4) be entering a U.S. accredited college or university as full-time, degree-seeking freshmen; (5) have demonstrated leadership abilities through participation in community service, extracurricular, or other activities; and (6) meet the stated federal Pell Grant eligibility criteria.

The Hispanic Scholarship Fund

Web site: www.hsf.net/scholarships.php

Overview

The Hispanic Scholarship Fund (HSF) is the nation's leading organization supporting Hispanic higher education. HSF was founded in 1975 with a vision to strengthen the country by advancing college education among Hispanic Americans, the largest and fastest growing minority group in the U.S. population. The mission of HSF is to double the rate of Hispanics earning college degrees. To reach this goal HSF provides the Latino community more college scholarships and educational outreach support than any other organization in the country.

Notes

Scholarship programs are available to high school seniors, community college transfer students, undergraduate students, and graduate/professional students. An extension of the program, the HSF/Pfizer, Inc. Fellowship Program, is available on a competitive basis to Hispanic graduate students at selected universities and in selected majors. The 2007 fellowship includes a $10,000 award for the academic year, and a paid summer internship working at the New York headquarters of Pfizer, a leading pharmaceutical company. A renewal award of $10,000 for a second year is contingent upon successful completion of the summer internship.

The Native Hawaiian Health Scholarship Program

Web site: www.nhhsp.org

Overview

The Native Hawaiian Health Scholarship Program provides financial support for Native Hawaiian students pursuing careers in selected health professions. The program aims to increase the number of Native Hawaiians in health professions and improve the availability of primary and preventive care services to Native Hawaiians in the State of Hawaii. Scholarships are awarded to students attending an accredited course of study leading to a health professional degree.

Notes

In 2007, scholarships were directly paid to selected students using monthly stipends of $1,065. These funds are earmarked for payment toward reasonable educational expenses (books, supplies, equipment, and equipment rentals, etc.). In addition, benefits include payments to the participants' school of the actual billed tuition and ancillary fees required of all students for the academic year enrolled in the same academic program. Support may be continued through graduation for a maximum of four years, provided appropriate funds are available and students remain in good academic standing. In return for each year of support, program participants agree to provide a year of full-time clinical or nonclinical service. This service commitment begins after completion of the professional course of study funded by the scholarship program and any approved deferment of service to pursue advanced clinical training (e.g. residency, internship, etc.).

Program for Minority Research Training in Psychiatry (PMRTP)

Web site: www.psych.org/research/apire/pmrtp5302.cfm

Overview

The PMRTP program is designed to increase the number of underrepresented minorities in the field of psychiatric research. Research training offers the opportunity to engage in exciting and pioneering scientific investigation across a full spectrum of disciplines, including basic neuroscience, genetics, pharmacology, cognitive and behavioral social sciences, clinical psychiatry, and mental health services research. Research exposure is designed help students and trainees develop sound skills for clinical assessment and treatment planning.

Notes

The program provides funding for short- and long-term training opportunities at three levels: medical school, residency, and postresidency. National competitions also enable qualified "mini-fellows" to attend research-oriented meetings of psychiatric organizations. Preference in selection is given to underrepresented minorities such as American Indians, Asian Americans, Blacks/African Americans, Hispanics, Pacific Islanders, or other ethnic or racial group members underrepresented in biomedical or behavioral research. The PMRTP is funded by the National Institute of Mental Health and administered by the American Psychiatric Association. Support from PMRTP falls into three categories: (1) stipends, (2) travel, and (3) tuition and fees. Stipends are based on the trainee's years of relevant experience and the length of the research training experience. During 2007 full-year equivalent scholarships amounted to $19,968 for medical students, $45,048 to $46,992 for medical resident students, and up to $51,036 for postresidency fellows. Stipends for shorter periods of time are prorated. Trainees cannot receive funds from another federal source at the same time; however, stipends may be augmented through nonfederal sources. Travel funds are available on a limited basis for full-time trainees and "mini-fellows" to travel to the annual meeting of the American Psychiatric Association or the American College of Neuropsychopharmacology. Limited tuition assistance is available for full-time trainees to attend specific courses that are required as part of their training.

SUPPORT FOR FELLOWSHIPS

American Association of University Women American Fellowships

Web site: www.aauw.org/fga/fellowships_grants/american.cfm

Overview

The American Fellowships Program at AAUW supports women doctoral candidates completing dissertations or female scholars seeking funds for postdoctoral research leave from accredited institutions. Candidates are evaluated on the basis of scholarly excellence, teaching experience, and active commitment to helping women and younger females through professional service. Candidates may apply for only one of the awards described below:

1. Postdoctoral research leave fellowships are available in the arts and humanities, social sciences, and natural sciences. One fellowship is set aside for a woman from an underrepresented group in any field. Limited additional funds may be available when matched by the fellow's academic or research institution.
2. Dissertation fellowships are available to women who will complete their dissertation writing within the designated funding period. To qualify, applicants must have completed all coursework, passed all required

preliminary examinations, and received approval for their research proposal or plan before the funding period. Students holding any fellowship for writing a dissertation in the year prior to the AAUW Educational Foundation fellowship year are not eligible. This fellowship is open to applicants in all fields of study, except engineering. Scholars engaged in research addressing gender issues are encouraged to apply.

3. Summer and short-term research publication grants fund female college and university faculty as well as independent researchers to prepare research for publication. This grant applies to a wide pool of applicants including tenure track, part-time, or temporary faculty as well as new or established scholars and researchers working at universities. At the time of submission, sufficient time must be available for eight consecutive weeks of final writing, editing, and responding to critical reviews. Funds cannot be used for undertaking research. Applicants must have received their doctorates by the application deadline. Scholars with strong publishing records are encouraged to seek other funding.

Notes

To be eligible for any of the AAUW fellowships, applicants must be a U.S. citizen or permanent resident. Postdoctoral fellowship applicants must also hold a Ph.D., Ed.D., D.B.A., M.F.A., or D.M. For the summer and short-term fellowships, applicants must hold a doctorate or M.F.A. degree. Applicants pursuing the dissertation fellowship must be enrolled in a program of study other than an engineering program, be in or entering the final year of dissertation, have their dissertation proposal approved by their graduate faculty committee, have all graduate coursework completed, and have passed all preliminary exams. Former recipients of these awards are not eligible to apply for additional AAUW American fellowships or publication grants.

American Educational Research Association (AERA) Minority Fellowship Program

Web site: www.aera.net/fellowships/?id=88

Overview

The Council of the American Educational Research Association (AERA) established the AERA Minority Fellowship Program in 1991 with a stated goal of improving the quality and diversity of university faculty and encourages outstanding minority doctorates to pursue careers in education research. This program offers doctoral fellowships with the goal of enhancing the competitiveness of outstanding minority scholars for academic appointments at major research universities. The program strives to assist minority faculty through provision of research support and by providing mentoring and guidance that will help candidates complete their doctoral studies. AERA will award up to three doctoral fellowships every year. Each fellowship award is for one year and is nonrenewable. Fellowships are awarded for doctoral thesis research conducted under faculty sponsorship in any accredited university in the United States.

Notes

Applicants must be U.S. citizens or native residents of a territory of the United States. Applicants must also have advanced to candidacy and successfully defended their doctoral dissertation research proposal (Ph.D./Ed.D.). Applicants must work full time on their dissertation and course requirements. This program is targeted for members of groups historically underrepresented in higher education (i.e., African Americans, American Indians, Alaskan Natives [Eskimo or Aleut], Native Pacific Islanders, Filipino Americans, Mexican Americans, and Puerto Ricans). Data from 2007 indicate that fellows will receive a one-year stipend of $12,000 and up to $1,000 in travel support to attend the AERA annual meeting. Fellowships may be supplemented by campus or department awards and tuition waivers.

American Psychological Association Minority Fellowship Program

Web site: www.apa.org/mfp/

Overview

The goal of the American Psychological Association's (APA) Minority Fellowship Program is to increase the knowledge of issues related to ethnic minority mental health and improve the quality of mental health treatment delivered to ethnic minority populations. To achieve this objective, financial support and professional guidance is made available to individuals pursuing doctoral degrees in psychology and neuroscience. APA has several minority fellowships available, including the Mental Health and Substance Abuse Services Fellowship, the Mental Health Research Fellowship, the HIV/AIDS Research Fellowship, the Substance Abuse Research Fellowship, and the Diversity Program in Neuroscience.

Notes

Eligibility for funding is unique to each of the aforementioned fellowship programs. For more information about the programs please visit the organizational Web site.

American Society of Criminology: Graduate Fellowships for Ethnic Minorities

Web site: www.asc41.com/minorfel.htm

Overview

Fellowships sponsored by the American Society of Criminology are designed to encourage African American, Asian American, Latino, and Native American students to enter the field of criminology and criminal justice. Interested applicants must be accepted into a program of doctoral studies to be eligible for consideration.

Notes

On average three fellowships in the amount of $6,000 are awarded each year. A complete application must contain up-to-date curriculum vita; indication of race or ethnicity; copies of undergraduate and graduate transcripts; statement of need and prospects for financial assistance for graduate study; a letter describing career plans, salient experiences, and nature of interest in criminology and criminal justice; and three letters of recommendation. Interested applicants do not have to be a member of the American Society of Criminology.

American Society for Microbiology: International Fellowship Program

Web site: www.asm.org/International/index.asp?bid=2778

Overview

The American Society for Microbiology (ASM) International Fellowship Program supports international collaborations in microbiological science research and training. Two different types of fellowships are currently available for minorities within this program:

1. The ASM International Fellowship for Latin America offers fellowships to young scientists from any Latin American or Caribbean country working in any of the microbiology disciplines to visit a host scientist residing in the United States or Canada.
2. The UNESCO-ASM Travel Fellowship offers fellowships to promising young investigators throughout the world for travel to another country or a distant site to obtain expertise in a method, procedure or specific topic. Such knowledge should not be available in their own laboratories and should be required to conduct or accelerate studies and advance knowledge in their own laboratories and countries. The award is not intended to provide travel to obtain a degree at the host institution.

Notes

The program requires a joint application from two partners—the investigator and the hosting scientist. A minimum of six weeks is required for participation in the program. The applicant is allowed to extend his/her stay with the host scientist for up to a maximum of six months if other sources of support are available. All fellowships provide an award of up to $4,000 to a visiting scientist. Preference will be given, in order of importance, to the following:

- Investigators who have not had the opportunity to travel outside of their own country
- Investigators who can demonstrate three years of membership in ASM or any other national microbiology society
- Applications that have additional sources of funding, which would enable the applicants to maximize their collaborations

The American Sociological Association: Minority Fellowship Program

Web site: www.asanet.org/page.ww?section=Funding&name=Minority+Fellowship+Program

Overview

Through its Minority Fellowship Program (MFP), the American Sociological Association (ASA) supports the development and training of minority sociologists in the field of mental health and drug abuse research. Funded by a training grant sponsored by the National Institute of Mental Health (NIMH) and the National Institute of Drug Abuse (NIDA), ASA's goal is to attract talented doctoral students to ensure a diverse and highly trained workforce in the field of mental health and drug abuse research.

Notes

MFP fellowships funded by ASA through the NIMH and NIDA training grant are designed for minority students sufficiently advanced in their Ph.D. program to demonstrate their commitment to a research career focusing on research relevant to the portfolios of NIMH and NIDA. MFP applicants must be enrolled in a Ph.D. program in sociology departments that have NIMH and NIDA relevant research programs and/or faculty who are currently engaged in research supported by NIMH or NIDA. Fellowship applicants for the MFP may be early in their graduate career but must be accepted into a Ph.D. program in sociology at the time the fellowship begins.

The Commonwealth Fund/Harvard University Fellowship Program in Minority Health Policy

Web site: www.mfdp.med.harvard.edu/fellows_faculty/cfhuf/index.htm

Overview

The Commonwealth Fund/Harvard University Fellowship in Minority Health Policy is designed to prepare minority physicians for leadership roles in formulating and implementing public health policy and practice on a national, state, and/or local level. Under the auspices of the Minority Faculty Development Program at Harvard Medical School, five one-year fellowships are awarded per year. Fellows will complete academic work leading to a master's level degree and, through additional program activities, gain understanding of the major health issues facing minority and disadvantaged populations. The goal of the fellowship is to support the development of a key group of leaders in minority health who are well trained academically and professionally in public health, health policy, health management, and clinical medicine, as well as committed to pursuing careers in public service.

Notes

The fellowship provides a wide range of support for selected applicants including: a $50,000 stipend, full tuition for a master's level degree, health insurance, books, travel and related expenses, and financial assistance toward the support of a practicum project. To be eligible to apply, applicants must be physicians who have completed their medical residency and preferably have additional experience beyond residency, such as chief residency. Potential applicants must have an interest and experience in dealing with, the health needs of minority populations. The applicant must also show strong evidence of past leadership experience, especially as related to community efforts and health policy. The applicant must have the intention to pursue a career in public health practice, policy, or academia. Lastly, the applicant must have U.S. citizenship.

Ford Foundation: International Fellowships Program

Web site: www.fordfound.org/news/more/11272000ifp/index.cfm

Overview

The Ford Foundation International Fellowships Program (IFP) provides opportunities for advanced study to exceptional individuals who aspire to become leaders in their respective fields, furthering development in their own countries and greater economic and social justice worldwide. The IFP provides support for up to three years of formal graduate-level study leading to a masters or doctoral degree. Fellows are selected from countries in Asia, Africa, the Middle East, Latin America, and Russia, where the Ford Foundation maintains active overseas programs.

Notes

U.S. nationals are not eligible, although fellows may study in the United States. To be eligible for the fellowship, applicants must demonstrate superior achievement in their undergraduate studies and hold a baccalaureate degree or its equivalent; have substantial experience in community service or development-related activities; possess leadership potential evidenced by their employment and academic experience; propose to pursue a postbaccalaureate degree that will directly enhance their leadership capacity in a practical, policy, academic, or artistic discipline or field corresponding to one or more of the foundation's areas of endeavor; present a plan specifying how they will apply their studies to social problems or issues in their own countries; and commit themselves to working on these issues following the fellowship period. IFP selects fellows on the strength of their clearly stated intention to serve their communities and countries of origin, and expects that they will honor this obligation.

The Harry Frank Guggenheim Foundation: Dissertation and Postdoctoral Fellowships

Web site: www.hfg.org/df/guidelines.htm

Overview

The Harry Frank Guggenheim Foundation (HFG) welcomes dissertation fellowship proposals from individuals studying any of the natural and social sciences and the humanities. HFG places a high priority on research that emphasizes an increased understanding of the causes, manifestations, and control of violence, aggression, and dominance in the modern world. In addition to a program of support for postdoctoral research, dissertation fellowships are awarded each year to individuals who will complete the writing of the dissertation within the award year.

Notes

To date, the dissertation fellowships average $15,000 each and are designed to contribute to the support of the doctoral candidate to enable them to complete the thesis in a timely manner, and it is only appropriate to apply for support for the final year of Ph.D. work. Applications are evaluated in comparison with each other and not in competition with the postdoctoral research proposals. Applicants may be citizens of any country and studying at colleges or universities in any country. Particular questions that interest the foundation concern violence, aggression, and dominance in relation to social change, the socialization of children, intergroup conflict, interstate warfare, crime, family relationships, and investigations of the control of aggression and violence.

L'Oréal USA for Women in Science Fellowship Program

Web site: www.lorealusa.com/_en/_us/

Overview

Created by L'Oréal and UNESCO in 1998, the goal of this fellowship program is to promote women in scientific research by creating the "For Women in Science" partnership. The program is built around three priorities. The first priority promotes excellence through the L'ORÉAL-UNESCO Awards, the founding act of the program. These prestigious annual distinctions are awarded to five leading women researchers, one per continent, identified as exceptional women who serve as role models for the generations to come. The second priority recognizes talent through the international UNESCO-L'ORÉAL Fellowships. Granted annually since 2000 to 15 promising young women scientists, doctorate or post-doctorate, these fellowships encourage international scientific cooperation and the development of cross-cultural networks. The third priority of the fellowship program seeks to develop diversity (i.e., cultural competence) through the L'Oréal National Fellowships using support from the UNESCO National Commissions, which anchor the "For Women in Science" program in countries around the world.

Notes

On a yearly basis fellowship recipients are selected based on (1) intellectual merit; (2) academic records; (3) accepted requisites for scholarly scientific study, including ability to plan and conduct research; (4) ability to work as a team member or independently; and (5) ability to interpret and communicate research findings. Applicants are also judged on scientific excellence and appropriateness of proposed research or a clearly articulated plan of study. Reference letters, choice of host institution (postdoctoral students), and the potential for career enhancement of the proposed research also play an important role in the selection of award recipients.

Open Society Institute

Web site: www.soros.org/grants/application/grant_apply_step_1_view

Overview

The Open Society Institute (OSI) is a private foundation whose goal is to shape public policy to promote democratic governance, human rights, and economic, legal, and social reform. On a local level, OSI implements a range of initiatives to support the role of law, education, public health, and the growth and development of independent media. At the same time, OSI works to build alliances across borders and continents on issues such as combating corruption and human rights abuses. To that end, OSI provides a number of grant and fellowship opportunities to minorities and international researchers.

Notes

OSI has numerous grant and fellowship opportunities listed on their Web site. Applications may be submitted electronically online.

Ruth L. Kirschstein National Research Service Award Research Training Grants and Fellowships: NIH Predoctoral Fellowships (F31, F32 Awards)

Web site: grants.nih.gov/grants/guide/pa-files/PA-00-069.html

Overview

The National Research Service Award Predoctoral Fellowship for Minority Students provides up to five years of support for research training leading to a Ph.D. or equivalent research degree, a combined M.D./Ph.D. degree, or other combined professional degree and research doctoral degree in the biomedical, behavioral sciences, or health services research. These fellowships are designed to enhance the racial and ethnic diversity of the biomedical, behavioral, and health services research labor force in the United States.

Notes

Support is not available for individuals enrolled in medical or other professional schools unless they are also enrolled in a combined professional doctorate/Ph.D. degree program in biomedical, behavioral, or health services research. NIH particularly encourages institutions to identify individuals from racial and ethnic groups that have been shown to be underrepresented in health-related research nationally. In addition, the applicant must be a U.S. citizen or permanent resident, must be from an ethnic/racial group(s) that have been determined by the applicant's graduate institution to be underrepresented in biomedical or behavioral research. The applicant must also currently be enrolled in a Ph.D. or equivalent research degree program, a combined M.D./Ph.D. program, or other combined professional doctorate/research Ph.D. graduate program in the biomedical or behavioral sciences, or have been accepted by and agreed to enroll in such a graduate program in the academic year for which funds are sought. The sponsoring institution may be private (profit or nonprofit) or public. The applicant must identify an individual who will serve as a sponsor or mentor and will supervise the training and research experience.

Social Science Research Council: Fellowships

Web site: www.ssrc.org/fellowships/

Overview

Social Science Research Council (SSRC) fellowship and grant programs provide support and professional recognition to innovators within the fields of social science. SSRC has previously funded the work of more than 10,000 researchers and junior scholars from around the world. Funded works include a range of themes from African youth and globalization to public spheres in the Middle East and North Africa, from human sexuality to memory and repression in Latin America, from the social role of information technologies to the causes and consequences of international migration. Most programs target the social sciences, but many are also open to applicants from the humanities, the natural sciences, and relevant professional and practitioner communities. Although SSRC fellowship and grant programs take a variety of forms, they share the goals of supporting innovative knowledge production and of building research capacity in areas of critical social importance. Priority is given to younger researchers and new investigators whose work and ideas will have longer-term impact on society and scholarship.

Notes

Most support from the council goes to predissertation, dissertation, and post-doctoral fellowships, offered through annual, peer-reviewed competitions. Some programs offer summer institutes, advanced research grants, and grants for professionals and practitioners to conduct basic or applied research. Most grants support individual researchers, rather than groups or institutions.

UNCF-Merck Science Research Fellowships

Web site: www.uncf.org/merck/programs/grad.htm

Overview

This program offers fellowships for undergraduate, graduate, and postdoctoral students and is designed to increase the number of African Americans engaged in biomedical science education and research.

Notes

To be considered for the UNCF-Merck Graduate Science Research Dissertation Fellowships, applicants must be African American (black), enrolled full-time in a Ph.D. or equivalent doctoral program in the life or physical sciences, engaged in and within one to three years of completing dissertation research, and a U.S. citizen or permanent resident.

Vietnamese Education Foundation Fellowship Program

Web site: www.vef.gov/

Overview

The Vietnam Education Foundation (VEF) is an independent federal agency created by the U.S. Congress and funded annually by the U.S. government. The VEF Fellowship Program is one of the key components of VEF's mandate to enhance bilateral relations between the United States and Vietnam through international educational exchange programs that help improve Vietnamese Science and Technology capacities. VEF provides fellowships to the most talented Vietnamese for graduate study in the United States in science and technology.

Notes

The fellowship is open to all qualified citizens of Vietnam and awards are made on a competitive basis. Ph.D. candidates, who are recent university graduates, including young college faculty, are strongly encouraged to apply for this fellowship. Working experience or government affiliation is not required.

The Wenner-Gren Foundation for Anthropological Research, Inc.

Web site: www.wennergren.org

Overview

The Wenner-Gren Foundation for Anthropological Research offers professional development international fellowships that are intended for scholars and advanced students from countries in which anthropology or specific subfields of anthropology are underrepresented. Interested applicants who seek additional training to enhance their skills or develop new areas of expertise in anthropology can apply to one of three types of awards: (1) predoctoral fellowship for study leading to a Ph.D., (2) postdoctoral fellowship for scholars wishing advanced training, and (3) library residency fellowship for advanced students and postdoctoral scholars within five years of receiving their doctorate to travel to libraries with outstanding collections in anthropology.

Notes

Applicants to predoctoral and postdoctoral fellowship programs must be prepared to demonstrate the lack of availability of such training in their home country, their provisional acceptance by a host institution that will provide such training, and their intention to return and work in their home country upon completion of their training. As of the date for publication of this book, predoctoral fellowships amount to $15,000 per year. Fellows may apply for up to three renewals, the last of which must be solely devoted to writing up the results of dissertation research. Current postdoctoral fellowships amount to $35,000 for one year, with the possibility of one renewal. Former predoctoral grantees are not eligible for a postdoctoral fellowship. Applicants with a degree from outside their home country are not eligible to apply. Applicants for library residency fellowships must be prepared to show that travel to a library is necessary for preparing a research proposal or completing a project designed to advance teaching and scholarship in the home country. Current library residency fellowships include up to $5,000 and can be obtained for a maximum period of three months. These Fellowships are not renewable.

SUPPORT FOR RESEARCH

The Bill and Melinda Gates Foundation

Web site: www.gatesfoundation.org/ForGrantSeekers/

Overview

The Bill and Melinda Gates Foundation awards the majority of its grants to international not-for-profit organizations and other tax exempt organizations identified by foundation staff according to the objectives of our four program areas: global health, education, global libraries, and Pacific Northwest. The foundation favors preventive approaches and collaborative endeavors with government, philanthropic, private sector, and not-for-profit partners. Priority is given to projects that leverage additional support and serve as catalysts for long-term, systemic change. Grants are not awarded to individuals and will not be awarded to projects that serve an exclusively religious purpose.

Notes

To apply for funding, applicants are instructed to visit the program Web site to determine eligibility, funding availability, and current foundation priority interests.

Department of Education: Research Grants

Web site: web99.ed.gov/GTEP/Program2.nsf

Overview

In response to the No Child Left Behind Act of 2002, the U.S. Department of Education (DOE) sponsors a range of awards related to education research. The wording of this legislation outlines strict guidelines to ensure that every child in the nation, regardless of ethnicity, income, or background, receives a quality education. The DOE currently makes awards to minorities via two programs, which are described in greater detail below.

Notes

The Traditionally Underserved Populations (OSERS) Program   Web site: www .ed.gov/programs/rsatup/index.html

The purpose of the Office of Special Education and Rehabilitative Services (OSERS) program is to grant awards to minorities and American Indian tribes for research, training, and technical assistance. This program also makes awards to states, public or private nonprofit agencies, and organizations, including institutions of higher education and American Indian tribes, to promote the participation of minority entities and Indian tribes and to enhance their capacity to carry out activities under the Act. A "minority entity" is defined by Section 21 of the Act as a historically black college or university, Hispanic-serving institution of higher education, an American Indian tribal college or university, or another institution of higher education whose minority student enrollment is at least 50%.

Minority Science and Engineering Improvement Program (OPE).   Web site: www.ed.gov/programs/iduesmsi/index.html

The Office of Posteducation (OPE) program assists predominantly minority institutions to improve science and engineering education programs and increase the flow of underrepresented ethnic minorities, particularly minority women, into science and engineering careers. The program awards are normally used to implement design, institutional, and cooperative projects. The OPE also supports special projects designed to provide or improve support to accredited nonprofit colleges, universities, and professional scientific organizations for a broad range of activities that address specific barriers that eliminate or reduce the entry of minorities into science and technology fields. OPE awards range from $20,000 to $500,000 (estimated average $99,195) for new awards and from $25,000 to $365,000 (average $83,000) for continuation awards.

The Harry Frank Guggenheim Foundation: Research Grants

Web site: www.hfg.org/rg/guidelines.htm

Overview

The Harry Frank Guggenheim Foundation (HFG) welcomes proposals from individual researching any of the natural and social sciences and the humanities with the goal of increasing understanding of the causes, manifestations, and control of violence, aggression, and dominance. Priority is given to research that can increase understanding and amelioration of urgent problems of violence, aggression, and dominance in the modern world. Particular questions that interest HFG concern violence, aggression, and dominance in relation to social change, the socialization of children, intergroup conflict, interstate warfare, crime, family relationships, and investigations of the control of aggression and violence. Priority will also be given to areas and methodologies not receiving adequate attention and support from other funding sources.

Notes

As of the publication date for this book, average HFG awards range from $15,000 to $30,000 a year for periods of one or two years. Applications for larger amounts and longer durations must be very strongly justified. Proposals should contain the budget for the entire period of the project and requests for support in future years will be limited to the amount projected for that year. Requests will be considered for salaries, employee benefits, research assistantships, supplies and equipment, fieldwork, essential secretarial and technical help, and other items necessary to the successful completion of a project. HFG does not award grants to institutions for institutional programs.

Minority Access to Research Careers Branch

Web site: www.nigms.nih.gov/minority/marc.html

Overview

The Minority Access to Research Careers (MARC) Branch offers special research training support to four-year colleges, universities, and health professional schools with substantial enrollments of minorities such as African Americans, Hispanic Americans, Native Americans (including Alaska Natives), and natives of the U.S. Pacific Islands. The branch's goals are to increase the number and competitiveness of underrepresented minorities engaged in biomedical research by strengthening the science curricula at minority-serving institutions and increasing the research training opportunities for students and faculty at these institutions.

Notes

The MARC program consists of several programs and awards including the following:

Undergraduate Student Training in Academic Research (U*STAR) Awards. Institutional training awards (T34) provide support to undergraduate minority students as a means of further preparing them for graduate training in biomedical research. As of 2007, awardees receive annual student stipends of $10,956, and additional funds may be requested for tuition, fees, and research supplies for trainees, limited travel for trainees and faculty, and program evaluation.

Ancillary Training Activities.   Ancillary training grants provide funding for institutions or organizations to conduct meetings, trainings, seminars, workshops, and so forth, that align with the mission of the MARC Branch and seek to increase minority involvement in biomedical research.

Postbaccalaureate Research Education Program (PREP).   An institutional R25 award provides support to biomedical research students with baccalaureate degrees. The program is intended to strengthen the research skills and competitiveness of participants pursuing a graduate degree while at the same time stimulating their interest in addressing the health problems that disproportionately affect minorities. PREP awardees receive a salary of $21,000 per year as of 2007.

Predoctoral Fellowships.   MARC predoctoral fellowships, also known as F31 grants, are available to successful graduates of the U*STAR programs to further assist minority graduate school candidates toward completion of their degree in biomedical research. The annual stipend for MARC predoctoral fellows in 2007 is $20,772. A maximum of five years of support is available. An additional NIGMS will provide funds for tuition, ancillary fees, and up to $4,200 per 12-month period to the predoctoral fellow's sponsoring institute.

Faculty Predoctoral Fellowships.   MARC faculty predoctoral F34 fellowships are awarded to faculty at minority serving institutions. These fellowships are provided to allow non-Ph.D. faculty to pursue degree studies and a research doctorate. Annual stipends for faculty predoctoral fellowships may be requested in amounts that equal the applicant's annual salary, but cannot exceed the stipend of a level 1 postdoctoral fellow ($38,976 as of 2007). Similar to the predoctoral fellowship, a maximum of five years of support is available, and the applicant may request funding for tuition and ancillary fees. An additional institutional allowance in the amount of $4,200 is also available.

Faculty Senior Fellowships.   MARC Senior Faculty Fellowships (F33) are awarded to faculty at minority serving institutions with an interest in updating research skills or moving into a new area of research. Fellowships are available for one year and are nonrenewable. A stipend equal to the faculty salary and that does not exceed the stipend for a level 7 postdoctoral fellow (currently $51,036) may be awarded. The applicant may also request an institutional allowance of $7,000 a year to be used for expenses directly related to the training.

Visiting Scientist Fellowships.   MARC Visiting Scientist Fellowships (F36) are awarded for periods of up to one year to support outstanding scientist-teachers serving as visiting faculty at eligible minority institutions. Stipends are determined on an individual basis.

Minority Biomedical Research Support Branch

Web site: www.nigms.nih.gov/Minority/MBRS/

Overview

In an effort to increase the number of researchers who are members of minority groups that are underrepresented in the biomedical sciences, the Minority Biomedical Research Support (MBRS) Branch at NIH awards has established a series of grants. Grants are awarded to two- or four-year colleges, universities, and health professional schools with substantial enrollments of minorities. These grants support research by faculty members and are intended to strengthen the institutions' biomedical research capabilities and provide opportunities for students to work as part of a research team.

Notes

The MBRS program consists of three components: the SCORE program, the RISE program, and the IMSD program, each of which is explained briefly below.

Support of Continuous Research Excellence (SCORE) Program. Web site: grants.nih.gov/grants/guide/pa-files/PAR-04-001.html

SCORE grants are institutional grants awarded to biomedical research faculty at minority-serving institutions who are committed to increasing the number of underrepresented minorities engaged in biomedical research.

Research Initiative for Scientific Enhancement (RISE) Program. Web site: grants.nih.gov/grants/guide/pa-files/PAR-05-127.html

The purpose of the RISE program is to enhance the research environment of minority-serving institutions. While the overall goal of RISE is to increase the interest, skills, and competitiveness of students and faculty in the field biomedical research, the program offers support for institutional staff, faculty, and student development activities. Example of appropriate activities might be: workshops held on or off-campus, specialty courses, travel to scientific meetings, and re-search experiences conducted at on- or off-campus laboratories.

Initiative for Maximizing Student Diversity (IMSD) Program. Web site: grants .nih.gov/grants/guide/pa-files/PAR-04-001.html

IMSD grants are made to domestic, private, and public educational institutions with a goal of increasing the number of students from underrepresented groups in biomedical and behavioral research who attain of a Ph.D. degree. Institutions seeking to place candidates in this program are responsible for selecting student recipients of the IMSD awards. While nationally, African American, Hispanic American, American Indian, and Pacific Islander groups are regarded as un-derrepresented in these fields, it is incumbent on the applicant institution to determine whether a group is underrepresented in biomedical and/or behavioral research fields in establishing his/her institutional objectives.

Minority Institutions' Drug Abuse Research Development Program (MIDARP)

Web site: grants.nih.gov/grants/guide/pa-files/PAR-05-069.html

Overview

The National Institute on Drug Abuse (NIDA) provides support to increase the research capacity of minority institutions to conduct research in addictions and drug abuse. Grants are provided to foster the career development of racial/ethnic minority faculty, students, and staff who are underrepresented in drug abuse research, and to enhance research infrastructure at minority institutions.

Notes

As of summer 2007, funding is available in the amount of up to $350,000 per year in direct costs. Because the nature and scope of the proposed research vary from application to application, the size and duration of each award also will vary. The total amount awarded and the number of awards made will depend upon the number, quality, duration, and costs of the applications received. Institutions eligible for this award are domestic minority academic institutions. Applicants must demonstrate either (a) minority designation or (b) minority status and research capacity development need. Eligible program directors (principal investigators) must be faculty or staff at the applicant institution. The program director should have research experience as evidenced by peer reviewed publications. Only one application per institution is allowed. Foreign institutions are not eligible.

The National Science Foundation

Web site: www.nsf.gov/funding/aboutfunding.jsp

Overview

The National Science Foundation (NSF) funds research and education in most fields of science and engineering. Annually, grants and cooperative agreements are awarded to more than 2,000 colleges, universities, K-12 school systems, businesses, informal science organizations, and other research organizations throughout the United States. NSF accounts for about one-fourth of federal support to academic institutions for basic research. NSF also supports cooperative research between universities and industry, U.S. participation in international scientific and engineering efforts, and educational activities at every academic level. Details for individual funding opportunities appropriate for minority candidates and that are provided by NSF are listed below.

Notes

Louis Stokes Alliances for Minority Participation (LSAMP) Bridge to the Doctorate.   Web site: www.nsf.gov/funding/pgm_summ.jsp?pims_id=5477

The goal of this program is to increase the quality and quantity of students successfully completing science, technology, engineering, and mathematics (STEM) baccalaureate degree programs and increasing the number of students interested in, academically qualified for, and matriculated into programs of graduate study. LSAMP supports a goal of increasing the number of students who earn doctorates in STEM fields, particularly those from populations underrepresented in STEM fields.

Minority Postdoctoral Research Fellowships and Supporting Activities.
Web site: www.nsf.gov/funding/pgm_summ.jsp?pims_id=13454

NSF offers Minority Postdoctoral Research Fellowships (and funding for related support activities) as a means of increasing the participation of underrepresented groups in selected areas of science in the United States. These fellowships support training and research at the postdoctoral level at a host institution in the areas of biology and social, behavioral, and economic sciences supported by NSF. Supporting activities are travel grants to graduate students to visit prospective sponsors, starter research grants for fellows, and an annual meeting of fellows and their mentors.

Research Centers in Minority Institutions (RCMI) Program

Web site: www.ncrr.nih.gov/resinfra/ri_rcmi.asp

Overview

The Research Centers in Minority Institutions (RCMI) program was developed by NIH to enhance the research capacity and research infrastructure at minority colleges and universities that offer doctoral degrees in the health sciences. In order to be eligible to apply for an RCMI grant, applicant institutions must have one or more underrepresented minority groups that comprise 50% or greater of their student body representation and offer doctorate degrees in the health-related sciences. RCMI grants provide funding to recruit established and promising researchers, acquire advanced instrumentation, modify laboratories for competitive research, fund core research facilities, and other research support. Because many investigators at RCMI institutions study diseases that disproportionately affect minorities, National Center for Research Resources support serves the dual purpose of bringing more minority scientists into mainstream research and enhancing studies of minority health.

Notes

Information regarding application guidelines, eligibility, requests for applications, program announcements, and notices are located on the RCMI program Web site.

Russell Sage Foundation

Web site: www.russellsage.org/about/whatwedo/howtoapply/awards/

Overview

The Russell Sage Foundation (RSF) makes a limited number of annual awards supporting basic social science research within programs announced and highlighted on its Web site. Awards primarily support data analysis and compilation of findings, but RSF occasionally considers larger awards for data acquisition projects highly relevant to the RSF's program goals.

Notes

RSF's major awards in 2007 range between $50,000 and $500,000. Applications for external awards should generally be preceded by a brief letter of inquiry to determine whether the foundation's present interests and funds permit consideration of a proposal for research. Letters of inquiry concerning research projects should summarize the project's objectives, the work plan, the qualifications of persons engaged in the research, and an estimated budget. Additionally, the president of the foundation makes a limited number of small awards each year. The budget for these awards must be $35,000 or less.

The Wenner-Gren Foundation for Anthropological Research, Inc.

Web site: www.wennergren.org.

Overview

In addition to its support for professional development fellowships, the Wenner-Gren Foundation offers grants for dissertation fieldwork, post-Ph.D. grants, and Richard Carley Hunt Postdoctoral Fellowships. These grants and fellowships are available for basic research in all branches of anthropology. Dissertation and post-Ph.D. grants are designed to seed innovative approaches and ideas or to cover specific expenses or phases of a project. The foundation is particularly supportive of projects employing comparative perspectives or integrating two or more subfields of anthropology. A small number of awards are available for projects designed to develop resources for anthropological research and scholarly exchange. The foundation also offers international collaborative research grants to assist anthropological research projects undertaken jointly by two or more investigators from different countries. The purpose of the program is to encourage new collaborations in which the principal investigators bring different and complementary perspectives, knowledge, and/or skills. Both investigators must work together at the research site.

Notes

In 2007, grants were available in amounts up to $25,000 for dissertation fieldwork and post-Ph.D. grants and $17,500 for International Fellowships (renewable for a total of four years of funding). Short-term Fellowships are available for up to three months in the amount of $5,000. The South African Fellowship is available to black students from South Africa who wish to study anthropology or archaeology. The South African Fellowship is a $15,000 award renewable for up to four years of funding. International collaborative research grants were available for amounts up to $30,000. Priority is given to new collaborations, but an independent project stemming from an ongoing, long-term collaboration will be considered. Projects must involve at least one principal investigator from outside the United States, Canada, Western Europe, Australia, or New Zealand. Both investigators must meet the qualification for postdoctoral grants.

TIPS FOR OBTAINING RESEARCH FUNDING: PRIORITIZE, IDENTIFY, QUALIFY, AND OBTAIN

Up until this point, this chapter has focused almost exclusively on providing detailed information regarding where to obtain access to information on grant and fellowship opportunities. By so doing, the chapter acts as a unique compendium of data resource for minority and international investigators. Unfortunately, access to this information is only the first necessary step on the road to procuring funding. Information alone provides only limited guidance with regard to construction and development of grant or fellowship applications. Moreover, while it is important to be aware of the available resources (otherwise receipt of funding would be nearly impossible), awareness is only one part of the funding equation. There are many additional and critical pieces of the funding puzzle that are missing and deemed essential for minority or international applicants to successfully compete for grants and fellowships. Chapter 3 discussed at length some of these requisite skills and in this respect should be highly useful. Many of the criteria used by reviewers to synthesize the "contents" of an application are implemented regardless of whether the application is submitted to NIH or a foundation.

The remainder of this chapter provides some additional and more refined insight on the essential skills required to assemble and produce a grant or fellowship application. It is probably best to read this material in conjunction with chapter 3 outlining the essentials of grant writing. With both sets of material in hand, and knowledge of where to apply for fellowship opportunities, applicants should be well prepared to construct high-profile, well-synthesized, successful grant and fellowship applications.

As we explore the details of preparing applications, it is important to note that funding opportunities are constantly changing and evolving. Over the course of a year or several years, programs offering grants or fellowships may grow or diversify along several fronts (thematic or financial), thus increasing the number of opportunities available, or the size of awards. New programs may be established while others are reduced in size or removed from the foundation's funding portfolio. As a result, minority and international researchers must establish a system that enables them to identify current and appropriate funding opportunities. We provide the following guide to help shape these efforts.

Phase 1: Prioritize Individual Goals and Related Financial Needs

Before you can research funding opportunities and submit applications for educational training, fellowships, or research grants, it is imperative that you identify and prioritize your research goals. Make a list of your current and future research goals. Prioritize them in terms of importance and/or urgency. For example, perhaps you are an established researcher in your native country of Belgium. At this time you would like to obtain funding to conduct a study with the University of Bangkok to examine the impact of substance abuse on HIV risks among commercial sex workers in Thailand. With these goals in mind (and written down on paper), it's time to prioritize! Based on the above example, your goals might include:

- Participation in a cross-country research collaboration
- Facilitation of a cross-country research collaboration
- Conducting international research
- Conducting international research in Thailand
- Conducting research specific to substance abuse, HIV, commercial sex workers, or all of the above
- Becoming an expert on HIV prevention among commercial sex workers in Thailand
- Obtain funding to cover 50% of stated salary

As part of your prioritization, it is important to consider both long- and short-term goals. You may want to keep a running list of your research goals and priorities so you can continually monitor your achievements and challenges. Or, you may choose to create a list of research goals each time you set out to obtain funding. Either way, once you have established your short- and long-term goals, you can prioritize them. Goals should be prioritized in order of importance and urgency. Your most important goal should be ranked first, the least important goal should be ranked last. This ranking system will allow you to identify funding opportunities that are most in line with your priorities and most adequately meet your current needs, as you will see below.

Phase 2: Identify Sources of Funding—Tuition, Fellowships, Research Support

Once you have identified your personal research goals and priorities, you are prepared to commence phase 2. During phase 2 of your quest to obtain research funding, you will initiate the process of obtaining funding by doing more research! Using the research priorities you identified in phase 1, you will spend a significant amount of time researching organizations, agencies, and institutions to identify potential sources of funding. To do this, you may want to start with some of the funding sources outlined above, or you may want to start a search of your own. To start a search of your own, you may want visit one of the Web sites below, all directly linked to databases of funding opportunities and inclusive of search engines to locate funding. By searching for funding opportunities using key words from your phase 1 priorities list, you will identify funding mechanisms closely aligned with your current goals. Sample sites you might search using key words from your phase 1 priorities list include:

U.S. Department of Health and Human Services, National Institutes of Health Grants and Funding Opportunities: grants.nih.gov/grants/

Research Assistant Funding: www.theresearchassistant.com/funding/index.asp

Centers for Disease Control and Prevention, National Information Network Funding: www.cdcnpin.org/scripts/locates/LocateFund.asp?SearchType= Advanced

If you are familiar with organizations or government agencies with research interests closely aligned with your own, we encourage you to go directly to those agency and organizational Web sites. The goal of your search should be to identify 5–10 potential funding opportunities. You should learn how to review opportunities to determine their overall appropriateness given your stated goals, research priorities, skills, time frames, resources, and your eligibility.

Phase 3: Qualify by Determining Eligibility and Competitive Fit for Identified Funding

When you have identified 5–10 opportunities that seem to have potential as sources of funding, it is time to read the "fine print." Print the program summaries, guidelines, applications, requests for proposals, and any other materials related to each of the 5–10 opportunities you identified. If these materials are not available online, call the funding agency, institution, or organization to request the materials be sent to you directly. Once you possess the necessary materials, read them in their entirety and read them very carefully. Then review the materials again, asking the following questions:

Am I Eligible to Compete for This Opportunity?

Do you meet *all* of the eligibility requirements? Can you find a partner or co-investigator to ensure you meet all of the requirements? If yes, proceed to the next question; if not, discard or file the materials for another time and move on to the next opportunity.

What Are the Application/Proposal Requirements?

Does the opportunity require the development of a 50-page, full-scale research proposal, a 10-page capabilities statement, a letter of intent, a resume, or some combination of the above? If the proposal requirements are unclear, ask questions and obtain clarification from the funding agency. If you have the research skills/qualifications and resources to complete the required documentation, proceed to the next question; if not, discard or file the materials for another time and move on to the next opportunity.

When Is the Application/Proposal Due?

Do you have enough time to develop and submit a quality application/proposal in the time frame available? If yes, set this opportunity aside for a brief period of time as you peruse more funding opportunities. You may decide after reviewing all of the opportunities that this one is best suited to your stated goals.

Continue to review all of the opportunities you identified in your phase 2 search, asking the three questions above. When you have reviewed all of the opportunities, you should have two sets of documents. One set will include opportunities to be discarded or responded to at a later point in time, and the other set will include opportunities for which you have qualified and deserve more immediate attention. In the event that you do not have any opportunities in this second set, you will need to return to phase 2 to identify additional opportunities. However, most likely you have one or two options that you will be able to pursue. At this point, you will choose to complete applications for some or all of these options. If you have the resources and time to complete high-quality applications for all, we recommend you do so. Your chances of getting funded increases with the number of applications you submit. If you have the time and resources to complete only one application, you must further narrow the identified opportunities. To choose one opportunity, review the materials one more time, keeping in mind your current research priorities—most likely, one opportunity will stand out as most appropriate and most aligned with your goals. If you are still unable to make a decision, conduct a review of the funding organizations. Examine their missions, goals, existing programs, recently funded projects, and anything else that will help you gain insight into how they make selections for funding. This information will help you to determine which funding agencies is best aligned with your research and personal interests and help you to make a decision about the opportunity for which you are best qualified. This information will also come in handy during the application preparation process and dovetails nicely with phase 4: obtain funding.

Phase 4: Obtain Funding by Providing Convincing Documentation of Your Ability to Perform Research Functions at the Highest Level Possible

During phase 4, you channel all of your energies into capturing, winning, or obtaining funding. While there are a variety of mechanisms through which you can obtain funds, the research community is competitive, and it is important to devote a considerable portion of your time to the development of grant or fellowship applications. This means preparation of the necessary documentation that demonstrates your ability to perform research as necessary to meet not only your personal goals, but the goals of the funding agency or institution. This documentation may be a full-scale proposal, a capabilities presentation, or simply a letter of intent accompanied by a resume or curriculum vitae. Regardless of the documentation required, as an applicant you only have one chance to make a first impression and you want that impression to be the best possible.

Before you begin development of your winning proposal, we recommend you do two things. First, you should prepare an application checklist, outline, and timeline. These items will keep you organized and focused on a reasonable schedule. Your checklist should detail each piece and/or requirement of the application. The outline should at a minimum include the specific application requirements, but also may include ancillary activities outside of the immediate submission procedure (i.e., getting community organizations to participate as data collection sites). However, the more detailed your outline, the more prepared you will be to complete the application. Your timeline should highlight the due date for completion of each application requirement and the person (if other than yourself) responsible (i.e., contracts and grants for signatures, institutional review board for human subjects approval, and obtaining the departmental chair or dean's signature). When developing the timeline, you want to be sure to include time for objective review of the finished product and for editing and production (printing, collating, or online submission). As necessary, you should include time to coordinate a team, partners, advisors, consultants, experts, and so on. More often than not, the inclusion of partners can improve your chances of obtaining funding.

The second thing you should do before you begin writing your proposal is schedule a face-to-face meeting with the decision makers at the organization from which you are requesting funds. There is a possibility that you will have a formal interview as part of your application for funding, but by taking the time to meet with organizational leaders prior to your submission, you demonstrate your initiative and commitment to your application. Meeting with decision makers also provides them with the opportunity to gain some insight into your skills, abilities, knowledge, and passion and to entertain discussion about your research vision. A face-to-face meeting provides you with the chance to establish personal connections and gives you the opportunity to highlight your research goals and showcase how they are aligned with the portfolio of the granting agency. If an agency has money for one of two equally qualified applicants, they often reward familiarity and pick the more seasoned applicant. While this nepotistic maneuver seems unfair, the agency possesses insight regarding your competitor's track record, and such familiarity may breed favorable reviews. It is important to meet with the funding agency as early in the application process as possible. In many cases immediately following solicitation for proposals or applications, funding agencies will scale back on the number of these meetings so as not to create the hint of any impropriety or to give unfair advantage to one applicant over another. Furthermore, in some instances, meeting with the decision makers at an agency may not be an option. This is often the case for international researchers who would have to travel a great distance for such a meeting. In this instance, we recommend making introductions or establishing a rapport/relationship with decision makers via phone or email. Regardless of how your make your introduction, in person or via phone or email, name recognition at the funding organization can only help your application.

After you create your checklist, outline, and timeline and schedule a meeting with your preferred funding agency, it is time to develop your application. Using your outline and timeline, proceed through your application checklist. Be sure to follow all directions and to allocate enough time to respond to each section of the proposal thoroughly. Do not spend all of your time on one section or requirement of the proposal, thus forcing yourself to hurry through others. You want your entire proposal to evenly showcase your research skills. As you complete your proposal, be sure to include your understanding of the funding organization's goals and missions and weave in how your proposed research will contribute to those goals. When you have completed your proposal, have it reviewed and carefully edited by a colleague or mentor. Make any recommended editorial changes and conduct a very thorough review of your product. There should be no typographical errors, no missing references, no information mentioned or tabled and then not included. Ensure that you have responded to all the requirements of the application without exceeding the stated page limit. Based on your knowledge of application requirements, produce your proposal as necessary for submission online, via fax, courier, or other delivery means. Be sure to follow all submission requirements carefully, as one simple error can result in your application being deemed nonresponsive and thus ineligible for funding. Be certain to maintain a copy of all materials submitted as part of your application package, as well as a file that includes contact information for each organization in the proposal selection process. Finally, submit your application for funding, take a breath, reward yourself for this professional milestone, and do it again and again and again until you reach the pinnacle of success you originally set as your funding goal.

8

R01 Grants: The Investigator-Initiated Cornerstone of Biomedical Research

WILLIAM L. DEWEY & MICHELLE R. HOOT

When one has finished building one's house, one suddenly realizes that in the process one has learned something that one really needed to know in the worst way—before one began.

—FRIEDRICH WILHELM NIETZSCHE, *Beyond Good and Evil*

THE NIH WAS created to maintain the health of the American people and society in general. Biomedical research and the resulting advances in medical treatment generated by the NIH is the most important component of maintaining the long term health of our society. NIH promotes biomedical research through a host of investigator-initiated research grant mechanisms. There are a number of different types of grants available for scientists to use to seek the financial support necessary to carryout their scientific investigations. This edited volume explores a wide range of these mechanisms and covers a lion's share of the most popular and in some cases the most competitive types (no one book could conceivably cover all the mechanisms).

A careful reading of the chapters in this book will show that individual and institutional training grants are available for trainees during graduate school or as postdoctoral fellows. As several chapters in this book describe in great detail, junior faculty (or less seasoned grant writers) often apply for an R03 grant, which has a maximum of $50,000 a year and can extend over two years of funding. There are other small grant mechanisms, as well, exploratory and developmental grants, a host of different fellowship mechanisms, and alternative roads to research independence. One important grant mechanism, which is the focus of the present chapter, is the research R01 grant, a highly sought after and competitive grant funding mechanism usually awarded to scientists of the highest caliber who meet strict scientific standards of excellence.

Support through an R01 usually signifies a higher level of science and greater prominence of the researcher in the scientific community. Because of its competitive nature and greater scientific accord, the R01 grant signifies a higher level of research independence. At the heart of an R01 mechanism is recognition by one's peers for scholarly work and the potential to advance science and knowledge. As a result of their stature within the research community, R01 grants carry a much heavier weight during review, undergo greater (and more rigorous) scrutiny, and demand a "higher" standard from program staff during their execution. From a logistic standpoint, R01 grants can be funded for longer periods of time and receive greater financial support compared to fellowships, small grants, or R29 first awards (R01 grants usually have a maximum of $250,000 a year, can extend over five years, but can exceed these limits with institute approval). The R01 is the most widely used grant to fund biomedical research in this country and therefore is the most important funding opportunity for the advancement of knowledge in the biomedical sciences.

All R01 grants stem from an investigators program of research that is carefully designed around a well-crafted set of research hypotheses. The point of embarkation in a successful R01 grant is the statement of these hypotheses in terms of Specific Aims and testable hypotheses (these sections of the grant are covered in depth in chapter 3). Therefore, most investigators who successfully apply for R01 grants carry with them a solid track record of performance, including publications, professional service, and a history of scholarly work for which they have been educated and trained (this is why the synthesis of training presented in an application is such a critical point during review).

Importantly, R01 grants provide a foundation on which to build other larger funding mechanisms including P-series centers, R37 merit awards, T32 training grants, and Small Business Innovative Research initiatives, to name a few. The R01 represents a "gold standard" or barometer that can be used to gauge an investigators' success. Scientists who lead program projects, cores within centers, or are directors of centers have proven their ability to lead a research team by being a successful principal investigator of at least one R01 grant. On the NIH ladder of success, the ability to secure R01 funding is the basis on which many larger funding opportunities are determined.

The R01 mechanism truly is an amazing opportunity for scholars to compete for funds to test their ideas. Despite the promise associated with obtaining an

Roi, they are incredibly competitive and demand a very high level of scholarly work. Roi funding is limited to investigators who possess ideas that will advance the specific field of research and who can present their ideas in a cogent manner, in effect, writing a very clear, succinct, and scholarly application. This chapter does not delve into the principles of innovation and idea generation, since that is more philosophical and less concrete than the overall focus of this book (although it makes for good conversation among Roi investigators). The focus or intent of this chapter is rather to provide step-by-step guide to help investigators present their ideas in a manner that will enhance their opportunity to obtain Roi funding.

EVENTS THAT TRANSPIRE PRIOR TO WRITING AN R01 APPLICATION

A quick and dirty poll of the contributors to this book would show that most regard their own grant writing success as a reflection of long, arduous, and often tedious work that transpired over a very long period of time. None of us reached our position in the university, think tank, or business community overnight. In fact, our work could best be described as demanding and in many cases "consuming," or at the very least, requiring a high level of professional and personal commitment. Notwithstanding, we all also recognize that this work, the path we traveled, and subsequent route through NIH represents a very select way to secure the necessary funding needed to jump-start our research careers. The very close and almost sycophantic relationship between investigators and the federal government is aptly described in both chapters 1 and 2. The authors of both chapters maintain research investigative careers but have chosen to work inside the federal government as a means of advancing science.

As all of us recognize implicitly, the only reason to ever write and submit a grant application is to obtain the necessary funding to perform independent scholarly work. In essence, the commitment to seek federal dollars for research support represents a commitment to conduct scholarly work of the highest caliber. The aims, research hypotheses, study design, experimental procedures, and protocols must meet the highest standards during peer review. Writing Roi grants is a significant step in any career and involves meeting these standards not just to obtain tenure or seek promotion but also to advance scientific inquiry and contribute to the fund of human knowledge. When grant applications contain an element of "discovery" and are written in an impeccable (erudite) manner, their review, scoring, and ultimate funding decision represent a milestone for any scientist's career.

In this respect, there are certain bits and pieces of information that should be useful to scientists as they begin the process of constructing an Roi and, in essence, constructing a career. While many of these pieces of information can be found embedded in numerous other chapters found in this book, it is worthwhile to quickly list them at the outset of this chapter. First and foremost, investigators should familiarize themselves with NIH guidelines. There should be no question regarding whether the application was constructed according to published guidelines. Next, all investigators are encouraged to establish a dialogue with the appropriate program staff member at NIH and ensure that their research goals and hypotheses are consistent with the institute's or center's current research portfolio, mission, and program goals.

Next, it is important to be aware of the three (newly revised) deadline dates for the submission of R01 applications each year (table 1.6 summarizes deadline dates for this and other award mechanisms). Currently, submission dates for R01 applications are February 5, June 5, and October 5 for new applications and March 5, July 5, and November 5 for resubmissions. Applications that do not arrive at NIH by these dates are held over until the next deadline. Note that if the submission date falls on a Saturday or Sunday or federal holiday, applications are accepted on the Monday immediately following the intended submission date. Applications are accepted via courier or delivery via an authorized delivery agent. They are no longer accepted via hand delivery by the principal investigator or any other person who is not a licensed delivery agent. Chapter 17 in this volume goes into great length to discuss the expected dates for electronic submission of R01 applications.

In addition to these concerns, it is critically important to read and understand the latest version of instructions for the particular grant mechanism in question, since a violation of the PHS instructions can cause an application to be returned without being evaluated. NIH has written and often revises very detailed instructions for the preparation of each of its grant mechanisms. It is absolutely essential to read and follow the latest version of these instructions before writing an R01 grant application. Appendix 1 contains the appropriate Web site addresses at NIH for obtaining instructions for an R01 application (www.nih.grantsinfo.com). If an investigator is really unsure whether he or she possess the latest version of the PHS instructions, a quick call to program staff at the appropriate institute or center will clear up this matter. All aspects of the instructions are important, including submission dates, page limitations, font size, margins, and form requirements. Other important tips include placement of materials in appendices, size of tables, figures, and pictures (diagrams), and appropriate lengths (suggested) for each of the major sections in a grant application.

One of the major reasons why these instructions have been developed is to aid reviewers in their work. A basic rule of writing any competitive grant, and especially an R01, is to ease the job of the reviewer as much as possible. The written format of an R01 grant should be as clear and concise as possible. Tables, figures, diagrams, reports of empirical findings all need to be self-contained, self-explanatory, and uncomplicated. Not only is this an essential component to scholarship, and an effective means to standardize presentation of grants, but reviewers must be able to grasp the concepts or data being presented inside the grant in a very short period of time.

Funding and Program Staff

The decision to fund a particular application is made by the institute staff based on the advice given by the initial review group (study section) and the institute advisory council (this dual review process is elaborated in chapter 1). Since the program staff of the institute makes this very important decision, it is to the benefit of the applicant to involve these staff in every step of the way. This means starting with a discussion of the core scientific ideas that will be articulated in the grant even prior to the initiation of grant writing. It is advisable for even the most seasoned scientist who is contemplating the submission of an Ro1 application to contact a program official at NIH who is responsible for the area of concentration for the proposed application. Program staff at the various institutes and centers has the responsibility to allocate funds provided by Congress in such a way that the health of the citizens is enhanced. Program staff members hunker down after council and consider a wide range of factors before funding a grant. At the heart of their deliberation is always the public health agenda, the current climate of scientific inquiry, and the mandate of their institute or center. In many respects, program staff members are the most knowledgeable source to determine whether a slate of proposed research is a priority at that specific time.

Understanding that the goal of the Ro1 grant program is to encourage investigator-initiated projects, program staff may be reluctant to discourage an idea unless there is good reason to do so. Yet, it is important for the investigator to know that a grant dovetails with the overall research agenda of the institute or center before spending the required time to compose and submit an application.

A concern of many potential grant applicants, especially young investigators, is that they would be putting the program staff in conflict if they discussed their intended plans for an application. Due to changes in recent years that have clearly separated the responsibilities of program staff and review staff within the institutes and centers, this matter should no longer be a concern. At this point in time, it is inappropriate for program staff to affect the evaluation of an application. The program staff members have the responsibility to ensure that the slate of congressional funds appropriated to their particular institute is used to fund the best program(s) of research available. In fact, it is a part of their job to interact with scientists who have good ideas to advance the research agenda of their respective Institute. It has been our experience that the program staff members at NIH institutes are anxious to meet with and provide important hints and be very helpful to prospective principal investigators.

In conclusion, the program staff members at the appropriate institute are very helpful in informing principal investigators as to the interest of the particular institute in the specific area of research being proposed. Obviously, they cannot inform an investigator whether a particular idea is fundable or not, but they have the greatest knowledge about the interests of the institute in the proposed project at this specific point in time. As many other chapters in this book reinforce, following grant preparation and submission guidelines represents only one part of the puzzle of successful grant writing. Connecting with program staff is highly recommended, but there exist other important outlets and promising mechanisms to consider.

Colleagues and Collaborators

A very rich and informative method involves presenting newly generated grant ideas to trusted colleagues prior to the actual writing of an application. This can be done in either an oral or a written form and using either informal meetings or structured grant review seminars or research meetings. There is no set practice to handle this type of internal review, and many options exist. Grant ideas can be initiated during cafeteria lunches between faculty members, at regularly scheduled cross-departmental meetings, during athletic events involving collaborators (e.g., institute softball picnics), walks across campus, phone calls, informal lunches, or grant reviews held in the Washington and Baltimore area (reviewers often become colleagues, as evidenced by this book, where many reviewers met at NIDA-K meetings). Regardless of the site or nature how they begin, these conversations are an integral part of the refining process that helps grants move from the chalkboard to the preparation stage immediately preceding submission.

There are certain advantages and disadvantages associated with each method of informal and formal review. In the informal method using an oral review among colleagues, a colleague may feel inclined to challenge a controversial issue, and this prompts further scrutiny and discussion. Younger colleagues often pay deference to more senior colleagues, but the overall receptivity of senior colleagues to criticisms offered by younger "sharks" may be lower. An investigator writing a grant may feel attacked or "miffed" by his colleagues but gets a chance to see how the grant is received prior to actual submission. Sometimes, your own colleagues form a very neatly packaged peer review system and save you time and money. Grants cost money to produce (time is money in the research world), and costly savings can be had by submitting a grant to informal "friendly" review prior to actual submission at NIH (which takes roughly nine months from submission to funding decision). There is a certain cost savings associated with obtaining an immediate opinion from respected colleagues, and this can save time and money in the overall scheme of things.

Also be aware that some reviewers may not back down from their conceptual, theoretical, or methodological position (or they are just pure antipathetic to a grant) and hence can block scoring or at the very least offer resistance during the review. The investigator who has a solid grasp of the field, has conducted a thorough literature review, is current on the techniques used (methods or laboratory procedures), and has examined the composition of the internal review group using the NIH Web sites for study sections and will have a "feel" for which reviewer has at least published in the field, or who may publish in related disciplines, or has a "working" knowledge of the grant. The investigator then has a choice how to "handle" this situation (making a weakness into a possible strength). The solution is perhaps the oldest trick in the book: Pick up the telephone and ask the individual who sits on the internal review group study section to be a consultant. At the very least, this would pose a conflict if this person is a consultant on your grant and then is asked to review your grant (or be present in the room during the review). The NIH peer review conflict guidelines stipulate that this individual cannot be present in the room during review of your application. More detailed information on the conflicts policies at NIH can be found at grants1.nih.gov/grants/policy/coi/index.htm. The long and short of this strategy is that you should "make your enemy your friend." You can do this with colleagues who can strengthen your grant and who may be potential peer reviewers, or request participation on your grant by leading thinkers in the field who can assist you to learn new techniques or laboratory procedures. You can add rivals who have developed contrasting or opposing interventions, treatment strategies, or laboratory procedures but who would strengthen your advisory board and embellish the grant.

Should the Grant Be an R01?

Another issue that often arises during an informal oral review is whether a grant merits the time and energy necessary to apply for funding. Colleagues may suggest that an R01 is not the appropriate mechanism given the developmental or exploratory nature of the proposed research. For instance, a young investigator may have accumulated a body of scientific findings, present this at an informal research seminar, and then receive feedback with respect to whether the findings are "strong" enough to merit an R01 application. Other R01 level investigators (or in some cases even a center director) can then indicate whether the body of scientific findings is pointing in the direction of a strong Preliminary Findings section. This type of discussion also helps an investigator clarify and develop a more complete set of Specific Aims (which often herald the contents of an application). Following this type of discussion, a more concerted set of research hypotheses can be developed, and the various experimental procedures and protocols can be hashed out in greater detail. Again, the mechanism of an informal research seminar provides a nifty way to size up findings and openly discuss their merit.

An informal review that occurs during a seminar or gathering of colleagues also can help an investigator to grapple with whether the research is significant. Since significance is such a critical point during review and is weighed very heavily by both peer reviewers and council, it should by necessity jump off the page. Hearing one's colleagues forthrightly state, "This is a significant piece of research that should be further explored," helps jump-start any inclinations to assemble and construct a grant.

Formal reviews provide a means for colleagues to sit down and pretend for awhile that they are conducting a peer review. In effect, the reviewer mentality comes to bear on the research ideas, and a colleague will draft a formal review document usually based on the given review criteria (chapter 3 covers the formal peer review criteria in detail). Receiving a written review with all the trimmings will help an investigator grapple not only with the research ideas but also with the manner or style in which they are presented (again reinforcing the importance that an investigator possess stellar writing skills!). This added level of review helps investigators attend to the grammatical and scholastic components of grant construction that might not crop up during an informal review.

As we discuss in greater detail below, the criteria for review of R01 grants relate to the significance of the project, the approach being taken, whether the work is innovative, qualifications of the investigators, and suitability of the environment (other grant mechanisms include additional layers of review criteria, and these are discussed in their respective chapters). Therefore, it is important to ask colleagues how your ideas would be perceived in relation to these five criteria. Going back to using colleagues for phantom reviews, what is most essential in this exercise is honesty. It is detrimental, rather than helpful, for a colleague to encourage a prospective principal investigator to write a particular grant unless he or she is convinced that the project has merit. It is much better to hear criticisms from a colleague prior to writing the application than to do all the work and not be competitive for funding. Obviously, the final decision to go forward is up to the principal investigator, but it is always better to proceed with the knowledge that other competent scientists believe that the chances of success are reasonable. Further, we propose that the principal investigator solicit input from as many learned colleagues as to the potential of the project as reasonable. Honesty rather than false praise is the most valuable contribution from a colleague.

A BRIEF GUIDE TO R01 REVIEW CRITERIA

It is useful to learn as much as possible about the review process prior to initiating the writing of the application. Reviewers are provided written guidelines by the scientific review administrator for their study section. These review guidelines help shape reviewers' comments both in their written summary statements and during any discussion. It is a means to keep the reviewers on task. In this respect, it is not surprising that the actual written reviews share a number of commonalities. The ability to incorporate the essential underlying points that constitute review criteria into the body of the grant will result in a much better application. Chapter 3 delves into the five review criteria in considerable detail; however, it is worthwhile to provide a brief synopsis of each review criterion and perhaps offer an alternative view from a seasoned grant writer (and an investigator who also plays curmudgeon reviewer).

The significance of the work is perhaps the most important review criterion. Significance regards how the proposed research will advance knowledge in a particular field. It is essential that investigators consider two things with regard to significance: (1) that the work is significant if it will have a pronounced effect on the field of research or if it will provide the stimulus for others to contribute along with the principal investigator to important advances in the field; and (2) that such significance can be appreciated in "incremental" or baby steps and need not be a radical change or gross alteration to current thinking.

Sometimes a minor refinement or tweaking of the current zeitgeist will be regarded as significant. This is particularly valuable if the investigator is using a particular laboratory technique and wants to add a slight modification or use a different testing apparatus to learn more about a process at the microcellular level. Baby steps often help us gain a more refined picture of processes and mechanisms that can be then used to paint the broader picture as science accretes knowledge from different laboratories. In this respect, there have been numerous Ro1 grants funded for relatively small amounts of money to engage a new scientific apparatus or testing procedure and where the work possesses incredible significance but is not costly or does not take an enormous amount of time to unfold.

Virulence or lethality of the focal topic is not necessarily a guarantee that a grant will be well received during peer review. Even if a new drug of abuse pops up on the radar screen (e.g., black tar heroin) and narcotic experts who monitor illicit street drugs (e.g., police, FBI, epidemiologists, trafficking experts, treatment providers, and street informants) notice increase trafficking, it is not enough to swing the public health pendulum. There have to be noticeable changes in the costs to society for prevention, treatment, and interdiction. The message of lethality needs to be reinforced by hospital statistics detailing emergency department mentions with reported drug abuse and increases in treatment numbers dictating any concerted public health response. There has to be a modicum of interest by the media and congressional input on the problem. Once these pieces are put into place, the next step usually involves a request for applications from one or more institutes or centers focusing exclusively on the new street drug (e.g., fentanyl, and the club drugs including MDMA, ecstasy, GHB, ketamine, and rohypnol are all examples of street drugs that appeared on the market and caused spikes of interest at numerous levels).

Despite the increased media attention and call for grant applications, it is important that investigators not assume that the nature of the disease (or drug) being studied will assure the potential success of the grant. A poorly written and loosely conceived grant formulated in a knee-jerk reflex will not be evaluated as favorably as a well-constructed grant with a tight focus that advances the field forward. It is of utmost importance to convey to reviewers just how the research proposed will move the field forward in significant and meaningful ways. Grants written in haste to be the first on the docket responding to a virulent problem and that pay no attention to significance (or any of the other four review criteria) will face an uphill battle during review.

A second important criterion for evaluating an R01 grant is the approach that will be used to test the hypotheses. The experiments must be well thought out and utilize state-of-the-art techniques. Each technique must be valid, have some familiarity among reviewers, and be feasible (if not cost-effective). Evidence from the literature as to how the investigators have previously used the techniques to generate important data provides reviewers with the confidence that the proposed experimental procedures and methodology rest within the expertise of the investigators. The series of proposed experiments must follow a logical progression with each one adding to the knowledge generated by the previous one (this is an example of scientific accretion or refinement). Additionally, the experimental data must be scrutinized with appropriate statistical analysis. Chapter 3 devotes considerable space to making this point under the approach section. Chapter 4 also weighs in on the choice of test statistics and computation of power as essential grant ingredients.

The third R01 review criterion concerns innovation. At the very least, the laboratory or research techniques used need to be outright forward thinking, and if not, then the grant must combine several techniques in a unique manner to be innovative. That is, either the techniques must be innovative or the way in which routine techniques are used to test a particular hypothesis must be novel. Up to this point, and taken all together, an investigator needs to present a project that will significantly move an important aspect of the field forward using an innovative approach that will provide important information using state-of-the-art analyses.

It is essential that the application provide convincing evidence to the reviewers that the principal investigator and the entire team of investigators that will be involved in the project are well qualified to carry out the proposed research. If the description of the work to be done is excellent but appears beyond the ability of the investigators, it will not receive a favorable evaluation from the reviewers. The previous history of the investigators using the techniques being proposed is important. This can be achieved by citation of previously published works and, more important, by the inclusion of preliminary data (R01 applications, unlike R21 exploratory grants, require inclusion of preliminary data). There is no better way to convince a review committee of your qualifications than including empirical findings that cast no doubt on your ability to master, implement, and make headway with the proposed laboratory procedures or experimental techniques.

Although the principal investigator has the responsibility to oversee all aspects of the project, that same individual need not be expert in every aspect of the described experiments. It is important that collaborators and/or consultants be recruited to assist and conduct research that may not rest within the purview of the principal investigator. Ro1 grants often include large-scale field trials or laboratory techniques that necessitate careful logistical planning and utilization of team approaches to science. The integration of a broad range of skills from different people requires the principal investigator possess administrative, managerial, and interpersonal communication skills and know how to implement research from a collective team framework. The application needs to address these issues to reinforce the investigator is capable of spearheading and running the project (i.e., leadership). The time commitment of co-investigators and/or consultants must be enough that their input is not considered "window dressing" but rather that they can make a meaningful contribution to the project. Reviewers are not impressed with the inclusion of a big name in the field if that individual does not make it clear in a letter included in the application that he or she will devote enough time and commitment to the proposed project to accomplish all of the stated aims and goals.

Reviewers have the responsibility to evaluate whether the environment is appropriate for the proposed experiments. Reviewers must be convinced that there is sufficient laboratory and office space available. In addition to a commitment of physical space, it should be clear that all necessary equipment for the proposed experiments is readily available for the investigators or that appropriate funds are requested in the application for its purchase (cost accounting is a large issue, and chapter 15 is devoted to the intricate nature of putting dollars to science). It also is important to convince the reviewers that the environment of the department, university, and institution is supportive of the type of research described in the application. One needs to ensure that appropriate release time exists for faculty to carry out the scholarly work proposed and that any significant obstacles such as teaching, student advising, or university service will not interfere with the execution of the grant in a timely manner.

In conclusion, an investigator considering submission of an Ro1 grant needs to become familiar with these five review criteria. While the additional effort may make the initial process of writing an Ro1 grant more time consuming, it can only serve to help you in the end.

MAJOR CRITICISMS EXPRESSED BY R01 GRANT REVIEWERS

The preceding sections of this chapter outline some compelling steps that can be taken to prepare a grant using in-house collegial review and also briefly address the five peer review criteria. In addition to prewriting preparation and familiarizing yourself with the review process, it is helpful to be aware of some of the most common pitfalls and major criticisms expressed by R01 grant reviewers. From our own experience and those of our esteemed colleagues, reviews of these applications usually follow a pattern. The reviews of the best applications are usually a series of statements that are very descriptive in nature. The descriptive tenor usually arises because the reviewer can find little fault with the application and opts to give an overview of the science to familiarize the review group.

Criticisms of grants with poorer priority scores follow certain patterns, including a consensus among reviewers the grant is unfocused, overly ambitious, poorly written, or not likely to produce significant advancements in the field. These recurrent themes crop up because of three essential oversights: the investigators constructing the R01 grants have (1) not learned to be focused, (2) not addressed the five review criteria in the "evolution" or construction of their grant application, and (3) have not submitted their grant for prereview by colleagues.

Let us expand on these three issues to see how they occur and whether there are specific remedies. One of the most frequently noted criticisms lodged during peer review is that a grant is unfocused. What does this mean? It is very important that the amount of work being proposed be realistic and in keeping with the proposed budget. The time period set aside for the grant and the timeline need to be configured so that the science can proceed unfettered. The amount of support needs to be sufficient to sustain the research over the duration of the study. The grant should not "wander" but rather be streamlined, tight, and cogent. Sections should feed into each other, as should paragraphs (one leading to another). Points made earlier in the grant should be taken up later and addressed fully. The aims should be tethered to the hypotheses, which should be tied to the analytic strategies and the goals of the science contained in the grant.

From a conceptual point of view, it is not in the best interest of the applicant to propose a group of experiments that are not related to each other even if they are in the same general area of research. The overall goal of the work should be hypothesis driven and contribute to the growing knowledge base in a specific area. Each specific aim also should be hypothesis driven in itself but also be directed toward advancing knowledge toward a more specific aspect of the overall goal of the work. Tying all these disparate piece of the grant together helps it to be more focused and seamlessly integrate the different sections. Some investigators propose discrete aims that are not linked with each other but are linked to the overall systematic research goals. Others include linking or branching aims, using one aim to fuel another. Once one aim is satisfied, the findings are used to support another aim.

Aims can also sit side by side and address two different sides of the same coin. For instance, in randomized control field trials (drug abuse prevention studies) that include a minimal or no-contact control group, there are etiology aims that sit side by side with the overall focus on evaluating the efficacy of the intervention. The no-contact control group represents normative growth absent the intervention effect and is a standard requirement for prevention studies. But the no-contact control group also represents an opportunity to explore normative development unfettered by the intervention (in the event the intervention does contribute to "change"). At the very least, some member of the investigative team should be examining development in the no-contact control group, and there should be an aim suggesting this important source of data and information is worth mining.

Under the general rubric of focus, another frequently encountered criticism is that the grant is overly ambitious. In this respect, it is advisable to present a well-thought-out series of experiments that are directed specifically toward testing the stated research hypotheses and do not include every experiment that comes to mind, even if they are related to the overall goal of the grant. Linkages and refinements of this nature make the grant look more packaged and afford a greater level of salesmanship.

The writing style used is another frequent criticism of grants that receive lower priority scores. A very dense style that is hard to comprehend is not in the best interest of the applicant. Again, make it as easy as possible for the reviewer. It is unnecessary to include everything that one knows on a topic. If the specific concepts are difficult to follow because the applicant has taken the tactic to be comprehensive, as opposed to thorough, or because the writing style is dense, reviewers will find it difficult to make meaningful linkages in the different sections of the application. When this occurs, reviewers will interpret this event as the absence of clearly defined objectives and the inability to synthesize the grant application.

As we mentioned above, reviewers are encouraged to concentrate on the significance of the grant. A common criticism that is frequently mentioned during review is that the grant is descriptive and not mechanistic. That is, reviewers are less enthusiastic about proposals that describe a phenomenon rather than those that propose to determine the mechanism responsible for this action (this may be a reflection of the times and poses paradigmatic issues that may wane with changing winds of discovery). Many reviewers believe that in order for an investigation to be mechanistic one needs to apply reductionism. A series of experiments directed toward elucidating a mechanism are preferred over procedures that concentrate on the description of the effects. To wit, studies of school-based drug abuse prevention focus on elucidating the "active ingredients" of the program and offer very mechanistic explanations of behavior change. Equally compelling, of course, is whether the program induced behavioral change among youth exposed to the experimental treatment. However, obtaining and explaining change in the target risk mechanisms (i.e., skills) is important as a means of accounting for change in target behavioral outcomes. The difference is whether the outcomes are proximal or distal and whether linkages exist between the different layers of cause and effect. Again, there are philosophical and theoretical issues that pervade any focus on active ingredients (this is true of studies focusing on pain analgesia, mechanisms of transport and storage for brain neurochemicals, and neuropharmacological studies emphasizing brain chemistry and behavioral drug effects). The truth is that both explanation and mechanisms are needed to account for behavior at the microscopic and more macroscopic levels.

In summary, reviewers evaluate proposals more favorably if they are directed toward elucidating the mechanism of an effect rather than proposals that describe a new effect. Also, proposals that are overly ambitious, unfocused, or poorly presented are not evaluated with the same high regard as proposals that are clearly written, focused on a particular important scientific problem, and realistic in relation to what is proposed in the budget and time constraints presented.

We cannot stress enough that the grant application needs to curry favor among the reviewers by fully addressing the five review criteria. One suggestion is for the investigator to review each criterion and locate in the bowels of the grant the specific text that addresses each criterion. Coupled with this effort is the use of "phantom" reviews by colleagues who also scratch notes on the grant noting whether all five criteria are addressed responsively. Taken together, the renewed emphasis on focus, on addressing the five criteria, and holding prereviews will help applicants more fully prepare for an actual peer review of their application.

WRITING THE FIRST DRAFT

Now that the appropriate steps have been taken to sufficiently prepare yourself, you should begin the process of writing your R01 application. In this section we discuss some tips and guidelines for writing particular aspects and sections of the grant. This focus is intended to help your grant receive the appropriate placement within a study section and increase your chances of receiving a fundable score.

At the NIH, an official assigns all grants to a study section based on information supplied by the principal investigator. An option available to all principal investigators is to include a cover letter attached to the front of the grant and use this letter to suggest a particular study section (internal review group) for review. One would opt for this strategy in cases where the principal investigator believes a particular study section contains members who are familiar with the work proposed in the application and that other study sections are less inclined to have experts in this substantive area. However, it is more likely that attention will be paid to requests that the grant not be assigned to one or more study sections. In order for this request to be seriously considered, the principal investigator must present a convincing argument that the published rosters of those particular study sections do not include scientists whose area of expertise is close enough to their own to adequately evaluate the subject matter of the application. Even if you feel that you have made a convincing argument for the placement of your R01 grant, it is important to bear in mind that there is no guarantee that these types of suggestions will lead to placement within your desired study section. For more on cover letters, see chapter 1.

Title and Abstract

Without a cover letter, the next source of information used to assign the application to the best of many possible study sections is the title of the grant. Since the title usually gets the grant assigned to a study section, it is most important that the title be chosen with great care and to accurately represent the contents of the application. If the title does not provide the necessary information for assignment, the abstract is the next best source of information. Like the title, the abstract should be prepared with great care and accurately reflect the contents of the grant. It is not reasonable to expect that all members of a study section will read every grant submitted to that review committee. Most review committees have at least 60 or more grants (and may have upward of 100) to evaluate at each of their three meetings a year. Each reviewer is assigned anywhere from 5 to 10 or more grants to read and must prepare a written evaluation and orally present these evaluations to the committee. This is a very time-consuming task that takes reviewers away from their own scholarly pursuits, teaching, and other responsibilities.

Remember that study section members are very busy scientists who agree to set aside their own research pursuits to evaluate a large number of grants for their respective study section. It is for this reason that the abstract should be prepared with great care. Members of a study section who are not assigned as reviewers of a particular grant (whose content may lie outside their professional expertise) often read the abstract while the reviewers are communicating their evaluation of the grant to the rest of the study section. This quick reading helps shape their opinion regarding the value and significance of the grant while the assigned reviewers are making their presentation to the review committee. Countless numbers of times members of a particular study section comment that the abstract gave short shrift to the actual contents of the grant application. In many cases the actual physical space set aside on the PHS 398 form for the abstract was not prudently used. If the box set aside on the form for the abstract can fit 500 words, then fit in 500 words that cover the significance of the study, a one- or two-line statement regarding the experimental design, a quick overview of the analytic plan, sample methods, and a closing statement regarding implications of the study if it achieves its stated goals. Investigators are well advised to maximally use the available space, since following receipt of a notice of grant award the grant abstract is also represented on CRISP, a public domain database (crisp.cit.nih.gov/).

Background Section

It is essential that the principal investigator have a thorough understanding of current trends and findings in the field of investigation. The background section of the application is the portion of the application that should convey to the review committee that the principal investigator has a solid grasp of the relevant literature in the field. One of the more serious mistakes that a principal investigator can make in this regard is not to include certain reported findings in the background section and then propose to repeat a set of studies based on a lack of familiarity with the available evidence in the field. The guidelines offered in the PHS 398 booklet outlining the different grant sections suggest that the background section be no more than three pages. Therefore, although a comprehensive review is not possible, it is essential that the principal investigator demonstrate a thorough knowledge of the literature most pertinent to the proposed experiments. Review articles should be referenced for publications peripherally related to the specific objectives of the grant, and primary references should be used to demonstrate how the proposed experiments would contribute to current knowledge and dovetail with recent advances in the field. If the field is flush with scientific evidence, use the Vancouver style of referencing so that space is conserved (this style uses superscripted references rather than embedding author names in the text, as in APA style [i.e., Jones & Smith, 2003]).

Clear presentation of excellent ideas is absolutely of paramount importance since funding for R01 grants is always highly competitive. An excellent idea is one that is unique, creative, and innovative (chapter 3 goes into greater detail with regard to the basic composition of innovation). Obviously, the idea has to be novel in terms of what has been accomplished in the field. Even more important, the idea proposed in the grant should advance a particular field and significantly increase the current fund of knowledge. This is particularly true at this time when NIH staff is telling reviewers of R01 grants that the most important aspect of the grant review should be to evaluate its significance. That is, the reviewers are instructed they need to focus on the significance of the research in terms of advancement of the field, not the severity of the disease being studied.

It is also essential that the goals of the application and each of the Specific Aims be hypothesis driven. Even if investigators have preliminary data to support their Specific Aims, reviewers will scorn an application that seeks to generate information without testing specific hypotheses. In fact, applications of this nature are often considered hunting expeditions, or the analogy is used that the investigator is fishing with very large nets and not using specific bait. A very serious oversight by many applications is the view that generating enough useful data will produce new information that can augment our current knowledge base. In many cases, reviewers will regard this attempt as lacking any true direction and also not being hypothesis driven. Generating data for the sheer pleasure of data snooping rather than to test a set of specific hypotheses is not the best use of limited funds and has a low potential to produce significant advances in biomedicine.

Attention to Detail

After writing the text of the application, it is important to ensure that it has been prepared with care and presented with clarity. It is customary for reviewers to assume that if the application is prepared with little attention to detail, then the research will be carried out in the same manner. Spelling errors and poor grammar, although not a good predictor of scientific ability, often may be interpreted as a lack of care for detail that might be transcribed to careless scientific work of the principal investigator. Figures and diagrams must be large enough that the details can be perceived without the use of a magnifying glass. Legends need to be presented in such a way that the reviewer does not have to search through the text to determine what message the figure or diagram is intended to convey. Another consideration is the use of abbreviations and acronyms. Usually one would spell out the word in full the first time that it is used and present the abbreviation or acronym in parentheses to the right of it. Often this works well, but in an application where many abbreviations are used, it is very tedious and time consuming for the reviewer to continually go back and find the reference for the abbreviation within the text. It is highly suggested that one construct a table of all abbreviations and acronyms that are used.

Tables, Diagrams, Figures, and Inserts

There are no hard-and-fast rules about use of tables and figures in R01 grants (or for that matter in any R-series grants). Figures can be useful to graphically portray charts that explain or summarize preliminary findings, but there is still a need to draw inferences or make connections when using figures. Imagine if the reviewer does not extract the correct information from the table and comments in their review that critical supporting evidence seemed to be missing from the application. Sure, the reviewer did not understand the table, but the onus is on the principal investigator to explain the contents of the grant and not assume that the reader will grasp tabulated materials. The NIH guidelines are quite clear on whether tabled information or figures and pictures should be included as an appendix. If the material is germane to reading the grant and allows the reader to obtain clear evidence of the scientific rigor of the proposed study, they need to be included in the 25-page limits. However, if the material supplements or "augments" the text and is not considered essential to reading the grant (and therefore would not hurt the overall reading and evaluation if these materials were "lost"), then these materials can be included as an appendix.

Nowadays, given the competitive nature of grants and the fact that many reviewers have complained about reams of text included as appendix material that should have been synthesized and synopsized in the text, investigators submitting R01 grants are choosing to include their tabled and graphic material in the text. This decision is also made easier by the rapid advances in word processing technology and the ability to port text from Adobe Acrobat, Microsoft Word, Excel, MathType, PowerPoint, or other proprietary word processing software programs that enable one to embed figures, pictures, charts, equations, and tables in text. The bottom line is that the creativity of the investigator will either be evident in the manner chosen to include tabled material or the application will be perceived as "dense" and difficult to follow, thus lowering the priority score.

A good rule of thumb is to include in the appendix materials all surveys, supporting manuals for psychiatric or psychological assessments, laboratory manuals, diagrams or protocols for machinery, and nonessential materials that would not hurt the review process if they were missed or lost in transport to reviewers. Flow charts on patient recruitment, psychometric data on key measures, literature sources for key measures, machine benchmark performance standards, laboratory procedures for handling sensitive data or conducting experiments, and other key items that help reviewers follow a particular study should be included in the 25-page limit, usually in Experimental Methods (section D).

Administrative Concerns

In addition to the various components of the R01 application discussed above, there are administrative issues that need to be prepared with the same attention to detail. These include the care and use of vertebrate animals and human subjects as well as whether the requested budget is appropriate for the work proposed. Chapter 15 goes into great detail on the various considerations in preparing budgets for R01 and other related grant mechanisms (P50 centers). Cost accounting of science and the means by which investigators properly consider their scope of work in terms of dollars (expenditures for labor, materials, and professional services) is a very delicate art, and chapter 15 is essential reading before you prepare the R01 grant application.

Chapter 16 attends directly to issues pertaining to use of human subjects, inclusion of women, children, and minorities, and the unfathomable institutional review board procedures. The directions for the completion of the portion of the application related to the proper use of vertebrate animals and human subjects are clearly presented on the NIH Web site grants1.nih.gov/grants/policy/hs/index.htm. Additional and more extensive information regarding the federal regulations on human subjects are located on the Office for Human Research Protections Web site: www.hhs.gov/ohrp/humansubjects/guidance/45cfr46.htm.

Additionally, we recommend that investigators become familiar with the federal regulations regarding research involving human subjects, which can be found in the *Code of Federal Regulations* (Title 45 CFR Part 46) and can be downloaded from www.hhs.gov/ohrp/humansubjects/guidance/45cfr46.htm.

In this day and age, with the passage of the Family Educational Rights and Privacy Act of 1974 (Buckley Amendment) and the Health Insurance Portability and Accountability Act (HIPAA) of 1996, investigators need to keep abreast of the latest regulations concerning use of human subjects (for more on the Buckley Amendment, see www.epic.org/privacy/education/ferpa.html; for HIPAA, see www.hhs.gov/ocr/hipaa; full text of HIPAA can be found at 45 CFR Part 160 and subparts A and E of part 164). Of particular concern are applications that claim exemptions that are not eligible for this status. Justifications for exclusions are appropriate for studies involving adults that require participants to be older than 18 years of age and therefore do not include children (some valid reasons for exclusion would be, e.g., the study's irrelevance to children, laws or regulations barring participation by minors, that the knowledge being sought in the research is already available for children, that separate age-specific studies are being conducted or planned, factors related to the occurrence of a particular disease in children, the lack of similar developmental processes, or absence of data to judge risks to children).

It is essential that these regulations be followed to the letter because funding is contingent upon assurances that all aspects of the governing regulations in these areas are being followed even though compliance with these guidelines is not considered in the scoring of the application. It is not enough that the institutional animal care and use committee at the university level approved the use of vertebrate animals or that the institutional review board approved the use of humans in the research; the study section and all other levels of evaluation also must be assured that all the regulations are being followed to the letter. Nothing but a clearly presented total compliance with these regulations is acceptable. Any concern raised during review will present a stopgap to funding and needs to be reconciled prior to program staff releasing a notice of award. Guidance for treatment and handling of specimens and data storage can be found at www.hhs.gov/ohrp/policy/index.html.

Another important aspect of the review of R01 applications is the evaluation of the budget proposed in relation to the work required to carry out the work. The NIH recently has changed the format of the budgets for R01 grants that request direct costs of $250,000 or less a year. The funds requested must be in $25,000 increments unless the total direct costs requested per year are in excess of $250,000. This is now referred to as the modular format for R01 budgets in this cost range. Strong justification is required for the budget to be in excess of the quarter of a million of dollars per year. Notwithstanding, it is very important to justify the budget no matter what size it may be. Justification is required even if the new modular format is being used (a budget justification page accompanies the budget even when modular format is used).

Enough funds must be requested to carry out the work proposed, but it is equally important that the budget not be inflated. Salary must be justified for each of the investigators, and their percent effort and therefore the salary being requested must be appropriate for them to contribute sufficiently to the project. Sufficient funds must be requested for all the expensive reagents, tissue cultures, animal models, and other supplies needed. It is equally important that good justification for these costs be included. If a less expensive procedure or methodology would produce equally conclusive results, it should be proposed.

In essence, the budget must be reasonable for the experiments being proposed. In many cases, reviewers have noted the budget costs estimated for subject compensation appear too low given the duress or amount of work required by participants. Studies that assess students in schools need to provide incentives to students (i.e., movie tickets or cash rewards) and compensate teachers, as well (i.e., classroom supplies). Both strategies boost participation rates. Subjects responding to surveys sent by mail should be compensated at a level commensurate with the amount of work required to fill in the survey, and return the materials using postal services. Even a new investigator has the responsibility to accurately estimate the cost of the experiments proposed. It is not the responsibility of the reviewers to spend time determining the cost of the potential experiments. The principal investigator must do the homework to determine the realistic costs of the proposed experiments and request adequate, but not excessive, funds so that they can be carried out. There have been cases where grants receive poor priority scores because the costs of tracking subjects longitudinally were not realistic given the current climate of locating people using the Web, outside vendors who track people professionally, and credit card history information or personal identifying information (i.e., using Equifax or TRW to track people is very cost effective).

To summarize, it is important that the title and abstract accurately reflect the contents of your R01 grant to ensure the most favorable placement of the application. Also, it is paramount that the reviewers be convinced that your ideas are innovative and will produce significant advancements in your field. Furthermore, the application should be presented in a clear and concise manner, with proper justification of material, methods, and budget concerns. Following these guidelines should help you to prepare the best application possible.

WHAT HAPPENS AFTER THE FIRST DRAFT IS WRITTEN

When the first draft of the R01 application is complete, it is important to have all the co-investigators and the collaborators, if possible, critically evaluate it in its entirety. This activity ensures that their areas of expertise are correctly presented. The first draft of the grant also should be given to at least one, and preferably multiple, trusted colleagues who work in a related field but are not involved in this project. This ensures that the grant is well prepared and is easy to follow. Actually, the more individuals the principal investigator can have read the grant, the better.

Obviously, it is important to give the readers enough time to carefully review the draft. They have their own obligations and time commitments, and the principal investigator is asking them to take time from their own work to evaluate his draft. It is suggested that an agreement be reached where various scientists read one another's grants. This way the group is working as a team and everyone's draft is being read. Graduate students are an excellent choice to read the draft of an advisor's grant. Students learn a great deal about grant writing from the process and also have much to gain from being associated with a successful grant submission. Graduate students are knowledgeable of the research area, are familiar with many of the techniques to be employed, and most important, share the responsibility with the head of the laboratory to obtain the resources necessary for the continuation of the scholarly activity of the laboratory.

The readers must be honest with the principal investigator and indicate all areas that may be unclear or presented in an illogical fashion. The readers should critically assess the significance of the work proposed, evaluate the appropriateness of the methods being used to test the hypotheses, and determine whether the project is sufficiently innovative. It is essential that these colleagues can thoroughly evaluate the quality of the grant and that these individuals think that the grant is well presented because they are in the same position as the reviewers of the grant. Peer reviewers can be colleagues who also are scientists working in related fields and have agreed to perform these evaluations for the granting agency.

Another consideration not to be overlooked in reviewing a grant for a colleague is to bring the principal investigator's attention to spelling, grammar, syntax, organization, or other portions of the grant that should have further evaluation before the grant is finalized. As mentioned above, a sloppy grant will be viewed unfavorably and will irritate the reviewers. The reviewers will conclude that the principal investigator did not devote enough attention or effort to prepare a high-quality application and will assume that the research will be given the same level of attention and care.

While it is not expected that each suggestion made by a reader of the draft of a grant will end up as a change, each suggestion should cause the principal investigator to give the issue some thought. Even if suggestions do not result in a change, the principal investigator should decide whether he or she can improve the presentation or eliminate that portion of the application.

RESUBMISSION OF AN R01 GRANT

In the current climate, very few projects are funded following the first submission of a new grant application. This is not to say that it is not possible to prepare a grant application that will be funded following the first submission, but at this time the rate of success for first-time submissions is well below 10%. An unsuccessful first-time applicant as well as a seasoned investigator who has submitted an application that receives an unfundable score should revise the application and pay close attention to comments made by the reviewers. Good advice about the preparation of a revised application is presented in chapter 18. The guidelines of care, clarity, and conciseness are as important for resubmissions as they are for first submissions. Of course, one should not expect that a resubmission would get a more favorable review just because it is a resubmission. The submission dates for a revised R01 application also have been changed recently (see grants2.nih .gov/grants/funding/submissionschedule.htm). The new dates effective at the time of publication of this book are March 5, July 5, and November 5. With revised resubmissions, the applicant has the advantage of the prior review and should use this information to present a revised application that embodies significance and utilizes an approach that will provide a valid test of the hypotheses presented in an innovative manner.

SUMMARY

In summary, R01 grant applications should be prepared with adequate time and great care. To aid in the process of preparation, there are a number of steps you can take, such as familiarizing yourself of guidelines, establishing dialogue with appropriate members of NIH, presenting your proposal to trusted colleagues, and making yourself aware of review criteria and common criticisms. When preparing the application, the proposal must be hypothesis driven, and the work proposed must result in significant advances in the field of research. The approach must be appropriate to obtain conclusive results, and the sequence of experiments and the proposed techniques should be innovative. Most important, the research proposed must be significant in that it will advance the field of study. Convincing preliminary data are necessary for a first submission, and impressive progress is required for a competing renewal application. Proof must be provided that the investigators are well qualified to carry out the proposed experiments and that all guidelines for the proper use of subjects are being followed. After the application is complete, it is critical to allow yourself adequate time to review, and to have others review, the application to ensure that your ideas are represented in a clear and appropriate manner. While the advice in this chapter can only aid you in the writing process, it is hoped that these suggestions can increase your opportunity to gain funding.

9   P50 Research Center Grants

Steven Sussman, Jennifer B. Unger, & Alan W. Stacy

Knowledge is like money: to be of value it must circulate, and in circulating it can increase in quantity and, hopefully, in value.

—Louis L'Amour, *Education of a Wandering Man*

SOMETIMES RESEARCH GROUPS desire to capture a "big picture" in a particular area of research. The goal is not just to solve one very specific problem, but rather to serve as a driving force for grappling with several different sides of the research structure that can solve a general problem. That is, research groups may wish to support several projects focused on a specific problem that contribute to the big picture, to support future researchers who can move the general arena forward, and to create (and maintain) a home base for stable, continued work in the designated arena. In this respect, P50 grants provide a vehicle or mechanism to support a multidisciplinary set of projects and cores that are centered on a common theme. This chapter describes the structure of P50s, outlines a few pertinent issues to consider when applying for a P50, and briefly describes an example of a successful funded P50.

WHAT IS A P50 CENTER?

From the term "center," one might think that a P50 is a building or at least a floor of a building. However, in NIH terms, a "center" is a collection of researchers, projects, and resources, rather than a physical place. Accordingly, a center may exist within a single university department, across several departments of a university, across several universities, or across various types of organizations such as research institutes, community-based organizations, and/or nonprofit businesses. A center may even be a "virtual center" or "center without walls" that is composed of researchers residing in numerous locations who collaborate on research projects by sharing data files over the Internet and communicating by email. A center gets its identity from its members and their collaborative research projects, rather than from a specific physical address.

The purpose of NIH centers is to advance knowledge about a health topic by establishing a structure to promote research integration through the sharing of personnel, facilities, equipment, data, and ideas. The rationale behind funding centers rather than numerous individual projects is that that the amount, quality, and breadth of the research resulting from a P50 should be greater than the research that would have resulted if each individual project had been performed in isolation. The old adage that the whole is greater than the sum of its parts is appropriately used to think about centers and the rationale behind funding centers from the government's perspective. Centers represent more than a critical mass of resources (physical, logistic, personnel, or otherwise) and cannot be created merely by sewing a thread through individual projects. Table 9.1 shows that the NIH regards centers very highly in its overall portfolio of research mechanisms. The table shows, for instance, that research centers (including P60, P50, P30, P20, and P01 mechanisms) involve a substantial share of the overall monies allocated to the different funding mechanisms that make up the NIH budget. To further illustrate this point, table 9.2 shows a single institute under the umbrella of NIH (the National Institute on Drug Abuse) also values centers in its research portfolio. The sheer raw number of centers has increased over time, as has the percentage the centers represent in the overall budget for NIDA.

A P50 center is organized into several research projects and a given number of service cores. The research projects are similar to traditional R01 grants—they typically have Specific Aims and various research activities to address the Specific Aims. The service cores (usually somewhere between two and four, but no formal limit is given to the number of cores) provide collective and collaborative resources to the projects such as statistical analysis, laboratory analysis, data collection, and administrative or dissemination services. P50s typically are awarded for five-year periods and may be renewed for additional five-year periods through a competitive renewal process.

TABLE 9.1 Obligations by Selected Mechanism FY 1995–FY 2005 (Dollars in Thousands)

Mechanism	Research Project Grants	Research Centers	Other Research	Research Training	R&D Contracts	Intramural Research	Research Mgmt. and Support	All Other	Total, NIH
FY 1995	6,194,524	1,006,009	504,314	380,502	791,415	1,222,646	506,415	735,016	11,340,841
FY 1996	6,612,184	1,040,126	554,318	395,137	764,824	1,294,777	479,746	739,535	11,880,647
FY 1997	7,154,107	1,088,546	582,625	416,992	790,324	1,346,127	479,297	912,753	12,770,771
FY 1998	7,786,920	1,161,103	631,244	427,958	793,746	1,434,635	487,229	964,024	13,686,859
FY 1999	8,779,019	1,380,117	808,100	509,185	1,067,197	1,564,547	542,188	992,922	15,643,275
FY 2000	10,118,249	1,547,152	1,013,499	539,510	1,147,672	1,746,220	600,203	1,101,234	17,813,739
FY 2001	11,595,311	1,859,600	1,240,917	589,624	1,387,989	1,952,319	692,508	1,194,788	20,513,056
FY 2002	13,038,451	2,123,723	1,473,943	650,686	1,643,362	2,225,292	788,950	1,243,826	23,188,233
FY 2003	14,287,058	2,428,178	1,616,587	711,441	2,300,590	2,564,664	929,871	1,901,515	26,739,904
FY 2004	15,165,386	2,545,972	1,651,823	743,076	2,691,897	2,658,853	977,771	1,664,544	28,099,772
FY 2005	15,304,522	2,642,355	1,650,975	743,076	2,499,275	2,737,865	1,014,218	1,883,865	28,476,151

Source: National Institutes of Health (with permission). Information may be retrieved from officeofbudget.od.nih.gov/KFactFY06/Obligations%20by%20Selected%20Mechanism%201995%20-%202005.pdf.

TABLE 9.2 Number of Center Grants Funded at NIDA

Activity	1997	1998	1999	2000	2001	2002	2003	2004	2005
P01	14	13	15	14	16	19	23	19	18
P20	1	1	1	1	1		3	3	4
P30		2	4	4	4	6	7	7	10
P50	27	27	28	27	26	27	24	25	23
P60	2	2	2	2	2	2	3	3	3
Total	44	45	50	48	49	54	60	57	58
Total Grants Funded	1,232	1,299	1,424	1,514	1,668	1,754	1,855	1,867	1,853
% of Total Budget	10.4%	10.2%	9.8%	9.0%	8.2%	7.8%	7.9%	7.7%	8.1%

Centers and grants include P50, P60, P20, P30, and P01 grant mechanisms
Source: National Institute on Drug Abuse.

The P50 must have a well-defined central unifying theme that is not too specific (or too general). Each subproject must be clearly related to the central unifying theme, and each core must support two or more projects. The projects and cores should be designed in such a way that they enhance the progress of one another. Projects may address a similar research question with different methods, in different samples, or even in different species (e.g., mice and persons). Research projects and cores can focus on a different segment of the continuum ranging from basic research to intervention development and even include studies of implementation effectiveness and community-level dissemination.

Nowadays, most successfully funded P50s span several scientific disciplines, ranging from biological to social to environmental sciences. In fact, many of the recent requests for applications (RFAs) for P50s have specifically called for transdisciplinary research teams. Some examples of these transdisciplinary P50 RFAs are the Transdisciplinary Prevention Research Centers (TPRCs) and the Transdisciplinary Tobacco Use Research Centers (TTURCs). At least one P50 (the University of California, Irvine TTURC) even included a transdisciplinary core to facilitate communication across scientific disciplines, cross-train investigators in new disciplines, and study the evolution of the center from a collection of isolated investigators to a transdisciplinary team.[1]

As described in various chapters of this volume, there are several different types of NIH centers. A P50 center is created in response to a specific RFA from NIH, whereas the topic of a P01 is initiated by the applicant. Because NIH solicits P50s to focus on a key topic, the sponsoring institute generally maintains a high level of involvement with the center's research. If NIH funds multiple centers on similar topics, the sponsoring institute typically attempts to facilitate research collaboration across centers, as well as within centers. Toward this end, institutes may organize conferences bringing together teams from several P50s, organize workgroups across P50s, or host symposia at the NIH headquarters to showcase the work of a set of P50 centers.

PROJECTS EMBEDDED WITHIN A P50

Each project within a P50 is similar to a traditional R01 grant, with one or more investigators (the project leader and co-investigators), requiring elaboration of significance, aims, hypotheses, research activities to evaluate the hypotheses, preliminary findings, experimental methods, and a project timeline (that is coordinated with other projects to show logistical sharing and cost-effectiveness). Each project within a P50 must stand on its own scientific merit and will be evaluated during review based on its own merit and its contribution to the overall center goals. Consistent with an R01 grant application, a project within a center must be significant to the field, approach the research question in a scientifically rigorous manner, rate high on innovation, include qualified investigators, and be designed around a feasible budget. However, the individual projects also must contribute to the central theme of the center.

To highlight the contribution of each project to the theme, investigators sometimes include a section in the grant proposal about how the project addresses the theme, how it integrates with the other projects, and how it uses the resources of the cores. Interestingly, each project does not have to span the full five years of the center. For example, one project could conduct basic research in years 1 and 2, and then another project could begin in year 3 to translate the findings of the basic research into practice. Typically, but not necessarily, the budget of a center project is slightly less than an R01 budget, depending on the number of projects that are proposed or funded. The tailoring of budgets results from the cost-effectiveness built into centers that arise from sharing resources, people, laboratory space, and streamlining certain grant components such as data collection to service multiple projects. Thus, two cadres of data collectors do not need to be hired, trained, and sent into the field, when one reliable team can service multiple projects.

CORES CONSTITUTE THE BACKBONE OF A P50

A P50 typically contains one or more service cores to provide administrative and research support services to the projects within the center. Each core should serve at least two projects. The following materials briefly present some examples of cores.

An *administrative core* supports the center's administrative functions, such as organizing interdisciplinary seminars, maintaining the center's Web site, monitoring the center's budget, preparing publications and posters for conferences, and/or coordinating meetings. If the center has scientific and/or community advisory boards, these may be housed within the administrative core. An administrative core may also handle training, community relations, dissemination, and other charges related to promotion of scientific goals within the broader lay and scientific communities.

If the projects have similar data collection methodologies, the P50 could contain a *data collection core*, so that trained staff can move from project to project when needed. This eliminates the need for individual projects to hire and train data collectors during periods of heavy data collection and then find other unrelated work for them during the months between data collections (or, worse, lay them off and then hire and train a whole new group of data collectors for the next round of surveys).

A *statistical analysis core* typically includes one or more statisticians or biometricians, one or more data managers, and a computerized system for data entry, cleaning, management, and storage. The advantage of having a statistical analysis core rather than separate statisticians for each project is that a core can provide statistical support to each project during the months when statistical support is needed, eliminating the need for each project to employ a statistician full time. Statistical core members also can conduct methodological research and simulation studies to develop new statistical methods that will be useful to the projects. The statistical core works across projects, and thus the investigative staff working under the umbrella of this core benefit from familiarity with measures derived from core assessment strategies. In the case of centers that include an integrated platform of intervention and basic etiology work, the statistical core can examine statistical relations using etiology models that may uncover or assess the potency of "active ingredients" used in the intervention model. This was the case when NIDA funded the P50 Multiethnic Drug Abuse Prevention Research Center in existence for two five-year periods at Cornell University Medical College. The statistical core worked to assess program effects with data obtained from a school-based drug abuse prevention program and then modeled statistical relations among risk and protective factors using etiology data from the control (minimal contact) groups participating in a group-randomized field trial.

Likewise, a measurement core can help the investigators identify valid measures for inclusion on surveys or other assessments, as well as create and validate new measures if appropriate measures are not available. A central measurement core also can establish a bank of survey scales and assessment protocols that multiple projects can use, increasing the likelihood that measures will be comparable across studies. Such cost-effective data collection and testing are very exciting to reviewers who see the economy of scale and cost-effectiveness in the way the cores are structured and their inherent accessibility across projects.

A *training core* serves as a means of involving graduate students and postdoctoral students in work on the center, leading to future roles as independent researchers. The training core can support predoctoral or postdoctoral fellowships, sponsor educational seminars, coordinate research and paper-writing seminars for students, provide funding for investigators to attend special trainings (workshops and skills training), and provide seed money for pilot studies. Depending on the center's theme, a center also might include other cores such as tissue cores, genotyping cores, or demographics cores, to name a few examples. Before cores are written into a proposal, investigators should contact the funding agency to make sure each core fits current agency guidelines. For example, training cores may not always be allowable.

DEVELOPMENTAL PROJECTS

P50s typically include seed money for developmental or pilot research. Depending on the specifications in the RFA, the developmental projects can be described in the original application, and/or money can be requested to fund new developmental projects over the course of the grant. Developmental projects are typically a good method to attract new researchers to conduct work closely allied to the P50 theme, or support new investigators, postdoctoral fellows, or graduate students and help direct their early career interests toward the center's theme. The center works effectively with a critical mass of scientists but this mass must always be regenerated through attracting new investigators and carving out new areas of research inquiry that dovetails thematically with the center. Thus, a major effort is tied to instigating developmental studies that help bolster the center and provide new venues for empirical inquiry and scientific investigation.

DIRECTORSHIP

A P50 has one center director, though NIH is currently considering permitting multiple Directors. The center director should be an established scientist with a strong record of grants and publications, who is substantially involved in the scientific leadership, integration and administration of the entire center. The center director also may be a project leader or core director, but this is not necessary. Other key personnel in a P50 may include center co-directors, assistant directors, associate directors, project leaders, core leaders, and co-investigators on the projects and cores. Depending on the breadth of personnel available and the management style of a center director, cores may have investigators who take a lead role, and thus are considered core leaders. If the core is structured around measurement or statistics, the core leader is usually a psychometrician or statistician with extensive publications and professional acumen in this area.

Individual projects also may have investigators who take a lead role (the project may have initially taken shape as an R01 and then been folded into the center) and thus are investigators of a principal investigator stature. Project leaders may "run" a project if it necessitates field work (i.e., population surveys, school or community-based interventions, laboratory research necessitating patient contact). The project leaders report to the center director and have regularly scheduled meetings with core leaders, all of whom report to the center director on the status of their projects. The regularity of these meetings, stewardship of projects, and the leadership demonstrated at the core levels are all intrinsic features of a center grant application that will come under direct scrutiny during review. One of the quintessential questions raised during reviews of centers is who makes certain types of decisions and how the overall decision process unfolds with respect to leadership or management of personnel.

FUNDING

Traditionally, P50s receive up to $1 million per year in direct costs, although this allotment may decrease in the near future. The money available for P50s also depends on how many of the NIH institutes are actively sponsoring the RFA and their respective budgets for the fiscal year. Effective June 1, 2003, budgets for new P50 applications have been limited to $1 million per year direct costs. It is important for the investigators to keep these limits in mind when planning the projects and cores. Resources and staff may need to be shared across projects and cores to stay within this limit. Any retrenchment of federal dollars for NIH in the next few years could adversely influence the allotment of funds for centers.

P50 FUNCTIONING WITHIN THE CONTEXT OF A UNIVERSITY ENVIRONMENT

Sometimes it can seem as if the very structure and purpose of the P50 is inconsistent with the traditional structure of a university. P50s often span multiple scientific disciplines, which typically means they span multiple university departments or even schools (medicine, arts and sciences, etc.). This configuration raises basic questions about how the indirect costs from the center should be allocated, where the center's main office space should be, and whose students are eligible to be supported by the center. P50s are an ideal way to forge collaborations among researchers in different departments or schools who have similar interests, but the university's structure and reward system do not always encourage this activity. For example, a faculty member in a sociology department who begins working on clinical trials, or a bench scientist who becomes interested in qualitative research, may be viewed by their peers as being less successful and therefore less eligible for promotion. The research environment should be one in which data resources, data analysis resources, research facilities, and shared laboratory resources are clearly available that will enable the center to function with a very high caliber of operations, potentially making it a national resource. Regardless of how the end product is eventually configured, the university will be forced to develop a system of revenue sharing (particularly for indirect cost monies). The center director also will need to make clear at the outset where command and control is vested and how financial decisions for the center are made. This is particularly important if numerous top flight investigators are brought together to collaboratively form a center. Discussions need to be held at the outset how spending decisions are made, where training of pre- and postdoctoral students will occur, how decisions are made about which developmental projects will be funded, and how cost sharing will be decided. Involvement of university personnel from contracts and grants at the outset can help formalize these relations and make clear how a single pot of money can be shared across departmental, division, college, or university lines.

WRITING A P50 GRANT

It should come as no surprise that preparation of a P50 proposal is a major undertaking. Before preparing a P50 application, investigators can receive input from program staff to determine if their ideas are responsive to the particular RFA. Other chapters in this book highlight the importance of establishing clear lines of communication with program staff at the various institutes or centers of NIH. Moreover, a concept or draft paper can be circulated as a prelude to a full-blown center application. In many cases, program staff can help the center director shape their concept to meet the needs of the institute, making sure the center is both timely and satisfies the public health agenda. At the very least, the vision of the center put forth by the center investigators must map well to the research priorities put forth by the scientific leadership at the institute or center level. The RFA calling for centers may not be specific, or the proposed center may transcend the RFA and offer new conceptual and/or empirical avenues of scientific inquiry. Either way, discussion with program staff prior to formal submission is sometimes essential.

To begin the process, the center director must identify the projects and cores to be included in the proposal and ensure that they are integrated with one another. There are several strategies for accomplishing this. Some center directors decide on the theme of the P50 first and then recruit investigators to write project and core proposals that address the theme. Other center directors invite a wide variety of investigators to suggest ideas for projects and then allow a common theme to emerge. The general guide with respect to preparation is to have at least three and no more than five projects integrated thematically and that can serve the interests of the center. Once these projects are in place, they need to be thematically integrated and formatively shaped in the center application. There will be a place in the application that briefly describes each project and then states how they are integrated or service the interests of the center. The focus on "centeredness" has increasingly become a mandate for centers to the extent that center applications that do not meet the critical test of centeredness to not move forward in the review process.

WHAT DOES A P50 GRANT PROPOSAL LOOK LIKE?

A P50 proposal consists of multiple R01-type grants and multiple cores. Each project and core has a separate NIH PHS 398 (or SF424 with the new electronic submission) application, with separate face pages, budget pages, biographical sketches, and so on. All of these sections now can be transmitted electronically on the eRA Commons Web site. Most P50 applications also contain an overall introduction of approximately 5–10 pages in length, which summarizes the overall theme of the proposed center and describes how each project and core addresses the theme. Depending on the guidelines specified in the RFA, a P50 proposal also may include appendices, short summaries of proposed pilot studies, and potential long-range plans. P50 center applications in their entirety can be as large as 350 pages once all elements are written up.

EXPECTED OUTCOMES OF P50S

Recently, NIH has increased its efforts to evaluate the "success" of its P50 centers, to justify that the knowledge gained from centers is worth the large share of an institute's budget allocated to fund them. For example, NCI and NIDA engaged in a comprehensive evaluation process with the seven originally funded TTURC centers. This process included brainstorming and then categorizing the various criteria that could be used to measure "success" (e.g., number of publications and new grants produced by center investigators, number of publications that involved investigators from multiple scientific disciplines, number of times the center's publications are cited, number of students trained, number of new researchers and students attracted to study the center's central topic, prestige of the centers and their investigators as rated by other scientists, impact of the centers on public policy and public health). This exercise demonstrated what many of the investigators and NIH staff had expected from the beginning: that it is extremely difficult to define success of a research center and to devise objective rating criteria that will be applicable to all centers. However, the effort to evaluate centers continues, as the NIH program directors face continuing pressure to demonstrate that P50s contribute more than the sum of their parts (and therefore should continue to be funded).

Another way to operationally speak of a center's "success" is its investigators' and trainees' perceptions of the center's value added to their individual careers. There has been considerable ongoing debate about this issue. For senior investigators who become center directors, the P50 can lead to increased national and international visibility for their research, opportunities to collaborate with new colleagues with diverse points of view, and the opportunity to create a long-lasting structure to conduct research and train new investigators. However, a center grant also brings more administrative responsibilities and the responsibility to monitor all the projects and cores to ensure that they are productive and that investigators are collaborating well with one another.

For junior investigators, a P50 offers the opportunity to participate in large-scale research projects and network with numerous senior investigators early in their careers, as well as the opportunity to be trained in several scientific disciplines. However, there is also a risk of becoming completely immersed in the center and not experiencing any research outside the center, or attempting to learn so many new methodologies that one becomes a "jack of all trades, master of none." In addition, the number of researchers on any one activity or publication may result in a junior researcher becoming enmeshed within a group without an independent identity. This list of caveats represents only a few of the handful of issues that surface as part of center management from a day-to-day basis and over the long haul during its existence.

AN EXAMPLE OF A P50 CENTER: THE USC TRANSDISCIPLINARY DRUG ABUSE PREVENTION RESEARCH CENTER (TPRC)

One example of a multidisciplinary research center has been established at the University of Southern California that aims to translate basic research in memory and examine peer group dynamics into drug abuse prevention programs for adolescents. Under this program, researchers are seeking to understand drug abuse at individual and social levels of analysis. The TPRC as a whole is centered around its focus on preventing drug use among adolescents. The individual projects within the center approach this problem from the perspectives of multiple scientific disciplines. These disciplines include neurobiology of memory, epidemiological analysis, clinical psychology, prevention science, and social network analysis. Funded by a five-year, $6.5 million grant from NIDA, this center consists of three cores (administrative, statistical, and training) and two projects (associative memory and implicit cognition, and Project Toward No Drug Use Social-Networked). In addition, 10 small developmental projects are being conducted in numerous areas pertaining to substance abuse prevention. As a general statement, this center focuses on increasing our understanding of adolescent drug abuse through closer ties to basic research, ways to assess mediation of model program effects, and development of novel prevention strategies. Findings previously ignored in prevention but consistently documented in neuroscience, cognitive science, social and clinical psychology, and sociology are applied in the center. New integrations across areas are encouraged through multidisciplinary meetings, training activities, and research projects specifically designed to test integrations.

CONCLUSIONS

It goes without saying that because of their financial largesse, logistic requirements, and the amount of work that goes into preparation of center applications, P50s represent a monumental task and are difficult to get funded. At the very least, they must satisfy the basic tenor of one or more of the NIH institutes, be written in a manner that is concordant with the current political climate (i.e., the public health agenda), and address a pressing scientific need. In this respect, various changing winds may blow a center out of favor. Moreover, as political administrations change, priorities change and so too must the focus of a P50. Often, center directors will talk about the need for a center to "morph" or change responsively at every renewal period. If successful morphing occurs and is supported by the larger research environment, and if funding is available, the center will continue on. Thus, key problems may be addressed and solved, but in a context of competing demands from society, funding agencies, and the research community.

Despite the daunting task associated with creation, development, and implementation of centers, some of the most progressive and far-reaching scientific findings have sprung forth from research centers. Centers are leaders in thinking and able to coalesce the critical mass of scientists needed to push the envelope. Centers are responsible for training as much as they are for investigative development and, as such, have been havens for young investigators to build careers. At the heart of centers are two elements that must work together: people and ideas. Successful center directors are those who can manage people and create the necessary environment to foster a stable supply of creative juices. Centers by their very nature must be progressive in order to obtain successful funding. The tasks of centers is to keep their pulse on the nature of science, get a good reading of the future demands on science, and address these pressing concerns with the appropriate mix of people.

P20 and P30 Center Grants: Developmental Mechanisms

ROBERT J. PANDINA & VALERIE L. JOHNSON

All growth is a leap in the dark; a spontaneous unpremeditated act without benefit of experience.

—HENRY MILLER, *"The Absolute Collective"*

THE P20 AND P30 granting mechanisms are essentially special cases of the general P50 center grant mechanism discussed in chapter 9. The essential difference is that the P20 and P30 devices are intended to permit investigators to develop, enhance, or accelerate research in a particular problem area. These mechanisms provide greater flexibility than the P50 inasmuch as investigators may not be required to provide the same level of detail as required in the P50 or R01 application regarding the research protocols to be followed for the entire project period. Hence, these mechanisms are considered to be "exploratory," particularly in the "out years," that is, in the later years (e.g., years 3, 4, and 5) of the grant period. This is not to imply that "any thing goes" in the out years. Rather, the investigators have greater flexibility to make major modifications in the research plans to follow up on the initial discoveries from the more specific project activities proposed in the first two to three years of the center. P20 and P30 applications differ from one another in that P20 centers are expected to conduct at least exploratory research similar to what might be conducted under a R21 mechanism as part of center activities, whereas the P30 supports core activities for several investigative teams that may already be conducting separately funded research. In the P30 scenario, the activities of the center may be enhanced or experience significant synergy by being brought together under a single guiding research umbrella.

CLARIFYING THE PURPOSE OF A DEVELOPMENTAL CENTER

Developmental centers are typically intended to break new ground in a particular problem area that is of special relevance, requires immediacy, or has been understudied or neglected. While NIH institutes will certainly consider investigator-initiated P20 and P30 applications, it is more often the case that an NIH institute will issue a specific request for applications (RFA) focused on a particular well-specified problem area that uses the P20 or P30 mechanism as a method for accelerating research activity. Such proposal announcements usually include the expectation that the research activities to be multidisciplinary in nature and draw together researchers from differing, but relevant, ongoing programmatic research. The expectation is that a multidisciplinary approach may provide a viable novel alternative to a specific problem. Potential grantees are well advised to describe specific mechanisms that stimulate and sustain the interactions among investigators from different research traditions. Hence, the P20 mechanism may be employed to explore the feasibility of certain research activities.

For example, recently the National Institute on Drug Abuse (NIDA) issued an RFA for Transdisciplinary Prevention Research Centers (TPRCs) intended to launch the "next generation" of prevention research activities. The synthesis of these activities were structured in such a way they could combine basic laboratory research (either animal or human) in the etiology of substance abuse with promising yet possibly untested approaches to prevention intervention with human populations. The concept behind this effort was to bring together research teams from a number of disciplines that typically would not communicate on a formal, ongoing basis, to create potentially novel paradigms in prevention. The intention was to help propel the prevention field forward in a manner not possible with a more incremental approach using the R01 mechanism.

The National Institute of Environmental Health Sciences issued an RFA in 1998 for P20 applications that focus on identification of the unique health concerns of underserved populations. Likewise, the National Center on Minority Health and Health Disparities issued an RFA in 2002 and again in 2006 for P20 applications to develop Centers of Excellence in Partnerships for Community Outreach, Research on Health Disparities and Training (Project Export—Establishing Exploratory Centers). The focus of this RFA was the advancement of research and development of interventions directed to reduce or eliminate health disparities.

Similar research funding announcements have been and continue to be announced in the biological science areas, including genetics of specific diseases, the development of novel pharmacological interventions, and the combinations of behavioral and biologically based interventions for disease states (e.g., cigarette smoking, tobacco use). Perusal of the NIH Web site (www.nih.gov) provides a number of examples of these announcements using the P20 and P30 mechanisms and further serves to illustrate the diversity and utility of the purposes served by these mechanisms. Hence, the developmental center mechanisms are highly flexible tools typically initiated via an RFA by the NIH institutes for targeted purposes fostering growth in specific research areas. Scientists seeking to take advantage of the flexibility and unique opportunities afforded by the P20 and P30 mechanisms need to be aware of the intentions and priorities of the particular institute at NIH that is concerned with their substantive area.

Often, the initiatives that result in a research funding announcement calling for P20 and P30 applications may be in the institute planning process for 6–12 months prior to a formal announcement. However, the turn-around time for applications may be relatively short (e.g., three months). Investigators should keep abreast of developments within target institutes and be prepared for the daunting task of application development long before a formal announcement is made. If the P20 or P30 is the result of an RFA, you may also have the opportunity to submit a "letter of intent" to apply for such funding. The letter should be taken seriously because it will be the first formal contact you have with the review process. The letter will alert program staff of your interest and may permit you to conduct informal discussions with appropriate institute program staff as you prepare your application. The institutes and the Center for Scientific Review will also use the letters of intent to select the panel of reviewers for the batch of P20 and/or P30 applications that are eventually submitted and reviewed. Hence, even this initial step should be taken thoughtfully.

STRUCTURE OF P20 DEVELOPMENTAL CENTERS

The diversity and flexibility of the P20 and P30 mechanisms makes it difficult to provide comprehensive descriptions. This is partly attributable to the fact that the structure of a particular center is often carefully outlined, if not strongly influenced, by the sponsoring institute at NIH. It is especially important for applicants to study carefully the RFA, respond to the requirements as specified, and, if deviating from specifications, offer explicit rationale for changes. However, there are a number of common features that can be noted and that would be advisable to consider when applying for the P20 and P30 centers. The P20 resembles the P50 in general structure. Typically, developmental centers are housed within a university or, occasionally, a not-for-profit research entity and are expected to have clear administrative support and recognition from the sponsoring entity with strong potential to continue after the period of developmental funding.

The P20 contains an administrative core led by a center director (typically a senior scientist with a successful administrative history) and often requires additional administrative support (e.g., a full-time administrative assistant and at least part-time budget support personnel) to maintain hub activities, to facilitate communication among research programs, and to give credibility to the fact that a center entity has been clearly established. An advisory board, which is adjunctive to the administrative core, should convene at least yearly if not more frequently. The advisory board consists of members of the community who serve in the capacity of liaison to the center. Academicians, scientists, members of nonprofit companies, business leaders, civic representatives, religious leaders, educators, physicians, and foundation directors can serve on the advisory board, which helps provide an outside source of governance to the center. The advisory board helps keep the center in touch with the pulse of the community.

The administrative core should also include an active steering or coordinating committee composed of lead investigators from projects and cores to guide the work of the center. This is especially important for developmental centers inasmuch as scientific efforts will likely require substantial modifications across time and serious scientific and fiscal choices will need to be made and justified to center investigators and NIH institute sponsors. In addition, given the likelihood that project areas will house investigators from quite different research traditions, regular meetings by the committee will help develop a common culture and language for ongoing interactions. The steering committee should be convened on a set periodic schedule (at least monthly) to discuss progress and develop plans for any protocol changes. Ultimate leadership and decision-making responsibilities lie with the center director. However, it is advisable to rely heavily upon the steering committee members to build consensus on important issues. One area of concern, addressed in greater detail below, is that of a sound fiscal management plan whose ultimate responsibility for execution is that of the center director.

STRUCTURAL COMPONENTS AND DIVISION OF LABOR

The P20 may contain three to five broader project focal areas. Note that this differs somewhat from the P50, which contains specific research projects with well-defined scopes and research protocols similar in nature and definition to what are contained in an R01 application. The P20 affords a more flexible approach to defining projected activities. For example, the TPRC that is housed within the broader university institutional framework of our addiction center at Rutgers identifies three distinct program areas: (1) peer-based intervention during high school; (2) brief interventions for problematic behavior in college; and (3) the role of cognitive and affective processes in intervention strategies.

Each of the areas has several ongoing and complementary projects. For example, the high school project area contains component projects that include curriculum-driven, peer-led transitions programs and adult mentoring for identified problem cases. The college area contains brief intervention programs for identified cases, ongoing interventions for entering first-year students, and special programs for student-athletes and other high-risk targets. The cognitive/affective processes area features a series of rigorous laboratory experiments aimed at understanding basic principles that are postulated to drive changes in our interventions being designed and tested in other project areas. Interdisciplinary teams of scientists staff each of these project areas. While there are disciplinary seams in the scientific expertise across areas there are also significant overlaps within and across areas.

The TPRC has developed a common set of principles that serve a structural purpose and helps to guide all research activities. In addition, the TPRC has developed several mechanisms to stimulate cross-fertilization of ideas and generate new lines of research among investigators from all areas. These include monthly research audits attended by all faculty and students, as well as an annual structured retreat. P20s may contain other relevant core activities. In our case, we included a "resource core" that provided services such as methodological and statistical assistance for all projects and also serves to identify scientists from outside our institution who could provide specific expertise to expand the vision of our investigative team on a periodic basis. When other cores are included in a P20 application, it is necessary to carefully justify the cores by specifying not only the functions they serve but also the nature of the add-on value of such cores.

Although the P20 affords the opportunity of flexibility in altering the scientific agenda of a research program during the period of the center's funding cycle, it should be emphasized that the blueprint for the center activities in the "out" years must provide sufficient detail to assure the sponsoring agency that meaningful and directed objective can and will be achieved. Hence, an important and often overlooked aspect of the P20 application is the identification of a tight mechanism for reviewing and evaluating progress in various programmatic areas and specific projects. This effort is then coupled with a workable plan for altering and revising the initial research blueprint that has the promise of productivity in the later stages of the center. Should your own reading of your application leave you with the impression that your revision plan is "see what happens in year 3" or "then a miracle will occur and a burning bush will lead us," it would be prudent to think through your evaluation and forward-thinking process again!

Sponsoring institutes at NIH anticipate a number of outcomes for P20 centers. There is, of course, the usual expectation of scientific output and the hope that the flexibility and opportunity for creativity will produce new or fresh scientific perspectives. There is also the expectation of longevity, that is, life of the "centeredness" and continuation of the mission produced by the P20 effort after the initial funding cycle. The hope is that investigators drawn together under this mechanism will appreciate the value of their multidisciplinary interaction by following up with new research efforts. These would be manifested, in part, by the generation of R21 and R01 applications that build upon results of the P20 "feasibility" projects. Hence, it is important that the P20 center application include plans for generating future research opportunities. There is the expectation that the universities and agencies that house the P20 centers also acknowledge the productivity of center-supported scientist by providing a method for sustaining the mission of the center after the initial period of support. Thus, potential applicants should obtain and include tangible evidence of institutional support for the mission of their proposed center.

FISCAL COMPONENTS OF A P20 CENTER

Your application should anticipate the significant challenges involved in managing fiscal aspects of the P20. First, this effort is likely to involve several components (e.g., cores, program areas, and research projects within areas). Multiple investigators will be involved with components. All investigators will probably feel that their area will require "priority resource allocation" and an ongoing commitment for resources for the entire project period. The P20 director should have a clear plan for allocation of resources for each component in the initial years of the center and achieve an understanding with the principal investigator of each component about the need for fair and balanced allocation of resources for the initial project period (e.g., two years is not unreasonable and fits the profile established for feasibility or pilot funding such as is modeled by the R21 mechanism). The proposal should include a method for evaluation of research efforts of each component and a plan for review of resource allocation on a yearly basis.

It will be necessary to reach an understanding with investigative team leaders in advance about the possibility that after the first two years of the P20 cycle it may be necessary to reapportion support for some projects to assure that the P20 will successfully make progress toward its ultimate goals. Investigators should be encouraged to develop spinoff funding opportunities. Timing of these efforts is difficult to anticipate; however, it is not unreasonable to expect spinoff applications to be generated in the second half of the P20 funding cycle. Most experienced investigators will recognize the wisdom of this process and will seek out opportunities to extend the "pilot" outcomes through other funding mechanisms. In a sense, the P20 is providing a special opportunity to investigators to be creative, collect initial data, and have a "leg up" with a sponsoring NIH institute because of their participation in a significant federal agency initiative.

At this point in our understanding, a relatively quick review is in order. The P20 is generally regarded as a building block mechanism. The P20 is intended to provide a new and exciting platform for research in an understudied or emerging area of vital importance or to transform an existent paradigm in an exponential manner. It is not intended to push science forward in an incremental manner. Most often, the P20 seeks to draw scientists together from a wide range of disciplinary traditions to capitalize upon the synergy of diversity. Hence, the application should clearly identify the nature and extent of contributions of scientists to be included in the P20 and their individual roles in and commitment to the mission of the center. In most instances, it is advisable to include a clear mission statement and set of operating principles that guide research efforts and can lay the foundation for "centeredness."

Clearly outlined mechanisms and procedures need to be articulated that will facilitate interaction among center investigators. A solid blueprint guiding the initial research efforts is required. Remember, P20s permit flexibility and creativity in the pursuit of scientific endeavor. Be careful to attend to the specifics of the RFA issued by sponsoring agencies and match your creative blueprint to the RFA requirements. Flexibility does not, however, mean license; hence, a clear plan for the manner in which the center will manage alterations and modifications in the research agenda should be included. The application should anticipate, to the extent possible, the life of the P20 center after the initial period of support. It is unlikely that a P20 will be renewed by the sponsoring agency as another P20. However, a "successful" P20 is likely to produce a research platform that results in a number of rich opportunities for collaborative efforts (e.g., R21, R01, P30, and P50 grant mechanisms).

THE MECHANICS OF P30 GRANTS

A P30 center resembles a P20 in many regards. It, too, is a mechanism envisioned by sponsoring institutes at NIH for launching a platform of research in areas of vital importance or to transform or accelerate an existent paradigm. To that extent, the NIH institutes, through highly structured RFAs, offer P30 opportunities with specific criteria crafted to meet special articulated needs. Such centers are expected to be multidisciplinary in nature and to capitalize on the synergies achievable by uniting investigators with different research traditions and skill sets.

A P30 center differs from a P20 in a number of important ways. A major difference is that the scope and focus of the anticipated research accomplishments are typically much narrower for the P30, and the anticipated outcomes are more carefully articulated. In addition, the P30 mechanism is often viewed as a device for uniting existing research groups with ongoing funded research and similar interests in a specific problem area under a single umbrella for a circumscribed purpose. Hence, in this regard, P30s are often mission driven and more focused compared to P20s. The P30 device is used to support core activities more so than to provide resources for broad pilot or feasibility studies, although it would not be unusual for the P30 to provide some pilot funding directed to a well-specified objective.

Typically, a P30 would support an administrative core with many of the same responsibilities as those outlined for the P20 (e.g., scientific leadership, coordination of research efforts, fiscal management, and integration of research teams into a cohesive center). The P30 is designed to provide additional resources for participating research groups that would not normally be available to each group alone. For example, an RFA for a P30 focused upon advancing specific knowledge on the genetics of, say, autism or bipolar disease is issued by the appropriate institute at NIH. The successful applicant may come from a university-based consortium composed of a group of genetic researchers working on brain mechanisms using animal models, a behavioral research group (e.g., psychologists) working on drug abuse etiology, and an affiliated medical school clinical treating addiction or mental health patients. All groups could be united under the P30 mechanism to work jointly to gather and assess biological material from patients using highly promising protocols derived from animal models, test behavioral interventions in various patient subgroups, and determine the impact of novel treatment modalities and assess biobehavioral characteristics in a laboratory setting using prototypic assessment batteries.

Each group has developed independently but is united under the P30 with the intent of providing a unified scientific, theoretical, and administrative structure. The core funding can cut across various costs associated with subject recruitment, assessment, data analysis, laboratory procedures in a manner that no group could have accomplished independently. The opportunity also will facilitate cross-fertilization among existing groups of research to inform a specific biobehavioral health-related problem initiative of the NIH institutes involved. Furthermore, should the endeavor be fruitful, the nascent center could emerge as a "permanent" feature of the institutional structure and serve as a platform for more extensive research. This example paints only a brief picture of the potential uses of a P30 mechanism.

ADVANTAGES OF THE P30 FUNDING MECHANISM

The P30 offers some advantages in that established research groups already focused upon a narrow aspect with established skill sets can join their resources to create a new and more promising research vision. However, significant challenges are also associated with this funding mechanism. For example, each group is presumably well occupied with its own work; investigators would need to switch their focus for part of their time and yield some research autonomy. Moreover, working in such an environment would require careful coordination by the administrative core, and so on. With all of its considerations, however, such P30 centers work well when each group sees a clear scientific advantage of the work and a way of obtaining necessary resources not otherwise available, and views the center as a mechanism to move to a larger scientific stage.

REVIEW PROCESS FOR P20 AND P30 MECHANISMS

It is important to recognize that P20 and P30 applications are typically reviewed outside of the general external peer review process; that is, "special review groups" conduct the evaluation of the application. Nonetheless, the reviews are treated, administratively and scientifically, in the same manner as routine reviews of R01, R21, and K-series applications. The reviews are rigorous and use the same peer review scoring criteria as are typically applied (see chapter 3). However, there are typically additional criteria, including demonstration of "centeredness" and synergy (i.e., sum of the whole is significantly greater than the parts), interdisciplinary focus (i.e., not simply a collection of varying disciplines but also the manner in which true interactions will occur), leadership abilities (particularly scientific and intellectual leadership but also administrative skills), and likelihood of "creative" or innovative outcomes that would not other wise be possible if the grants were treated as separate entities.

It is often the case that applicants for P20 and P30 grants are disappointed following review, as are institute program staff that look to the promise of gathering teams of scientists under one roof. Many times, the RFA for these centers require reissuing and modification, resulting in another round of competition before a successful application is identified. Hence, it is important to understand that in some respects the competition for these awards may be more rigorous than for many other more usual forms of support. Should you choose to apply for one of these centers, you must brace yourself for the long haul and be prepared to be well prepared.

CONCLUSIONS

The developmental center program typified by the P20 and P30 mechanisms affords special opportunities for the scientific community. Prominent among these is the ability to move a new area of research significantly forward or to take an existing area and move it in novel directions. These mechanisms can be self-initiated by either scientists in a particular field or, more typically, used by NIH institutes to stimulate experienced scientists to join together to think in novel ways about existing or emerging problems of significant health concerns. To research scientists and the NIH institute sponsors alike, the ventures supported through these mechanisms are high risk and stand to have high potential gain. For scientists, breaking new ground is both exciting and challenging. Such efforts require creative vision, a tolerance of ambiguity, and willingness to invest substantial time with uncertain rewards.

It goes without saying that, for the NIH sponsor, these attempts to move a problem area forward represent a considerable investment and a degree of trust in senior investigators' desire and willingness to think outside the box. By no means, however, are the developmental efforts supported in this manner considered "shots in the dark." These efforts represent the time, effort, and commitment of the NIH program staff and administrators who are responding to special needs informed often by senior investigators at academic and research centers. Successful applicants are established investigators willing and committed to take on new challenges and who are able to see past the substantial, yet more incremental gains, of the more established R01 sources of support.

11 The K Award

An Important Part of the NIH Funding Alphabet Soup

FRANCES R. LEVIN

The secret of success is constancy to purpose.

— BENJAMIN DISRAELI

THE PROCESS OF applying for a K award is certainly a daunting task, particularly for a clinician who may not have a lot of experience writing papers, let alone constructing grants. One means to assuage these fears is to have a template or outline of what makes K awards highly meritorious during review. This was my thought or impetus when writing this chapter, that I would spill the beans and let readers know what made my K awards and those from grantees I mentor successful. In many respects, this chapter is not meant to replace the guidelines outlined on the NIH Web site (see appendix 1 at the back of the book for appropriate K sites). Rather, the chapter is intended to provide a jump-start to candidates thinking about writing a K award, help them differentiate between the different types of awards, and also clue investigators in on what makes K awards so daunting and challenging but also so rewarding.

NIH provides a wide range of K awards, including, among others, K01s, K02s, K05s, K08s, K12s, K23s, and K24s. The NIH K-series award requirements and scoring criteria are elaborated in table 11.1.

Surprisingly, the ascending sequence of these numbers does not necessarily co-incide with the seniority of the investigator. For example, a K05 award is intended for senior investigators, whereas both K01 and K23 awards are intended for more junior investigators. Some of the K-series awards are designed to launch the career of a junior investigator in basic preclinical research, whereas other K awards are designed to promote ongoing mentoring and research for senior scientists.

The best approach to decide which award matches your professional needs involves reading the specific NIH guidelines for each award. Then, if you have questions, it is best to contact the scientific review administrator at the appro-priate institute in order to discuss your training background and research in-terests (this point is also made in chapter 2). The scientific review administrator or program staff at the institute can help guide you in the appropriate direction and make sure you "fit" the specific K requirements before you apply. Therefore, the purpose of this chapter is not to tell you which K award is appropriate pending your individual background, but rather is to discuss some of the com-mon pitfalls associated with K award applications and provide some corrective advice and helpful hints. Nothing in this chapter should be taken as definitive with respect to published guidelines; rather, the suggestions provided are based on extensive experience as a reviewer on the NIDA-K committee as well as having received several K awards and mentoring other candidates for K awards. I hope that, by reading this chapter, physicians and doctorate clinicians will consider launching their research careers via the very rewarding K grant mechanisms.

WHY APPLY FOR A K?

There are several clear advantages to receiving a K award. First, for busy clinicians it provides the elusive "gift" of time. For most clinicians who work in academic or community settings, a substantial portion of their time is taken up providing clinical service, administrative duties, or providing supervision as part of a grad-uate training program. It is extremely difficult to devote time to research when faced with so many pressing time commitments and professional service obli-gations. Further, a physician mired in clinical and administrative responsibilities often does not have adequate exposure to experienced researchers who can help shape research ideas and stimulate the pursuit of research funding. Although there are some full-time clinicians who are able to have productive research careers, this is exceptionally difficult. The K award mechanism allows clinicians to turn this predicament around and capitalize on a fruitful opportunity. With a K award, a majority of time can be spent receiving research training and spearheading basic science research, with less significant amounts of time carved out solely for clinical and administrative duties.

Second, a K award allows the clinician time to explore new training areas and entertain new areas of research. Without the flexibility of a K award, it is often

TABLE 11.1 K Award Requirements and Scoring Criteria.

Type of Award	Purpose of Award	Requirements*,**
K01 – Mentored Research Scientist Development Award	The Mentored Research Scientist Development Award (K01) provides support for an intensive, supervised career development experience in one of the biomedical, behavioral, or clinical sciences leading to research independence. The proposed career development experience must be in a research area new to the applicant and/or one in which an additional supervised research experience will substantially add to the research capabilities of the applicant. The candidate must provide a plan for achieving independent research support by the end of the award period.	1. Must have a research or a health-professional doctorate or its equivalent, and must have demonstrated the capacity or potential for highly productive independent research in the period after the doctorate. 2. Must identify a mentor with extensive research experience. 3. Willing to spend a minimum of 75% of full-time professional effort conducting research and research career development during the entire award period. 4. Must clearly describe the need for intensive research supervision for a period lasting three, four, or five years leading to research independence. 5. Under some circumstances, may have been principal investigators on NIH research or career development awards, provided the research experience proposed in this application is in a fundamentally new field of study or there has been a significant hiatus in their research career because of family or other personal obligations.

(continued)

Table 11.1 K Award Requirements and Scoring Criteria (*continued*)

Type of Award	Purpose of Award	Requirements*,**
K01 – International Research Scientist Development Award†	This program supports U.S. postdoctoral biomedical, social, and behavioral scientists. It provides the successful candidate with a period of mentored research as part of an established collaboration between a U.S. sponsor and a leading developing country scientist at an Internationally recognized research institution in a developing country. The role of the IRSDA is to: • Attract new research talent to global health research and enhance multidisciplinary synergy among the research collaborators at the U.S. and foreign site; • Advance the career paths of exceptional junior U.S. scientists with mentored training in health issues of developing country population; • Extend the impact and reach of existing research and training support for developing country scientists and U.S. scientists committed to international research; • Provide opportunities for developing country institutions with significant potential to advance to higher levels of research excellence; and • Stimulate a more effective translation of the results of research on global health problems into practical public health actions.	1. Have demonstrated a commitment and competence in health and health-related research, as well as the potential to engage in independent and productive biomedical, social, behavior or epidemiological/clinical research in the period following the award. 2. Have mentors in the United States and in the eligible developing country where the proposed research will be performed, who are committed to both the research and training requirements of the candidate. 3. The two mentors for IRSDA applicant must have a recent or ongoing collaboration on a relevant research program or project. An enhancing factor for consideration is a funded collaboration between the mentors.

K02 – Independent Scientist Award	The Independent Scientist Award (K02) provides up to five years of salary support for newly independent scientists who can demonstrate the need for a period of intensive research focus as a means of enhancing their research careers.	1. Must have a doctoral degree and independent, peer-reviewed research support at the time the award is made. Some of the NIH institutes and centers require the candidate to have an NIH research grant at the time of application.
		2. Must be willing to spend a minimum of 75% of full-time professional effort conducting research and research career development during the period of the award.
		3. Must be able to demonstrate that the requested period of salary support and protected time will foster his/her career as a highly productive scientist in the indicated field of research.
		4. Scientists whose work is primarily theoretical may apply for this award in the absence of external research grant support.
K05 – Senior Scientist Award	The Senior Scientist Award (K05) provides stability of support to outstanding scientists who have demonstrated a sustained, high level of productivity and whose expertise, research accomplishments, and contributions to the field have been and will continue to be critical to the mission of the particular NIH center or institute. The award provides salary support for award periods of up to five years as a means of enhancing the individual recipient's skills and dedication to his/her area of research.	1. Must be a senior scientist and a recognized leader in the field with a distinguished record of original contributions.
		2. Must have a record of support from a funding institute or center.
		3. Must have peer-reviewed grant support at the time of the award.
		4. Scientists whose work is primarily theoretical may, depending on the policy of the institute or center, apply for this award in the absence of research grant support.

(continued)

TABLE 11.1 K Award Requirements and Scoring Criteria *(continued)*

Type of Award	Purpose of Award	Requirements*,**
K07 – Academic Career Award	The Academic Career Award (K07) support two types of activities: 1. The K07 provides up to five years of support for more junior candidates who are interested in developing academic and research expertise in a particular field, as a way to increase the overall pool of individuals capable of research or teaching in the identified area. During the period of the award, the candidate will become a successful academician in the chosen area. Teaching, curriculum building, research, and leadership skills are to be learned during the tenure of the award. 2. The K07 can also provide from two to five years of support for more senior individuals with acknowledged scientific expertise and leadership skills who are interested in improving the curricula and enhancing the research capacity within an academic institution. It is expected that support under this award will increase the visibility and the overall research support or academic capacity for the given field or research within the academic medical/health and research community.	1. Must have a clinical or research doctoral degree. Candidates for the Development Award must demonstrate the potential to develop into an excellent academician, in the field of interest to the NIH awarding institute or center. 2. Must be able to identify a mentor who is an expert in the research field of interest and has a record of providing the type of supervision required by this award. 3. Must also be able to devote at least 75% of full-time professional effort to the research and development programs required for academic development. 4. Candidates for the Leadership Award must have sufficient clinical training, research, or teaching experience in the academic area of interest to the NIH to implement a program of curriculum development which the applicant institution. 5. Must have an academic appointment at a level sufficient to enable her/him to exert an influence on the coordination of research, teaching, and clinical practice in an emerging field. 6. Must be in a position to devote at least 25% but not more than 50% effort to the program, a portion of which my include research.

K08 – Mentored Clinical Scientists Development Award	Mentored Clinical Scientist Development Award (K08) is to support the development of outstanding clinician research scientists. This mechanism provides specialized study for individuals with a health professional doctoral degree committed to a career in laboratory or field-based research. Candidates must have the potential to develop into independent investigators. The K08 supports a three-, four-, or five-year period of supervised research experience that may integrate didactic studies with laboratory or clinically based research. The proposed research must have intrinsic research importance as well as serving as a suitable vehicle for learning the methodology, theories, and conceptualizations necessary for a well-trained independent researcher.	1. Must have a clinical doctoral degree or its equivalent. 2. Must have a Ph.D. or other doctoral degree in a clinical discipline. Individuals holding the Ph.D. in a nonclinical discipline but certified to perform clinical duties should contact the appropriate institute concerning their eligibility for a K08 award. 3. Must be able to identify a mentor with extensive research experience. 4. Must be willing to spend a minimum of 75% of full-time professional effort conducting research and research career development.
K12 – Mentored Clinical Scientists Development Program Award	This Mentored Clinical Scientists Development Program Award is an award to an educational institution or professional organization to support career development experiences for clinicians leading to research independence. Under this award, newly trained clinicians are to be selected and appointed to this program by the grantee institution. Applications for this award should propose a research plan that (1) has intrinsic research importance and (2) will serve as a suitable vehicle for learning the methodology, theories, and concepts needed for a well-trained independent clinician-researcher. The program should be designed to accommodate research candidates with varying levels of experiences.	1. The applicant organization must have a well-established research and clinical career development program and qualified faculty to serve as mentors. 2. The research candidate, mentor, and institution must develop innovative programs to maximize the available research and educational resources. 3. Phase I, the didactic component; and Phase II, an intensive research experience under the guidance of a qualified mentor: During Phase I the candidate will acquire knowledge and research skills in scientific areas relevant to the career development goals of the research candidate. This phase must include relevant didactic and laboratory experiences that are consistent with the research candidate's prior experience and needs. During Phase II the candidates will carry out their research experiences.

(continued)

TABLE 11.1 K Award Requirements and Scoring Criteria (*continued*)

Type of Award	Purpose of Award	Requirements*,**
K18 – Career Enhancement Award for Stem Cell Research	The purpose of this program announcement is to encourage investigators to obtain the training they need to appropriately use stem cells in their research. The Career Enhancement Award for Stem Cell Research will enable investigators to change the direction of their research careers or to take time from their regular professional responsibilities to broaden their scientific background by acquiring new research capabilities, specifically in the use of human or animal embryonic, adult, or cord blood stem cells. Two types of applicants should consider applying for support: (1) independent junior faculty who wish to expand their research by the use of stem cells, and (2) more senior, established investigators who wish to redirect their research, in whole or in part, to include the use of stem cells. All applicants need to enlist a well-qualified stem cell expert, either within their own institution or elsewhere, to serve as a sponsor.	1. Must have a clinical or research doctoral degree and be actively engaged in research of interest to the NIH. 2. Should have completed at least three years of postdoctoral work prior to applying for this K18. Individuals from underrepresented racial and ethnic groups as well as individuals with disabilities are always encouraged to apply for NIH program. 3. Must be able to devote at least 50% effort to the proposed program of didactic and/or research training in stem cell research. One may devote full-time effort to the award.

K22 – The NIDA Scholars Program

This program provides an opportunity for outstanding new investigators to begin their independent research careers (the intramural phase) first within the collaborative and mentoring environment of the NIDA intramural research program and then to continue their careers (the extramural phase) at an institution of their choice. This program is also intended to continually enhance and invigorate the NIDA intramural community by providing a cadre of new, creative scientists who will interact with and expand the collaborative research opportunities of NIDA intramural scientists.

1. Must have a research or health professional doctoral level degree or equivalent and be recognized by their peers and mentors as exceptional, but have no more than 5 years of postdoctoral research training at the time of receiving the award.

2. Individuals who have been principal investigators on either PHS research grants (e.g., R29, RO1, P-mechanisms, or P-mechanism subprojects) or non-PHS peer reviewed research grants are NOT eligible for this award program. However, an exception is that recipients of R03 or R21 awards remain eligible.

3. Eligibility to apply for the extramural component (K22) of the NIDA Scholars Program will require (1) admission to the Scholars Program's intramural component and successful completion of two to four years of research in the intramural component, and (2) endorsement for continuation by the director of NIDA's Intramural Program. Postdoctoral fellows currently in the intramural program who apply for the intramural NIDA Scholars experience may, with the consent of the IRP director, count experience already gained there towards the requirement for two to four years of research in the extramural setting.

(continued)

Type of Award	Purpose of Award	Requirements*,**
K23 – Mentored Patient-Oriented Research Career Development	The purpose of the Mentored Patient-oriented Research Career Development Award (K23) is to support the career development of investigators who have made a commitment to focus their research endeavors on patient-oriented research. This mechanism provides support for three to five years of supervised study and research for clinically trained professionals who have the potential to develop into productive, clinical investigators focusing on patient-oriented research.	1. Must have a clinical doctoral degree or its equivalent. 2. Must have completed their clinical training, including specialty and, if applicable, subspecialty training prior to receiving an award. However, candidates may submit an application prior to the completion of clinical training. 3. Must identify a mentor with extensive research experience. 4. Must be willing to spend a minimum of 75% of full-time professional effort conducting research career development and clinical research.
K24 – Mid–career Investigator Award in Patient-Oriented Research	The purpose of the Mid-career Investigator Award in Patient-Oriented Research is to provide support for clinician investigators to allow them protected time to devote to patient-oriented research (POR) and to act as research mentors primarily for clinical residents, clinical fellows and/or junior clinical faculty. This award is primarily intended for clinician investigators who are at the Associate Professor level or are functioning at that rank in an academic setting or equivalent nonacademic setting, and who have an established record of independent, peer-reviewed federal or private research grant funding in POR. This award is intended to advance both the research and the mentoring endeavors of outstanding patient-oriented investigators.	1. Must have a health-professional doctoral degree or its equivalent. 2. Candidates with Ph.D. degrees are eligible for this award if the degree is in a clinical field and they usually perform clinical duties. 3. Applicants should be at the associate professor level, or are functioning at that rank in an academic setting or equivalent nonacademic setting and must have an established record of independent, peer-reviewed patient-oriented research grant funding and record of publications.

K25 –
Mentored
Quantitative
Research
Career
Development
Award

The K25 mechanism is meant to attract to NIH-relevant research those investigators whose quantitative science and engineering research has thus far not been focused primarily on questions of health and disease. Examples of quantitative scientific and technical backgrounds considered appropriate for this award include, but are not limited to, mathematics, statistics, economics, computer science, imaging science, informatics, physics, chemistry, and engineering.

The K25 award will support the career development of such investigators who make a commitment to basic or clinical biomedicine, bioengineering, bioimaging, or behavioral research.

1. Must have an advanced degree in a quantitative area of science or Engineering.
2. Must identify a mentor with extensive behavioral, biomedical, bioengineering, or bioimaging research experience.
3. Must take a commitment of at least 75% effort to research and research career development and the remainder of the effort must be committed to other career development activities consistent with the overall purpose of the award.
4. Former principal investigators on NIH research project (R01), program project (P01), center grants, FIRST Awards (R29), subprojects of program project (P01) or center grants, K01, K08 or K23 awards, or the equivalent are NOT eligible.

(continued)

Type of Award	Purpose of Award	Requirements*,**
K30 – Clinical Research Curriculum Award	The NIH developed this program to attract talented individuals to the challenges of clinical research and to provide them with the critical skills that are needed to develop hypotheses and conduct sound research. The Clinical Research Curriculum Award (CRCA) is an award to institutions. It supports the NIH's efforts to improve the quality of training in clinical research. This award is intended to: • support the development of new didactic programs in clinical research at institutions that do not currently offer them, or • support the improvement or expansion of programs at institutions with existing programs.	Core of knowledge and skills common to all areas of clinical research that should form the foundation of the well-trained, independent clinical researcher. Formal course work includes • design of clinical research projects • hypothesis development • biostatistics • epidemiology • legal, ethical, and regulatory issues related to clinical research

*Candidates must be U.S. citizens or noncitizen nationals, or must have been lawfully admitted for permanent residence by the time of award. Individuals admitted for permanent residence must be able to produce documentation of their immigration status such as an Alien Registration Receipt Card (I-551) or some other verification of legal admission as a permanent resident. Noncitizen nationals, although not U.S. citizens, owe permanent allegiance to the United States.

**This table provides some of the salient requirements, but does not include all necessary requirements for the award. Please refer to the specific program announcements for the more information.

†Eligible countries include those in the following regions: Africa, Asia (except Japan, Singapore, South Korea, and Taiwan), Russia and countries of the Former Soviet Union, Central and Eastern Europe, Latin America and the Caribbean, the Middle East (except Israel), and the Pacific Ocean Islands (except Australia and New Zealand). Applications for work in institutions in sub-Saharan Africa are especially encouraged. Awards may be delayed or denied by any state department restrictions in effect at the time of award.

quite difficult for clinicians to pursue new areas of training and establish collaborative relationships with mentors in areas that are not within their expertise.
Notwithstanding, it is almost "expected" that throughout the duration of the K
award mechanism clinicians will challenge themselves to creatively pursue new
areas and seek out the collaborative support that they need.

Third, the K award provides "financial freedom" that you might not have
obtained otherwise. Particularly in academic institutions, salary is often based on
"soft money"; that is, your salary is generated from funded grants (maybe one of
your own or from a colleague) or through provision of clinical and teaching services. Alternatively, there may be monies available from private practice revenues
or administrative services. It is rare that financial support will be provided while
you spend time developing research proposals. To offset this financial bind, the K
award provides up to five years of financial support to further develop and hone
research skills in an environment somewhat free from previous financial constraints.

Finally, the K award provides a substantial amount of prestige. This is no
small matter when one is pursuing an academic career. A K award "informs"
your colleagues that you are an exceptionally promising new or established investigator "worth" investment of salary and administrative support (i.e., a faculty
line) in order to pursue career and research goals. In other words, a K award
establishes that you are part of a very select pool of candidates, capable of obtaining independent funding and demonstrating the requisite skills and persistence to receive federal funding. It is one of the many defining "intangibles" in life
that can alter your career trajectory and also serve as a barometer or litmus test of
your own professional ambitions. You can certainly succeed as a clinical researcher
without a K award, but it provides the necessary "boost" that you might not
otherwise have experienced.

FINANCIAL CONSIDERATIONS WITH A K AWARD

Until recently, if your salary exceeded $126,000, in order to receive the "capped"
amount of $90,000, you would have to agree to spend 75% of your time on K-
related activities. However, this regulation has recently changed for individuals
who make less than $126,000. For a K01, K08, K23, or K02, you may request funds
for up to 100% of your salary as long as the total amount does not exceed
$90,000. Furthermore, the fine print on financial matters for K awards indicates
that individuals with income exceeding $126,000 can supplement their salary with
additional federal funds. This was always the case with the K24 award but is new
to the K01, K02, and K23 awards. Opening up new avenues for financial support
has greatly enhanced the desirability of the K award, particularly in settings where
salaries are partially supported by federal grants.

There is, however, one disadvantage to all this glowing news about money.
For clinicians whose salaries exceed $126,000, the $90,000 K award salary cap

means that over the three- to five-year award period, in order to receive a raise based on the entire salary, the academic institution needs to be willing to compensate the grant recipient with funds from other sources because the $90,000 cannot be further increased. Depending on your institution and individual situation, this may or may not happen. Finally, obtaining salary from different sources can have a negative impact on benefits and retirement. These factors are often not considered when a candidate applies for a K award and clearly need to be ironed out prior to submission. Although a number of my colleagues have received K awards, several of them have commented that they did not fully appreciate the financial ramifications prior to receiving the award. On the other hand, for most individuals, the positive aspect of having a K award far outweighs any financial downside.

MAKE SURE YOU ARE THE RIGHT CANDIDATE FOR A K AWARD

After digesting all of this financial brouhaha and thinking about your career aspirations, it may not be as simple as you think to decide whether or not you are an appropriate candidate for a K award. A good place to start is to consider whether you are truly interested in a research career. For the more senior K awards, this is less relevant from a career choice standpoint; however, junior investigators should engage in some introspection regarding whether they have the psychological constitution for a career in research. At this point, it is worth considering some of the less "attractive" components of a research career. For instance, being successful as a researcher requires a long delay of gratification, extreme persistence, detail-oriented behavior, and the ability to deal well with negative feedback. While, individually, many of these "traits" are laudable, it is their combination in the right balance that portends success in research. Naturally, there are individuals, tabbed as the "lucky ones," who write brilliantly, are tremendously creative and innovative (but not too innovative that grant review committees feel the work is too risky), and obtain funding with regularity and ease. However, most "mortals" do not fit into this mold. Some of the most successful researchers in the field have had unscored grants or rejected papers (other contributors to this volume also raise this same issue). Fear not, this is standard operating procedure in this business and requires a stiff chin. In many respects, maturity, conviction, and resilience are trademarks of success and will help any investigator bounce back from negative feedback provided on summary statements as well as criticisms of research proposals.

The trials and tribulations of a research career dictate that individuals seeking a mentored K award (more so for junior investigators) will encounter many ups and downs along the way. In order to obtain higher level K awards (mid or senior career), investigators first have to obtain independent funding. In the current research climate, or even in the best of research climates, this is not an easy feat. The three to five years of early K support is merely the first step in a long process of grant submissions that will provide a budding young scientist the necessary jump-start for an independent research career. Furthermore, in order to obtain future funding one needs to write well and write often. At first, particularly with the early career K awards, it is not expected that a young investigator has an expansive list of publications, but as with any career trajectory, greater attention is eventually paid to overall productivity (sheer number of papers published) and certainly with respect to quality (nature and prestige of journals).

Quite candidly, perhaps one of the hallmark issues faced by most scholarly researchers is getting over the hump or struggle of writing. Naturally, most of us find some joy in writing, a staple part of the profession. However, for many this task does not come easily. With this in mind, a good point to consider is that we don't need to write like Ernest Hemingway or F. Scott Fitzgerald (or Tom Wolfe!). Likewise, it is not imperative to maintain a level of prolific writing consistent with research "superstars" in your field. However, there are unspoken review criteria regarding number of publications, sequencing, and journal selection (and visibility) that collectively provide a basis for objective ratings of progress. All of this facilitates a reviewer's goal of evaluating whether an investigator is capable of successfully carrying out the proposed research and eventually publishing the obtained research findings. The caveat here is that all investigators must deal with writer's block at some point along the line, and we constantly evaluate our passion for writing. If you absolutely despise writing and or require a "cattle prod" to write, then a research career is probably not for you.

There are some other considerations worth noting. Although it is not requisite, it helps if you feel comfortable talking in public settings, giving prepared speeches, and engaging in open debate with a live audience. Other contributors to this book have highlighted the importance of connecting with NIH program staff and also advised that maintaining high visibility among your colleagues can benefit careers. I concur and suggest that you attend scientific meetings relevant to your work and present preliminary findings at poster sessions. Introduce yourself to senior investigators who you respect in the field. A persistent and pervasive theme in this book is to gain face recognition, which can occur through presentations, panel submissions at conferences, and just moseying up to well-known scientists and introducing yourself. Remember, ideally, senior investigators will be your future colleagues and can provide support and beneficial advice. If a senior investigator "blows you off" or disregards your collegial attempts, do not take it personally (this happens to even the most senior persons in a field and is just about personality).

Finally, no matter what your talents or accomplishments, humility is the single best approach. In other words, personality goes a long way in this profession. It will help you get along much better with your peers, and senior investigators will be more likely to lend a helping hand. Always credit your collaborators when speaking in public forums. It creates tremendous goodwill. Since I have been actively engaged as a clinical researcher, I have seen a number of researchers run into difficulties because they have had too many negative interactions with their colleagues. Even though our work is focused on science, it essentially comprises a human enterprise, and if you are someone who does not "play well in the sandbox," there can be dire consequences that are far reaching and ultimately hurt or diminish your career in some way. Successful research careers ultimately depend on collaboration and interpersonal and team-building skills.

GIVE YOURSELF ENOUGH TIME TO PREPARE THE GRANT

Once you decide that you possess the "right stuff" to engage a research career, your next activity revolves around submission timelines and grant preparation. Here, the most important concern is to avoid being sloppy. Chapter 3, covering essentials of grant writing, and other chapters in this volume provide a litany of tips and strategies on grant preparation, all of which are incredibly useful regardless of type of grant mechanism. Moreover, these tips are informative whether you are a junior scientist seeking to jump-start your career or a more established senior researcher applying for a K05 award. Paying attention to detail and avoiding sloppiness might seem like an obvious fact, but I have been repeatedly surprised at how many candidates submit applications containing major grammatical errors, misspellings, and crammed (or dense) materials to the extent that reading the grant becomes a tremendous and onerous chore. NIH provides clear-cut regulations pertaining to recommended font, type size, and line spacing, all of which need to be followed carefully. Avoid angering reviewers by attempting to disregard these regulations. The grant should read smoothly and be absent any grammatical or typographical problems. In addition, failure to attend to detail will detract from the overall priority score. Moreover, this will signal to the reviewers that the grant was not adequately reviewed by colleagues. Given that the mentor and co-mentor should review an early K award prior to submission, a poorly written career award makes the mentors look bad (this point is also hammered home in chapter 6 on F-series grants, which also requires mentoring). In the case of a senior investigator, a poorly prepared application suggests that the investigator does not believe that he/she has to put much effort into the K proposal because other productivity and research endeavors are stellar and should stand on their own merit. While an investigator's track record will certainly warrant consideration, the absence of formality and close adherence to explicit rules in the grant construction process displays an arrogant attitude. Reviewers, after all, are only human, and this double-edge whammy can certainly influence the resulting priority score. These pertinent issues can be avoided if the grant is carefully reviewed and evaluated prior to submission. Moreover, candidates should provide sufficient lead time to prepare their best work and provide the "finishing touches" to the grant after internal review, routing through the department, contracts and grants, and consideration of feedback from colleagues.

SOME QUICK HINTS TO A SUCCESSFUL K AWARD

What are the essential points to consider if you decide to submit a K award? First and foremost, it is best not to try to write a K award in one weekend. It takes a considerable amount of time to formulate a research training plan, develop a sound curriculum in the event you decide to include coursework as part of the K training, and obtain approval from mentors (and line them up). Putting the finishing touches on a grant application as discussed in many chapters in this book requires routing to the administration to gain departmental or dean's approval, signatures from contracts and grants (also called sponsored research in some academic environments), and final institutional approval for submission. Leave at least three months for writing and grant construction, and plan to revise the grant several times as you solicit feedback from mentors and colleagues. Do not try to pack an incredible amount of prose into the page limits so that the grant becomes almost impossible to read. If you follow the NIH guidelines for characters per inch and lines per inch (and font and typeface suggestions), a grant should not offend the eye. Importantly, have a few colleagues preview the grant. After spending so much time writing on a single topic, you will think the grant is well organized, concise, and clear. This may not be the case. Therefore, a good piece of advice is to have more established investigators or colleagues who are not well acquainted with your substantive area read the grant. Their careful eye may pick up on typographical errors or materials that do not flow (segue) or lack coherence from a lay perspective. Further, do not have your application reviewed by colleagues the day before the grant is due; most likely, you will not have time to incorporate any recommended changes into the final product. Thus, the three-month timeline becomes more attractive and reasonable if you think about the different phases of grant production.

The next few sections of this chapter provide a more detailed breakdown of the various review and evaluation criteria for K-series grants. These evaluation criteria crop up during peer review, and you will find these reinforced in chapter 3, in its discussion of the five review criteria (i.e., the schema) used by peer reviewers. Appendix 11.1 at the end of this chapter encapsulates the specific NIH review criteria for each of the K-series grants. The section-by-section analysis of these evaluation criteria should help the reader to better prepare these different sections and more closely adhere to the cognitive framework applied during peer review.

THE CANDIDATE SECTION: BRAG BUT DON'T BE CONCEITED

The candidate section of the K award is the place to present your accomplishments. The point of this section is to demonstrate your professional appropriateness for this award. If you are applying for an early career award, it is not expected that you have 20 publications, but you need to demonstrate promise as well as the persistence and interest to pursue a research career. While it is important to highlight your awards, honors, and talents, it is important that you do not appear arrogant. Again, particularly with an early career award, focus on your strengths but recognize that you possess areas of weakness (these areas become the focus of the K award). Give credit to the individuals that have helped pave the road to your current success and influenced your thinking, if not your publication track record. It is not necessary to delve into the personal reasons why you choose your area of research (e.g., my father was an alcoholic and therefore I chose a research career studying treatments for alcohol dependence). Further, do not provide personal explanations of why you have not been productive (i.e., after my fellowship I did not write any papers because I was caring for a sick grandmother). Although some reviewers might be interested in why a candidate decided to seek out a research career and might be sympathetic if there were extenuating circumstances as to why an individual has not been productive, overall the review committee is not favorably inclined to applications that include these personal details. It is risky business to bring up personal matters and probably best to leave out this material from an application. Alternatively, material submitted by a mentor or contained in a reference letter that mentions personal issues will probably not harm and may help provide credibility to specific concerns raised during review about a hiatus or period of inactivity.

For mid-career or senior scientist K awards, it is important to highlight your accomplishments and explain how your work has helped advance the field. The issue of blending one's research into the larger scientific fold represents a critical point of review. Applicants should definitely address how their focus, their corner of the scientific edifice, has helped advance the field. The effort to illuminate one's work and gauge scientific progress in light of existing research and historical precedence can be accomplished in one of several ways: Highlight that your work presents an alternative view, extends current themes, opens new doors for examination, or provides an historical basis from which to evaluate the field's scientific credibility and social impact. Humility is quite germane for any applicant but nevertheless not as pronounced for senior investigators. However, using 20 pages to expound on accomplishments will probably be seen as "overkill."

THE TRAINING PLAN CAN DEFINITELY BE MORE IMPORTANT THAN YOU THINK

What distinguishes a career development award from an R01 or other research grants is the training plan. You can have a brilliant research plan, but your chances of getting a solid priority score might be sabotaged if your application contains a poorly thought-out training plan. It is critical that you carefully outline your training objectives and show how these objectives will be met (i.e., through coursework and/or meeting with mentor or colleagues). The research plan should serve as a vehicle for facilitating training objectives. Further, how your training objectives allow you to attain your short-term and long-term career goals needs to be clearly delineated. Unfortunately, it is not uncommon for candidates applying for K awards to leave out some of this information or provide this material in a confusing format. When this occurs, it negatively influences scoring by reviewers who find it difficult to discern how the training activities provide a vehicle for the investigator to attain their long-term goals over the course of the award. As a reviewer, it was always a relief when a candidate summarized their training plan with a well-constructed table that covers these key areas.

In addition to these concerns, you want to develop a training plan that is impressive but not totally unrealistic. No matter how enthusiastic you may be, it is unlikely that you will be able to take six courses at one time, spend 20 hours a week with mentors, submit 10 first-author publications each year, and carry out a research project using K award funds. As ambitious as this plan sounds, it would most likely require R01 funding to complete. Alternatively, the training plan should be comprehensive and challenging. If one of your colleagues reviews your application and asks, "Is this person for real?" or "Do you ever plan to sleep?" then you need to revisit your training plan and tone things down. Keep in mind, the individuals reading your application may have undertaken a similar career path, thereby possessing first-hand knowledge of the logistics behind a K award. Their experience will also harbor deeper knowledge regarding the implications of this award to your daily regimen of teaching, mentoring, clinical, and administrative duties.

As much as these few pieces of advice will help to clear your desk and get you "prepared" for the onerous task of constructing a K award, there are a few additional pointers worth noting. Do not forget to include in your training plan specific training in the ethical conduct of human research or, if applicable, animal research. Also, if you are applying for an early career award, do not bundle together an inordinate number of mentors. The appearance of a "crew" or frayed group of mentors lacking any unified purpose will give the appearance that the applicant is unfocused and unable to set realistic goals. On the other hand, the careful and methodical selection of appropriate mentors with adequate expertise matching areas outlined in the training plan should bode well for the applicant.

If you are applying for an independent or senior award, collaboration with other senior investigators is well regarded by reviewers. So, too, is emphasizing the importance of training and the "zeal" for continued learning (you *can* teach an old dog new tricks!). Even though a senior investigator has been conducting research for many years, everyone has something new to learn, and providing new venues in which you plan to expand your current line of research or develop new lines of research is viewed favorably. Moreover, adding coursework to the training plan, even with senior investigators, is regarded positively because it suggests that even the senior investigator feels that he/she still has new information to learn. Also, it is important for a senior investigator to present his/her accomplishments. If a previous K award has been received, the accomplishments attained during the past funding period need to be judiciously highlighted.

THE RESEARCH PLAN SHOULD NOT MATCH R01 STANDARDS

It is not expected that a candidate applying for an early career award will be conducting a research project that is as comprehensive and sophisticated as an R01. Alternatively, for an independent career award or senior scientist, it is expected that the research conducted during the K award period will be funded through an R01 mechanism. If not, the funding should be realized as a major project part of a center grant, with the candidate as the principal investigator of the R01 or center project.

One of the biggest problems that often occurs with research plans composed by more junior investigators is their hubris and ambitious goals. It is important that the research project be conceptualized as a program of empirical study that can be achieved within the required time frame of the award. This point needs to be underscored given that K-series grants have concurrent training plans that carry heavy time demands. Further, the research plan needs to be consistent with the training goals. For example, if the candidate wants to develop expertise in conducting clinical trials, then conducting a small clinical trial during the training award makes sense. However, basic laboratory research training may not be necessary.

Alternatively, if the research plan can be completed in six months during a five-year award, this may not be viewed as complex or demanding. From the perspective of a reviewer, the feasibility of the proposed research plan, the appropriateness of the methodology, the adequacy of the data analysis plan, and the data and safety monitoring plan are important sections for evaluation. Lack of attention to these areas can adversely influence an application's score. However, the review committee tends to be more generous (i.e., understanding) in its review of the research plan for an early career K award because reviewers understand that early investigators have yet to learn how to write a research plan at the level of an R01-funded grant—that is the purpose of the early K awards!

Further, unlike an R01, where there are 25 pages to expound on why the research is important, present preliminary data, and outline an appropriate methodology, a K award has to include these sections as well as a complete description of the candidate and training plan bound by the same 25-page limit. Thus, by necessity, less methodological detail is possible with a K award compared to an R01.

Although there are no strict guidelines regarding how long each section of a K proposal should be, a general rule of thumb is that the career development and training plan should be approximately 9–12 pages, and the rest of the 25 pages might consist of the research plan. Also, it is crucial that a junior investigator outline a framework for scientific papers that will be written during the course of the award. In the event that a candidate is planning to conduct a clinical trial for three years, it is not clear, given this time frame, how the candidate will produce more than, at most, one or two papers. Secondary analysis would provide one means to augment productivity in a defined time period, allowing for simultaneous conductance of a clinical trial. Often, candidates will state that their primary goal of their K award is to become an independent investigator. If the candidate writes only one or two papers during the course of the award, he/she may not be considered productive enough to merit being a principal investigator on an R01. This issue needs to be addressed head-on in the training and research plan by describing how and when papers will be written during the training period (this information can be presented in tabular form). Realize of course, a more conservative paper production schedule is not uncommon for new faculty or investigators joining a productive laboratory anyway. Senior investigators often will develop a timeline for paper construction using this as an objective gauge to evaluate productivity.

For an independent scientist award or a senior K award, the candidate is expected to present funded R01 or center grant program projects in which the candidate serves as principal investigator. The K grant application requires divulging this information in a systematic manner, albeit investigators often opt for different stylistic approaches. Some will provide brief summaries of the various R01 grants in which they serve as principal investigator. Other investigators who have one R01 will present the R01 in an abbreviated form or, if they have several R01 grants in which they are principal investigator, will choose to present one representative R01. Regardless of approach, it is critical that enough detail be presented so that reviewers have some idea of how candidates will be spending their time over the award period and how they plan to accomplish their research objectives.

Surprising, even with senior investigators, this section can be unnecessarily confusing. Often, too much consideration and deliberation is left to the reviewer's imagination. In some cases, applicants fail to provide specific details including grant title, funding period, agency, funding amount, and grant status (i.e., noncompeting continuation, pending, scored), even though this material is clearly required and critical for peer review (and can easily be presented in tabular form).

Clearly, it is understood that if a research plan focuses on an R01 funded grant, a training committee reviewer is not supposed to re-review the parent R01 grant and reassess the grant for scientific merit. However, it may appear arrogant or even sloppy if an applicant presents too few details. In the event that an applicant presents a slate of new research, inevitably this material will be carefully reviewed. Further, if the research plan is out of line with the training plan, this might cause some consternation during review. For the independent or senior investigator, it is important that there be a clear rationale for the current or future line of research.

CHOOSE YOUR MENTORS CAREFULLY AND WITH TACT

For all early career awards, the choice of mentors is crucial (chapter 6 emphasizing F-series grants also highlights this important concern). First and foremost, the primary mentor needs to demonstrate some key characteristics. The mentor needs to possess expertise in the areas of training the candidate wishes to pursue over the course of the award. However, it is not necessary for the mentor to have expertise in all of the candidate's proposed training areas; other mentors can provide additional expertise. Second, it is preferable that the candidate has an established professional relationship with the primary mentor. There may be situations where this is not the case; however, the applicant should clarify their choice in great detail to justify their selection. Such clarification should go to great extremes to show how the mentoring will work and provide the oversight required to execute the grant.

Third, and consistent with this latter point, if the primary mentor's office is located across town or in another city or state, this will require an even greater explanation of how the mentoring will work effectively. The length of the explanation is directly proportional to the office distances between the candidate and primary mentor. As a candidate, you might try to make a case that emails, telephone calls, and scheduled visits will make the apparent distance surmountable. However, this might not be easily done or believed. In the best of all possible worlds, it is a best to have a mentor who is easily accessible for face-to-face contact and whose advice can be solicited without scheduled appointments. At the very least, scheduled visits should be frequent (more than once a month). Along these lines, the primary mentor should have an established record obtaining independent funding. Surprisingly, there are applications submitted in which this is not made clear (i.e., the other support pages do not show any evidence of current or prior grant support in which the mentor is the primary investigator). Finally, a mentor who has successfully mentored other candidates, particularly guiding them toward independent research careers, is clearly an advantage, although not a prerequisite.

The co-mentors often provide additional support to facilitate the candidate's training and research plan. Choosing a mentor who has a national reputation in an area that the candidate is planning to gain expertise can enhance an application. Unlike the primary mentor, it may not be as crucial to meet weekly or be located within close physical proximity to the candidate. The candidate might outline a specialized area of training that requires travel to a co-mentors laboratory or clinic. Opting for this scenario might be viewed as a strength and improve an application's priority scoring. However, if the candidate plans to have 10 co-mentors and the candidate plans to meet with each of them on a weekly basis and spend 20 weeks a year visiting mentors, this is probably overkill and unfeasible.

Even after giving careful consideration to all these points, there are some additional issues to keep in mind. Most university-based faculty will consider it an honor to serve as a mentor on a K award. Notwithstanding, it is best not to choose faculty mentors simply because you like them or to avoid crossing paths and instigating problems. The mentor needs to have the necessary professional and personal characteristics that will ensure the success of your award. Also, the supporting reference and mentorship letter submitted by your mentor needs to be adequately detailed. If the mentor provides a perfunctory paragraph agreeing to serve a mentor, particularly if it is the primary mentor, this will probably detract from the application when it comes time for scoring. Alternatively, if the mentor can describe how often he/she will meet with candidate, the content of mentoring sessions, the candidate's strengths, and what areas need bolstering, this will surely enhance the application.

Although senior awardees do not need to have formal mentors, they may choose to collaborate with colleagues who have expertise in areas that will further promote or embellish their career and adequately bolster their research plan. If senior investigators can highlight new areas of training that they wish to explore through formal or informal collaborations, this is viewed positively since it demonstrates an openness to learn and grow intellectually. Alternatively, a senior investigator is expected to "give back" to the field and spend some time enhancing the professional lives of younger candidates. Although it not a formal criterion for some awards (e.g., a K02 award), ongoing mentoring and training junior investigators are viewed favorably by reviewers.

Again, the section detailing mentoring and, for senior career awards, how applicants will advance their careers requires "thought" and making some tactical decisions. For the younger applicant seeking to advance their career, choosing a great mentoring team will not assure that the application will be funded, but choosing a poor mentoring team can sabotage its chances of being funded. For the more senior applicant seeking release time from administrative duties and free "unfettered" time to pursue research activities, choosing to operate in isolation without true collaboration does not show great promise.

DON'T OVERLOOK THE IMPORTANCE OF YOUR INSTITUTIONAL ENVIRONMENT AND COMMITMENT

This section may seem a bit "pro forma," particularly if the candidate is carrying out his/her K award at a large academic institution. Most K grants are carried out in strong academic environments, but the candidate needs to emphasize the opportunities for collaborations and the availability of the necessary resources to carry out the planned career and research plan. It is crucial that if candidates plan to conduct research at certain clinics or laboratories, they obtain letters of commitment from the appropriate clinic or laboratory directors. These letters should highlight a working knowledge of the grant mechanics and specify the requirements or components needed at the laboratory/clinic. The commitment letter from the applicant's institution, usually written and signed by the department chairperson, represents a crucial component of the application. A strong letter outlines the candidate's achievements and how the institution will provide the necessary resources so that the career and research plan can be successfully executed. Often, reviewers are forced to plant the "kiss of death" when scoring K awards for junior candidates because a supporting letter did not make clear what will happen to the candidate if he/she does not receive the award. Even more egregious is when the letter states that a promotion to a faculty or research position is contingent on the successful attainment of a K award. Statements such as "there may be a faculty line" or "we may reduce teaching load" are not inconsequential and more damaging than one thinks.

Another, less common problem is when the review committee believes that the candidate has enough funding and does not need additional financial support in order to attain his/her training or research goals. Although a superb research environment and strong institutional support do not ensure funding, if excellent resources and study support are not crucial, the scoring of the application will reflect the committee's tenor. Remember to take the "environment" section seriously and do not consider this section an "afterthought."

THE OTHER STUFF IN THE APPLICATION IS IMPORTANT, TOO

Although the focus of a K award review rests on the career, research, training, and mentoring plan, careful attention needs to be paid to the human subjects section and the budget (chapter 15 details the importance of matching budgets to proposed scientific goals). If the budget does not fit with the requirements of the planned research or inappropriate personnel are chosen, the reviewers will notice this oversight and not be happy. For example, if a candidate is planning to carry out a clinical trial evaluating a new treatment for cocaine dependence, it is most likely that cocaine urine toxicological testing will be needed. Thus, if the budget does not include costs for urine testing, this will be seen as an oversight and viewed as something that the mentors (and applicant) should have identified. Keep in mind, the mentors are more accustomed to running a laboratory and have the "inside scoop" on what it takes to conduct empirical research. This includes developing a financial picture regarding cost for urine specimens, laboratory protocols for specimen storage and handling, data safety, and monitoring, to name a few items, all of which would accompany the study.

Further, if necessary sections in the human subjects section are missing or they are inadequately justified this may influence priority scoring. For example, if depressed substance abusers are enrolled in a treatment study, and there is no assessment for suicidal risk or plan for minimizing this risk in the human subjects section, this would be considered a major oversight (and likely raise the flag of a human subjects concern). Chapter 16 highlights the tremendously damaging nature of overlooking human subject concerns. If women are excluded for the study but there is no justification or an inadequate justification, this will be considered problematic. Even in the event of an outstanding priority score, funding for a grant with a "comment" will require a justification document be submitted to the human subjects group within the institute. Any "red" flagged application will not receive funding until the "flag" is removed, meaning that the justification page sent to the NIH institute or center argues convincingly what should have been included in the original submitted application (this entails another level of review by internal program staff).

Although it might not make intuitive sense, any study that involves human subjects and provides an intervention—even if it is not a treatment intervention—needs to have a data and safety monitoring plan. This plan does not need to be excessively long but needs to be reasonable and appropriate. Prior to submission, do ask your mentor to read this section. It has been my experience in mentoring young investigators that with the "crush" of putting the finishing touches on the other sections of the K award, the human subjects section often is written at the end, and there is little chance for senior investigators to read and review these materials. Although it might seem like a boring section to write and read, get your mentor to read it—it's his/her job to read your application from beginning to end. If you are a more established investigator submitting a mid-level or senior level K award, it is understood that the ongoing funded research that you are conducting has been reviewed by your institutional review board and contains an adequate human subjects plan. Chapter 16 goes to great length to showcase the proper features of an adequate human subject plan and also provides examples where failing to meet institutional review board requirements can be the death knell of an application. The best advice is to read chapter 16 in concert with the K award requirements to assure that you make progress solving these requirements.

TAKE A DEEP BREATH AND KEEP PERSPECTIVE IF YOUR GRANT IS NOT SCORED

In the event that you receive a summary sheet that details why your grant was "unscored," do not feel that this is the end of the world. Ideally, if you have the support of your institution, you will be able to continue working until you can revise and resubmit your application in the hope of an improved priority score. Chapter 18 details the requirements for revisions and resubmissions and how to handle the prose and structure responses to the reviewers. Keep in mind that, just as it is painful to have your grant unscored, it is also painful for the review group to unscore the application. Reviewers want to encourage young investigators and are fully aware that receiving an unscored application, even for a seasoned investigator, is extremely discouraging. During the grant review meeting, and as part of the new "streamlining procedures," the review group is repeatedly told that the bottom 50% of K applications have to be unscored. Often, unscored grants are very good, filled with scientific merit, and written by solid investigators who deserve a crack at career advancement through NIH support. At times, there is deliberation in the room how "unfair" and "unfortunate" the scoring process can be. Nevertheless, this conversation does not reverse the fact that the lower half of applications will be unscored.

Thus, if you have an unscored K, take a deep breath and read the reviews carefully. A good reviewer will provide a comprehensive critique outlining the essential problems and may even offer suggestions how to improve the application (although review instructions specifically ask reviewers not to offer suggestions of this nature). If you choose to resubmit the application, respond to each of the criticisms. Do not ignore the criticisms you do not like, and do not become too argumentative or defensive in your written response. You do not have to agree with all of the criticisms made, but if you disagree it is best done in a respectful tone with a clear justification of why you disagree. Also, if you disagree with all of the criticisms made by the reviewers, this will probably not go over well with the review group. Your application may or may not be read by the reviewers who reviewed the application the first time. Therefore, it is best to paraphrase the criticisms in your response and be aware (unfortunately) that new reviewers may have new concerns.

One of the key characteristics of a successful scientist is persistence. If you are able to respond to the criticisms in a thoughtful, reasonable way, even if it requires a couple of review cycles, the likelihood of getting a K award increases with each submission. Remember, most productive and highly successful batters in major league baseball end up with career batting records well below .300 (only a few memorable sluggers, e.g., Ted Williams, whose career batting average of .344 surpassed that mark). A K grant application that receives funding on the third submission is "batting" a .333!

Appendix 11.1   SPECIFIC NIH REVIEW CRITERIA FOR EACH K-SERIES GRANT

K01—MENTORED RESEARCH SCIENTIST DEVELOPMENT AWARD

Candidate

- Quality of the candidate's research, academic and (if relevant) clinical record
- Potential to develop as an independent researcher
- Commitment to a research career

Career Development Plan

- Appropriateness of the content, the phasing, and the proposed duration of the career development plan for achieving scientific independence
- Consistency of the career development plan with the candidate's career goals
- Likelihood that the plan will contribute substantially to the achievement of scientific independence

Training in the Responsible Conduct of Research

- Quality of the proposed training in responsible conduct of research

Research Plan

- Scientific and technical merit of the research question, design and methodology
- Relevance of the proposed research to the candidate's career objectives
- Appropriateness of the research plan to the stage of research development and as a vehicle for developing the research skills described in the career development plan
- Adequacy of the plan's attention to children, gender, and minority issues when human subjects are involved

Mentor/Co-Mentor

- Appropriateness of mentor(s) research qualifications in the area of this application
- Quality and extent of mentor(s) proposed role in providing guidance and advice to the candidate
- Previous experience in fostering the development of researchers

- History of research productivity
- Adequacy of support for the proposed research project

Environment and Institutional Commitment

- Adequacy of research facilities and training opportunities
- Quality and relevance of the environment for scientific and professional development of the candidate
- Applicant institution's commitment to the scientific development of the candidate and assurances that the institution intends the candidate to be an integral part of its research program
- Applicant institution's commitment to an appropriate balance of research and clinical responsibilities including the level of 75% effort proposed by the candidate

Budget

- Justification of the requested budget in relation to career development goals and research aims

K01—INTERNATIONAL RESEARCH SCIENTIST DEVELOPMENT AWARD

Candidate

- Commitment to an independent international research career including potential to contribute to knowledge that will address a major global health problem
- Potential to develop (or evidence of the capacity to develop) as an independent investigator pursuing international research
- Quality and relevance of prior scientific training and experience including detailed description of previous research, record of previous research support and publications

Career Development Plan

- Likelihood that the research and training in the plan will contribute substantially to the scientific development of the candidate, the achievement of scientific independence, and ongoing involvement in collaborative international research
- Appropriateness of the plan to the career goals of the candidate
- Appropriateness of the plan to increase conceptual and theoretical knowledge in the research area proposed
- Consistency of the plan with the candidate's prior training, research and academic experience and the stated career goals

- Clarity of the goals and scope of the plan and the need for the proposed research and training experience at the foreign site
- Adequacy of the proposed training for responsible conduct of research in an international context
- Clear description of the roles of the U.S. and foreign mentors in the training and research planned

Research Plan

- Usefulness of the research plan as a vehicle for enhancing existing research skills as described in the career development plan
- Scientific and technical merit of the research question, design, and methodology judged in the context of the candidate's previous training and experience
- Relevance of the proposed research to a major global health problem
- Relevance of the proposed research to the candidate's career objectives

Mentor/Co-Mentor

- Appropriateness of U.S. and foreign mentors' collaborative research and their other research and training qualifications for the proposed project
- The extent of the commitment of each mentor to supervising and guiding the candidate throughout the award period
- Adequacy of each mentor's previous experience in fostering the development of independent researchers highlighting persons involved in international research
- Adequacy of each mentor's research productivity and grant support related to the proposed project

Environment and Institutional Commitment

- Adequacy of the research facilities at the U.S. and foreign institutions
- Adequacy of the training opportunities and quality of the environment for scientific and professional development at the U.S. and foreign institutions

K02—INDEPENDENT RESEARCH SCIENTIST DEVELOPMENT AWARD

Candidate

- Capacity to carry out independent research
- Potential to become an outstanding scientist who will make significant contributions to the field

- Past and present research productivity as evidenced by contributions to the scientific literature, and success in obtaining independent funding
- Ability to conceptualize and organize a long-term research approach
- Evidence of current independent, peer-reviewed, research support
- Level of training, experience, and competence commensurate with the purposes of the award

Career Development Plan

- Likelihood that the award will contribute substantially to the continued scientific development and productivity of the candidate
- The extent to which the award will enable a candidate to devote full time (at least 75% effort) to research and related duties by release from teaching, administration, clinical work, and other responsibilities
- Consistency of the career development plan with the candidate's career goals
- Proposed collaboration with other active investigators and other opportunities for professional growth

Training in the Responsible Conduct of Research

- Quality of the proposed training or instruction in areas related to the responsible conduct of research

Research Plan

- Quality of research plan and potential for advancing the field of study
- Scientific and technical merit of the proposed research plan
- Adequacy of plans to include both genders and minorities and their subgroups as appropriate for the scientific goals of the research, and plans for the recruitment and retention of subjects

Environment and Institutional Commitment

- Institutional commitment to the development of the candidate as an independent scientist and assurances that the candidate will be an integral part of its research and academic program
- Evidence that the candidate's full-time effort (at least 75%) will be set aside to pursue research and career development activities
- Strength of the institution's commitment to scientific research

Budget

- Justification of budget requests in relation to career development goals and research aims and plans

K05—SENIOR SCIENTIST AWARD
(FOR THIS AWARD, CANDIDATE AND RESEARCH PLAN
ARE THE SAME REQUIREMENTS.)

Candidate

- A consistent record of outstanding research productivity including program research funding and record of publication of scientific reports, including publication of influential research papers or seminal theoretical papers
- Recognition as a leading senior scientist as judged by peers
- Leadership of a productive research program
- Ability to develop and maintain a high-quality environment for training and mentoring investigators
- The candidate's current involvement in science education, science researcher
- Quality and breadth of prior scientific training and experience
- Degree and extent of previous research support and publications considering the academic level of candidate

Career Development Plan

- Scientific and technical merit of the research plan
- Significance of the research plan and the probability of significant contributions to scientific knowledge
- Long-term substantive plan for future research
- Consistency of the career development plans with the candidate's career goals
- Quality of plans for mentoring and science education activities
- Conduct of research

Research Plan

- Goals of the research, and plans for the recruitment and retention of subjects will also be evaluated

Mentor/Co-Mentor

- Research project

Environment and Institutional Commitment

- Adequacy of the facilities and general environment as it relates to the proposed research and career development program
- Availability of collaborative opportunities with other investigators

- Reputation of the applicant institution and the candidate's department as a center of active, high-quality research
- Institutional support of the candidate's commitment to research and research training and departments
- Adequacy of the research facilities and training opportunities for this award

K08—MENTORED CLINICAL SCIENTIST DEVELOPMENT AWARD

Candidate

- Quality of the candidate's academic and clinical record
- Potential to develop as an independent researcher
- Commitment to a research career

Career Development Plan

- Appropriateness of the content, the phasing, and the proposed duration of the career development plan for achieving scientific independence
- Consistency of the career development plan with the candidate's previous training and career goals
- Likelihood that the plan will contribute substantially to the achievement of scientific independence

Training in the Responsible Conduct of Research

- Quality of the proposed training in the responsible conduct of research

Research Plan

- Scientific and technical merit of the research question, design and methodology
- Relevance of the proposed research to the candidate's career objectives
- Appropriateness of the research plan to the stage of research development and as a vehicle for developing the research skills described in the career development plan
- Adequacy of the plan's attention to children, gender and minority issues when human subjects are involved

Mentor/Co-Mentor

- Appropriateness of mentor(s) research qualifications in the area of this application
- Quality and extent of mentor(s) proposed role in providing guidance and advice to the candidate

- Previous experience in fostering the development of researchers
- History of research productivity
- Adequacy of support for the proposed research project

Environment and Institutional Commitment

- Adequacy of research facilities and training opportunities
- Quality and relevance of the environment for scientific and professional development of the candidate
- Applicant institution's commitment to the scientific development of the candidate and assurances that the institution intends the candidate to be an integral part of its research program
- Applicant institution's commitment to an appropriate balance of research and clinical responsibilities including the level of 75 percent effort proposed by the candidate

Budget

- Justification of the requested budget in relation to career development goals and research aims

K12—MENTORED CLINICAL SCIENTISTS DEVELOPMENT PROGRAM AWARD

Candidate

- Recruitment and selection processes are adequate to achieve high-quality candidates
- Accomplishments of named candidates and the quality of their planned research activities are appropriate to their level of experience and expected progress during the award
- Efforts to recruit candidates from racial or ethnic groups under-represented in biomedical, behavioral, or clinical research are adequate
- Competing continuations and supplements: current and past appointments show evidence of success at recruitment and training

Mentor/Co-Mentor

- The proposed program director is an acknowledged research leader/administrator with a track record of mentoring successful researchers
- The proposed co-mentors complement the skills and experience of the principal investigator, and their experience in research and prior success in training is appropriate to their role?

- Need for particular mentors is well justified by the aims of the program
- The mentoring team has committed sufficient time to ensure the success of the program

Environment and Institutional Commitment

- Existing facilities and resources enrich the potential of the proposed K12 award to provide strong research mentoring and development experiences for the candidates
- Support letters are available from individuals who control access to these resources that show their willingness to collaborate
- The institution indicates that the candidates will be provided a minimum of 75% time for the career development experiences and shows how they will be protected from other administrative, teaching, or clinical duties

Budget

- The reasonableness of the proposed budget and the requested period of support in relation to the proposed research

K18—CAREER ENHANCEMENT AWARD FOR STEM CELL RESEARCH

Candidate

- Evidence of excellence in academic, research, and, if appropriate, clinical activities
- Potential to become, or continue as, an outstanding investigator, teacher, resource person, and leader in research programs related to the mission of the appropriate IC
- Quality and breadth of prior scientific training and experience
- Degree and extent of previous research support and publications, considering your academic level

Training in the Responsible Conduct of Research

- Quality of the proposed training in the responsible conduct of research that has been, or will be, completed

Research Plan

- Scientific and technical merit of the research question, design, and methodology

- Relevance of the proposed research project to your own research interests
- Appropriateness of the research plan to your career level and as a vehicle for developing the research skills described in the career development plan
- Quality and feasibility of your training plan, including plans after completion of the award
- Relationship of the research training plan to previous research focus as well as future research plans
- An assessment of the value of the proposed training experience as it relates to enhancing your capabilities as an independent investigator

Mentor/Co-Mentor

- The stem cell expert's qualifications as well as prior experience and record of fostering academic growth and productivity
- The expert's history of research productivity and peer-reviewed research support
- Adequacy of active support for the proposed research project, if applicable

Environment and Institutional Commitment

- Adequacy of the research facilities and training opportunities for support of this award at the host institution, which may be the applicant institution or at another institution
- Clear evidence from your own institution that you will be given sufficient release time to complete the proposed training and research project
- Level of commitment from your institution in supporting your future plans to use stem cells in your research

Budget

- Justification of the requested budget in both time and amount, relevant to your research career goals and interests

K22—THE NIDA SCHOLARS PROGRAM

Candidate

- Capacity to carry out independent research
- Potential to become an outstanding scientist who will make significant contributions to the field
- Past and present research productivity as evidenced by contributions to the scientific literature, and success in obtaining independent funding

- Ability to conceptualize and organize a long-term research approach
- Level of training, experience, and competence commensurate with the purposes of the award

Career Development Plan

- Likelihood that the award will contribute substantially to the continued scientific development and productivity of the candidate
- The extent to which the award will enable a candidate to devote full time to research and related duties by release from teaching, administration, clinical work, and other responsibilities
- Consistency of the career development plan with the candidate's career goals
- Collaboration with other active investigators and opportunities for professional growth

Research Plan

- Quality of research plan and significance for contributing to the scientific literature
- Scientific and technical merit of the proposed research plan
- Adequacy of plans to include both genders and minorities and their subgroups as appropriate for the scientific goals of the research, as well as plans to include children and plans for the recruitment and retention of subjects

Budget

- Justification of budget requests in relation to career development goals and research aims and plans

K23—MENTORED PATIENT-ORIENTED RESEARCH CAREER DEVELOPMENT

Candidate

- Quality of the candidate's academic and clinical record
- Potential to develop as an independent clinical researcher focusing on patient-oriented research
- Commitment to a career in patient-oriented research

Career Development Plan

- Likelihood that the career development plan will contribute substantially to the scientific development of the candidate

- Appropriateness of the content and duration of the proposed didactic and research phases of the award
- Consistency of the career development plan with the candidate's career goals and prior research experience

Training in the Responsible Conduct of Research

- Quality of the proposed training in responsible conduct of research

Research Plan

- Scientific and technical merit of the research question, design and methodology
- Relevance of the proposed research to the candidate's career objectives
- Appropriateness of the research plan to the stage of research development and as a vehicle for developing the research skills as described in the career development plan
- Adequacy of the plan's attention to gender and minority issues associated with projects involving human subjects
- Adequacy of plans for including children, as appropriate, for the scientific goals of the research, or justification for exclusion

Mentor/Co-Mentor

- Appropriateness of mentor(s) research qualifications in the area of this application
- Quality and extent of mentor's proposed role in providing guidance and advice to the candidate
- Previous experience in fostering the development of more junior researchers
- History of research productivity and support
- Adequacy of support for the proposed research project

Environment and Institutional Commitment

- Adequacy of research facilities and the availability of appropriate educational opportunities
- Quality and relevance of the environment for scientific and professional development of the candidate
- Applicant institution's commitment to the scientific development of the candidate and assurances that the institution intends the candidate to be an integral part of its research program

- Applicant institution's commitment to an appropriate balance of research and clinical responsibilities including the commitment of 75% of the candidate's effort to research and research related activities

Budget

- Justification of the requested budget in relation to career development goals and research aims

K24—MIDCAREER INVESTIGATOR AWARD IN PATIENT-ORIENTED RESEARCH

Candidate

- Evidence of ongoing high quality patient-oriented research and the relationship of that research to this program
- Evidence of the candidate's capabilities and commitment to serve as a mentor for patient-oriented research
- Demonstration that the proposed program and protected time will relieve the candidate from non-research patient care and administrative duties and allow him/her to devote additional time to patient-oriented research
- Record of financial support for patient-oriented research

Research Plan

- Appropriateness of the research plan as a vehicle for demonstrating and developing skills and capabilities in patient-oriented research to prospective mentees
- Scientific and technical merit of the proposed research
- Relevance of the proposed research to the candidate's career objectives
- Availability of adequate resources to conduct the research program, including adequacy of plans for continued support of the research during the funding period of the grant
- Adequacy of the plant's attention to gender and minority issues associated with projects involving human subjects
- Adequacy of plans for including children as appropriate for the scientific goals of the research, or justification for exclusion

Mentor/Co-Mentor

- Adequacy of the plans for mentoring or supervising beginning clinicians in patient oriented research

- Adequacy of plans to integrate appropriate clinical research curricula, such as those offered by available K30 programs at the institution, into the mentoring plans
- Appropriateness of the proposed level of effort committed to the mentoring component
- Extent to which the career, research and mentoring objectives of the previous award have been achieved
- Justification of the need for an additional three to five years of support
- Evidence of leadership in patient-oriented research such as through being principal investigator on independent peer-reviewed research grants and providing high-quality mentorship

Environment and Institutional Commitment

- Applicant institution's commitment to the scientific development of the candidate and assurances that the institution intends the candidate to be an integral part of its research program
- Adequacy of research facilities and the availability of appropriate educational opportunities
- Quality and relevance of the environment for continuing the scientific and professional development of the candidate and for others pursuing patient-oriented research
- Applicant institution's commitment to provide adequate protected time for the candidate to conduct the research and mentoring program
- Applicant institution's commitment to the career development in patient-oriented research of individuals mentored by the candidate

K25—MENTORED QUANTITATIVE RESEARCH CAREER DEVELOPMENT AWARD

Candidate

- Quality of the research and academic record
- Potential to develop as an independent quantitative biomedical or bioengineering researcher or to play a significant role in multidisciplinary research teams
- Commitment to a career in quantitative biomedical or bioengineering research

Career Development Plan

- Likelihood that the career development plan will contribute substantially to the candidate's scientific development

- Appropriateness of the content and duration of the proposed didactic and research phases of the award
- Consistency of the career development plan with the candidate's career goals and prior research experience

Training in the Responsible Conduct of Research

- Quality of the proposed training in responsible conduct of research

Research Plan

- Appropriateness of the research plan to the candidate's stage of research development and as a vehicle for developing the research skills as described in the career development plan
- Scientific and technical merit of the research question, design and methodology
- Relevance of the proposed research to the candidate's career objectives
- Adequacy of the plans to include both genders, minorities, and children and their subgroups as appropriate for the scientific goals of the research when human subjects are used, as well as plans for the recruitment and retention of subjects

Mentor/Co-Mentor

- History of research productivity and support in the area of basic or clinical biomedical, bioengineering, bioimaging, or behavioral research
- Appropriateness of the mentor's research qualifications in the area of this application
- Quality and extent of the mentor's proposed role in providing guidance and advice
- Previous experience in fostering the development of researchers

Environment and Institutional Commitment

- Evidence that the institution is committed to the candidate's scientific development and assurance that the institution intends for the candidate to be an integral part of its research program
- Adequacy of research facilities and training opportunities (including access to such facilities or opportunities in other institutions)
- Quality and relevance of the environment for the candidate's scientific and professional development
- Institution's commitment to an appropriate balance of research and other responsibilities

Budget

- The requested budged must be appropriate in relation to the candidate's career development goals and research aims and plans

K30—CLINICAL RESEARCH CURRICULUM AWARD

The NIH developed this program to attract talented individuals to the challenges of clinical research and to provide them with the critical skills that are needed to develop hypotheses and conduct sound research. The Clinical Research Curriculum Award (CRCA) is an award to institutions. It supports the NIH's efforts to improve the quality of training in clinical research. This award is intended to:

- support the development of new didactic programs in clinical research at institutions that do not currently offer them, or
- support the improvement or expansion of programs at institutions with existing programs.

Core of knowledge and skills common to all areas of clinical research that should form the foundation of the well-trained, independent clinical researcher. Formal course work includes:

- design of clinical research projects
- hypothesis development
- biostatistics
- epidemiology
- legal, ethical, and regulatory issues related to clinical research

K99—PATHWAY TO INDEPENDENCE AWARD

Candidate Requirements

- Postdoctoral scientists who lack sufficient research experience or institutional authority to lead an independent research program
- No more than 5 years of postgraduate research experience
- Cannot have been on NIH or non-NIH research grants exceeding $100,000 direct costs per year
- Applicant must certify they: have research entirely funded by other investigator's grants; have research conducted in another investigator's space; do not hire or supervise postdoctoral fellows or graduate students; and lack rights and privileges normally accorded to faculty

- Evaluative potential based on experience, research training background, and evidence of research creativity
- Potential to become an outstanding, successful independent investigator
- Quality of pre- and postdoctoral research training experience

Career Development Plan

- Award must contribute substantially to candidate's scientific development
- Plan must fit with the candidate's goals and prior experience
- Established need for mentoring followed by up to 3 years as an independent scientist
- Evaluation plan covering mentoring progress and transition to the independent phase
- Plans for the transition to the independent phase

Training in the Responsible Conduct of Research

- Instruction in scientific integrity and responsible conduct of research

Research Plan

- Describe research prior to and during the mentored phase and planned for the independent phase
- Appropriateness of the specific aims and viability of research goals

Mentor/Co-Mentor

- Research qualifications, scientific stature, mentoring track record
- Support for all components of application
- Research training plan, career development activities, formal course work
- Provide annual evaluations of the candidate's progress

Environment

- Adequacy of the research facilities and educational opportunities
- Commitment of institution to foster candidate's career development

T32 Grants at the NIH

Tips for Success

Linda B. Cottler

We are not what we know but what we are willing to learn.

—Mary Catherine Bateson

Improvements in the quality of life, including better treatments for medical disorders, have derived from research efforts funded by the NIH. The NIH also has been the principal funding source for training in the areas of bioinformatics, genome sequencing, and other biomedical, behavioral, and clinical research. In order to continue making great strides in diseases affecting humankind, a trained workforce of scientists is imperative.

Training the scientific workforce has been a cornerstone of the NIH since it was established by the Ransdell Act in 1930. A single institute, the NIH was directed by federal mandate to offer fellowships in basic biomedical and medical problems. In 1937, with the creation of the National Cancer Act, a National Cancer Institute was established; it funded the first training program specific to one disease. In 1944, the Public Health Services Act merged the NCI with the NIH and expanded research and training programs. This Act also broke existing divisions into institutes, which then provided a means to develop individual training and research missions.

From the 1940s to the 1960s, annual increases in the NIH budget stabilized at about 40%, which concomitantly resulted in increased training budgets. In the late 1960s, the budget increases fell to about 6% annually. By 1974, the 11 institutes under the umbrella of the NIH were authorized to fund training in multiple areas. However, in that same year the NIH also proposed a phasing out of research training and fellowship programs. In this same year, Congress, in response to growing concern about a lack of a trained workforce, enacted the National Research Act (Public Law 93-348), which consolidated training into the NRSA program (National Research Service Award), one of the most important programs of the NIH. The Act set up guidelines for training, many of which are still in use today, such as years of support limitations, imposed service obligations, and payback requirements. Over the years, the Act has been revised to allow for training in nursing, health services, and primary care research.

Around the same the NRSA program was established, the NIH began an effort to increase the training of underrepresented minorities with the MARC program (Minority Access to Research Careers). In addition, the NIH introduced research supplements to allow principal investigators to mentor minorities by adding these individuals to their existing Ro1 grants. In the mid-1990s, to mandate a diversified training program, the NIH required training program directors to describe their plans for recruiting minorities in the body of the grant proposal itself. This directive resulted in a more than fourfold increase in the number of minority trainees recruited.

Numerous sources for funding mentored training are available through the NIH. They include training supplements to grants, K awards, F awards, and the Medical Scientist Training Program. Many of these award mechanisms are described in other chapters of this book. The present chapter discusses a research mechanism called the T32 grant, recently named the Ruth L. Kirschstein National Research Service Award (NRSA) Institutional Training Grant. The chapter is meant to be useful to mentors and directors alike by providing information on the background of training grants, the components of the grant proposal mechanism, and ideas for mentors and trainees.

The tips given in this chapter are the result of my own personal experience as training director for the National Institute of Mental Health T32 for some 15 years (the T32 is in its 25th year), the director of a National Institute of Drug Abuse T32 for seven years, the Director of a Fogarty International Center training grant for three years, and directing a master degree program in psychiatric epidemiology. Additionally, I have been a charter member of the career development review committee at the National Institute on Drug Abuse, charged with reviewing all of the institute's T32s. Naturally, I would appreciate any feedback to make everyone more successful in their next submission of the T32 grant proposal (emails are available in the List of Contributors located in the back of this book).

SIGNIFICANCE OF THE NRSA SINCE ITS ESTABLISHMENT

In the 30 years of the NRSA T32 program, more than 140,000 students and young investigators have been trained by more than 450 universities, institutes, and teaching hospitals. The number of training slots has increased 40% since 1980, from 5,884 predoc and 6,173 postdoc slots to 9,308 predoc and 7,457 postdoc slots in 2003. Although slots have increased in this time period, and likewise there has been a concomitant increase in the NIH budget, the overall training budget declined from 7.9% of the extramural budget in the early 1980s to 4.3% in 1998 and 3.8% in 2003. Institutional training grants receive 84% of the NRSA training slots. As shown in table 12.1, competition for T32 grants is steadily increasing. More grants are being submitted each year, and the success rate for funding is decreasing. Little variation in these statistics is seen across the 25 NIH institutes, with the exception of the National Library of Medicine, National Institute of General Medical Sciences, National Institute of Nursing Research, and the Fogarty International Center, which spend a higher proportion of their overall extramural budgets on training.

The President's FY 2006 budget request for the NIH was $28,740 billion; the proportion of that budget spent on training was 2.9% of the extramural budget. In FY 2007 (at the publication of this book), the budget is $28,587 billion and training was 3% of that amount. In addition, congress appropriated $15 million in

TABLE 12.1   Success Rates of T32 Grants

Fiscal Year	No. Reviewed	No. Awarded	Success Rate
1996	691	395	57.2
1997	666	413	62
1998	610	398	65.2
1999	713	424	59.5
2000	741	483	65.2
2001	671	417	62.1
2002	790	456	57.7
2003	872	459	52.6
2004	932	442	47.4
2005	1,096	469	42.8
2006	957	420	43.9

Source: grants1.nih.gov/grants/award/training/train9606.htm.

the Pathways to Independence program, providing increased support for new investigators. Postdoc slots comprise 40% of most training grants; predoc slots comprise the remaining 60%.

NRSA awards are an important funding mechanism at the NIH because they

- Attract talented investigators into biomedical research
- Help direct training into specific areas of research focus that are emerging or in need of increased workforce
- Develop training guidelines and standards
- Offer trainees a chance to interact with scientists from many areas and to explore new areas of interest
- Train all trainees, and involve mentors, in the responsible conduct of science
- Offer tuition funds and stipends to trainees

In addition, the impact of NRSA on productivity of scientists has been significant. In a 1998 review of NRSA trainees, some interesting statistical trends were noted for the biomedical sciences and similar results were found for the behavioral sciences:

- NRSA trainees spent less time enrolled in graduate school compared to non-NRSA-supported students.
- 58% of NRSA trainees versus 39% of non-NRSA trainees received their doctorate by age 30.
- 37% of NRSA fellows versus 16% of non-NRSA fellows held faculty positions seven to eight years after their degree.
- 87% of NRSA fellows versus 77% of non-NRSA fellows in the same department and 72% of fellows from departments without NRSAs were in research career positions.
- NRSA fellows received grants at a higher success rate than non-NRSA fellows (67% vs. 47%).
- NRSA fellows report more publications than non-NRSA fellows.

NRSA REPORT CARD AND THEIR RESPONSE

Since 1975, Congress has been mandated to evaluate the supply of the scientific workforce, and it has relegated this activity to the National Research Council, the umbrella organization overseeing the National Academy of Sciences (NAS), the Institute of Medicine, and the National Academy of Engineering. The National Academy of Sciences issued its 12th such report in 2000, titled "Addressing the Nation's Changing Needs for Biomedical and Behavioral Scientists." The report made a number of suggestions concerning the current and future supply of scientists, future demand, and overall production of research personnel. This report is available through National Academy Press or online at www.nap.edu

(appendix 1 provides brief descriptions of this and other useful Web sites mentioned throughout the book).

In response to the National Academy Press 2000 report, the NIH determined that it would follow a number of recommendations:

- Although the NAS report recommended no growth in the number of Ph.D. doctorates awarded in the basic biomedical sciences, the NIH felt that it was not in a position to control graduate enrollment. Rather, the growth of specific areas of enrollment would be left up to individual universities.
- The NAS suggested that support for NRSA training grants at the pre- and postdoc level should be gradually increased. The NIH felt that training grants were not to be used as a way to support students; rather, they are used to support training via research project initiatives. In addition, an unpublished report reflecting the power of T32 grants indicated that trainees who received at least nine months of NRSA support were more likely to attain a faculty appointment and to apply for and receive an NIH research grant compared to colleagues without NRSA support. The NIH agreed that universities should give all trainees adequate training and career development opportunities, faculty should frequently monitor progress, and there should be adequate channels for the resolution of grievances.
- The NIH agreed that the emphasis on multidisciplinary training should be expanded.
- The NIH agreed that tracking of trainees and fellows was of relatively high importance.
- The NIH agreed that stipends and compensation should be based on educational level and experience and should be adjusted reflecting changes in the cost of living.
- Training of foreign students is vital, and research grants should support such training in the mechanism available for such training.
- Training programs should expose participants to issues associated with health disparities according to the NIH Strategic Plan to Reduce and Ultimately Eliminate Health Disparities (www.nih.gov/about/hd/strategicplan.pdf).

Areas of training interest have recently been guided by the NIH Roadmap. That Roadmap was initiated by Elias A. Zerhouni, M.D., to address issues in medical science that no single one of the NIH institutes could tackle alone. Nearly 500 scientists developed the research vision statement that the NIH is following to address New Pathways to Discovery, New Research Teams of the Future, and Re-engineering the Clinical Research Enterprise. These areas of interest directly influence priorities for T32 funding.

A BRIEF DESCRIPTION OF THE NRSA PROGRAM

It is obvious that the NRSA program is vital to the overall mission of the NIH, in that it provides predoc and postdoc research training opportunities for individuals interested in research careers in biomedical, behavioral, and clinical research.

Purpose and Background Information

As described previously in this chapter, the purpose of the NRSA research training program is to train the next generation of scientists to assume leadership roles related to the current research agenda. This has been the role of the NIH since 1974, when NRSA legislation was passed. The most up-to-date information about NRSA programs may be found at grants.nih.gov/training/nrsa/htm. Training foci include basic biomedical and clinical sciences, behavioral and social sciences, health services research, and other disciplines relevant to the NIH mission.

The training program director (TPD) at an institute or university determines the aims and goals of the grant in a specific area, determines how trainees will be selected, and develops a curriculum of study and an evaluation component. The NIH allows for a competitive stipend, the cost of tuition (which includes fees and health insurance), and other allowable costs. The specifics of each of these are addressed in more detail below, along with some very useful tips for writing a competitive T32 grant.

Special Program Objectives and Considerations

Funds Available

Because each grant application varies considerably in scope and focus, the size and respective duration of each award is different. Training directors must follow the NRSA guidelines (grant.nih.gov/grants/policy/nihgps_2003/NIHGPS_Part10.htm) and comply with Circular OMB A21 guidelines. One of the things that must be determined at the time of submission is the level of each slot requested. If more experienced fellows are expected, the stipend levels will be higher, and the budget will be higher; however, there must be compelling justification for the number and level of each trainee slot requested. Additionally, some expenses are unallowable, and it is better to know this piece of information before the grant is written rather then right before it is about to be submitted. The individual institutes each have their own mission, program goals, and initiatives that govern the funding priorities. Since these foci change over time, it is important for individuals considering submission of a T32 to consult with the appropriate contact at that NIH institute before submission (chapter 2 reiterates this important point). In fact, some NIH institutes will reject submissions if the topic is not relevant.

Allowable Costs

According to the guidelines, stipends are awarded to the trainee to help defray the costs of living expenses during the research training experience; they are based on a 12-month

Save Time
It is a good idea to consult with the gifts and grants office or sponsored projects office at your institution before getting too far into the preparation of the application.

appointment. Recipients of stipends are not employees of either the federal government or the respective funding institute (or center), and this has implications for recruiting from one's own academic institution or research think tank. As a result of the NAS report, and regular surveillance of the training pool, the NIH has increased the level of stipends by 10% each year and will continue to do so until certain target stipend levels are reached; after that, annual cost of living adjustments are anticipated. In FY 2006 (at the time this chapter was composed), the annual stipend level for a predoc was $20,772. The FY 2006 range of annual stipend levels for postdocs was from $36,996 to $51,036. For postdocs, the annual stipend is based on the number of full years after the degree was awarded (for additional regulations concerning stipend amounts, see grants2 .nih.gov/grants/guide/notice-files/NOT-OD-06-026.html).

The NIH allows a set amount of tuition, fees, and health insurance per trainee. At the time this chapter was written, the NIH had just completed a survey of the field to determine whether policies should be revised for these costs. Currently, the NIH awards 100% up to $3,000 and 60% of costs in excess of $3,000 per predoc. Tuition at the postdoc level is limited to that required for specific courses identified in the application. The NIH tuition policy can be found on the NIH Web at grants.nih.gov/training/nrsaguidelines/nrsa_toc.htm.

Trainee travel costs are the same as they were at least 20 years ago; thus, in many respects they have not kept up with the economic times and cost of living. Travel funds may be used to attend scientific meetings and workshops necessary for a training related experience. Many directors of NIH training centers stipulate that trainees must be presenting at a conference in order for travel monies to be used. Amounts for trainee travel vary throughout the NIH.

The grantee also is allowed a standard NRSA training related expense per trainee, which in FY 2006 was $2,200 annually for predocs and $3,850 annually for postdocs. These funds can be used to support staff salaries, consultant costs, equipment, research supplies, more travel for trainees, and faculty/staff travel directly related to the research training program (additional information covering regulations for training related expenses can be found at grants2.nih.gov/ grants/guide/notice-files/NOT-OD-06-026.html).

Indirect rates, or facilities and administrative allowances, cannot exceed 8% of the direct costs (exclusive of tuition and fees, health insurance, and expenditures for equipment). Institutions are allowed to supplement funds to fellows over and above the stipends provided by the NIH. These additional monies may cover teaching efforts or additional research. However, the supplemented stipend cannot in any way interfere with, detract from, or prolong the trainee's program. Only nonfederal funds can be used to provide supplementation, and formally established policies must be used to determine the amount of the supplementation. Most important, the NIH restricts the amount of time that can be compensated to a part-time basis, separate from the normal full-time research training. A full description of the NIH policy regarding NRSA supplements is available at grants1.nih.gov/grants/policy/nihgps_2003/NIHGPS_Part11.htm.

Postdocs also may be eligible for the NIH Extramural Loan Repayment Program, and the guidelines for this are available at www.lrp.nih.gov/.

Program Eligibility

Eligible Institutions

Nonprofit organizations, public, or private institutions, such as universities, colleges, hospitals, and domestic institutions, are eligible to apply for the T32 grant. Under the current guidelines, foreign institutions may not apply. NRSA grants are meant to fund institutions with a high-quality research program that have the requisite staff and facilities for the administration of the training program.

Eligible Training Program Directors

TPDs should have the skills, knowledge, and resources necessary to direct the program; individuals from underrepresented racial and ethnic groups, with disabilities, and from disadvantaged backgrounds are encouraged to apply. Because the TPD must be responsible for overseeing the NRSA, he/she should be an established basic, behavioral, and/or clinical researcher with a successful track record training junior investigators and be able to document the resources to house such a program at the institution.

Travel

It is expected that although only $1,000 is awarded for travel, the mentor will sponsor the trainee for more travel opportunities from grants.

Other Employment

Trainees should not enter the T32 with the idea that they will be able to keep up another paying job because the traineeship is a full-time job in and of itself. However, if the trainee finds that periodically there is another pursuit that is time limited and can pay additional funds, he/she can be allowed to pursue it. Close monitoring is important to be sure that the trainee is not overextended.

Institutional Eligibility

It is also important that your institution be aware of information related to program eligibility, travel, and compensation before submitting the grant to avoid any disappointments later.

Trainees

Methods for appointing trainees to the program must be adequately described in the grant. Each trainee must be willing to commit 40 hours per week to the program. Trainees must be citizens or noncitizen nationals of the United States, or must have been lawfully admitted to the United States for permanent residence, that is, in possession of a currently valid Alien Registration Receipt Card (I-551) or some other legal verification of legal admission as a permanent resident. Persons on temporary or student visas are not eligible for the Ruth L. Kirschstein NRSA support. Additional eligibility criteria exist for predocs. Predocs must be individuals with a baccalaureate degree in training at the graduate level, who are enrolled in a Ph.D. or equivalent doctoral degree program. Health-professional students, graduate students in quantitative science, and postgraduate clinical trainees wanting to interrupt their studies for a year or more to pursue full-time research training before completing their formal training programs are also eligible. Postdocs who can produce official documentation that all degree requirements have been met are eligible. They must agree to specialized training in one of the areas that meet national research priorities in the biomedical, behavioral, or clinical sciences.

> ***Training Program Directors***
> The grant should elaborate substantially on the track record of the TPD. This is not the time to be bashful.

Some TPD request funds for short-term positions, during either the summer or other short periods, for medical, dental, or other allied health students. These monies also cover graduate students in the physical or quantitative sciences. These short-term slots provide students with a brief exposure period but are intended to attract them into the research area. Specific guidelines for short-term training, including the support timeline (8–12 weeks) can be found at grants.nih.gov/grants/guide/pa-files/PA-05-117.html.

Trainees cannot receive more than five years of combined NRSA support at the predoc level or three years of postdoc support, including any combination of support from any institutional training or individual fellowship awards (F awards). The Tax Reform Act of 1986 (Public Law 99-154) states that nondegree candidates are now required to report in their gross income all stipends and any money paid on their behalf for course tuition and fees required for attendance.

> ***Tip***
> The National Postsecondary Student Aid Survey (NPSAS) data for 2000 indicate that the average graduate student is 33 years old and that nearly one quarter (23%) of all graduate students are over 40. The result is that these older students have family responsibilities and bring prior work experience. These data can affect the recruitment and retention of trainees today who have important marital, family, and professional commitments. And yet, with funding levels at the NIH reduced, training positions become more attractive, especially among the older cohorts.

Degree candidates can exclude from their taxable income any expenses such as fees, books, supplies, and equipment.

As specified in the NIH Revitalization Act of 1993, Ruth L. Kirschstein NRSA awardees are mandated to a payback obligation for the first 12 months of postdoc support. However, the second year of training support fulfills the payback obligation.

Payback Obligation

TPDs must be sure postdoctoral students understand this criterion or else they may find people applying who just want to find something to do for a year while they search for a job opportunity, or reapply for a grant. They cannot just complete one year and move on without a significant financial penalty.

Application and Submission Information

Application

Applicants considering the NRSA grant should follow the current PHS 398 research grant application instructions and forms, which can be found at grants .nih.gov/grants/funding/phs398/phs398.pdf. Keep in mind that there are separate guidelines for T32s. The title and number of this funding opportunity must be typed on line 2 of the face page of the application form and the YES box must be checked.

Each of the NIH institutes has its own criteria for submitting a T32 grant, which are appended to the overall T32 guidelines; also, there are new standard dates for grant submissions in FY 2007, which can be found at grants.nih.gov/grants/guide/notice-files/NOT-OD-07-001.html.

Research Training Program

The write-up of the training program should include plans to provide both hands on apprenticeship-style training in the lab or clinic as well as formal didactic training. The NIH guidelines specifically state that this should include a plan for monitoring a trainee's progress to accomplish their training goals. Areas to cover include skills in understanding research, applying abilities to conduct research, identifying problems in the process of conducting research, raising questions, and

---

Tip

Applicants should follow the guidelines faithfully. If the guidelines state that a table on X or Y is needed, do the table exactly as the guidelines state it should be done. Reviewers will be looking for the required tables, in the stated format, and since many reviewers are TPDs, they are acutely aware of the requirements. The T32 requires numerous tables and many necessitate historical data from faculty that take considerable time to collect and prepare. It is prudent that applicants collect and collate these materials as early as possible.

proposing solutions to resolving problems. NRSA trainees should receive professional development skills specifically in grant writing, as well as instruction in laboratory and project management. The past record of the training program is also used to assess the merit of the application. The record usually describes the past training history of the program, management, leadership, and administrative qualities and performance of the program director and, likewise, the performance of the designated preceptors/mentors. The information contained in this portion of the application usually describes the current funding of the trainee, successful completion of educational or professional training programs, further career advancement such as receipt of fellowships, careers awards, training appointments, and related accomplishments. Evidence of successful careers includes competition for research grants, receipt of honors or awards, publication record, receipt of patents, nominations to committees, and current academic, university committee, or professional appointments (e.g., chair and/or leadership positions at various professional organizations).

Program Director

The TPD should have the scientific background, leadership, and administrative capabilities to direct a research training program. The TPD is responsible for determining the selection and appointment process for trainees, for the overall direction of the program, and for the program evaluation. Directors must complete the forms in a timely manner and inform the trainees of all requirements.

Research Environment/Resources

The grantee institution must document a strong research program in the area proposed with adequate mentors and preceptors to carry out the work. Additionally, the institution must document a commitment to the proposed research training program's goals, by providing assurance that the program will be integrated into its infrastructure.

Tip

Program directors should meet each and every trainee who is admitted to their program. They should also meet regularly with the trainees both together as a group and individually to build rapport and provide professional guidance. Monthly lunchtime or research discussion meetings represent a good way to keep in touch with the trainees in the program. Yearly meetings with the trainees individually are a good way to assess the progress of each trainee. It is a good idea for the mentor to rate the trainee, and likewise, the trainee should rate the mentor. The TPD should review the evaluations with the mentor and the trainee, separately. Such insight is useful for improving the program and helping evaluate the mentor's outreach to trainees beyond their immediate research skills.

Tip

Program directors should consider including in their application a statement from their chancellor, dean, and department head describing the financial or other logistical support for the program. These letters could include information on space given for the trainees and fellows, laboratory facilities and equipment, plans for curriculum development such as teaching the "art" of grant writing, publishing tips, release time for the program director and mentors, and any other resources to enhance the research training program. If there is other training programs in the department or located around the institution, it would be a good idea for the TPD, dean and other figurehead to explain how the interaction of the programs enhances the goals of the institution.

Evaluation and Tracking Component

T32 grants are now required to provide a detailed and well-defined plan outlining the methods used for evaluation and tracking trainees over time. Training directors must submit their system for tracking trainees for a period of 10 years after completing the program. This is one of the major benchmarks used to determine success or failure of the program. Thus, each trainee enrolled in the program must be able to provide to the director, for a period of 10 years, what articles they have published, what grants they have received, where they are working currently, and their positional title. These measures must be described in detail in the annual progress report, in future competing continuation applications, and as part of the final progress report.

Recruitment Plan

Training directors must submit a detailed plan for recruiting both local and nonlocal trainees. For each applicant, the director must track a number of criteria, including race/ethnicity. Directors also must report whether the trainee was offered admission, and if so, if the trainee accepted. For predocs, a number of other criteria are necessary, including Graduate Record Examination (GRE) scores. The GRE scores must be maintained on file for a number of years to report in the application. As described in the background section above, the NIH recognizes that minority recruitment has been seriously lagging, and this may

Tip

It is a great idea to ask trainees when they leave the program for "tracking and locating" data, just as one would do for study respondents. The most important question is: "What is the name and number of a person who will always know your whereabouts?" With this information, you can track and locate nearly all trainees for the period of 10 years. Also, it is a good idea to try to locate them annually for ongoing updates. It is also a good idea to encourage exit interviews to monitor the program and seek advice from trainees in order to improve the program.

contribute to health education disparities at the professional levels. As a result, the NIH determined that each program would need to provide details on how to promote diversity in the biomedical, behavioral, clinical, and social sciences workforce. While recent census figures show a growing diversity among the general population (12.9% of the population reports being black alone or in combination with one or more other races), 8.9% of the graduate school population reports being black. Similarly, 1.5% of the population in the 2000 census reported being American Indian or Alaska Native, while 0.5% comprises the overall graduate school population. Health problems among these underrepresented minority populations are increasing and thus these populations may be underserved if they cannot attract highly trained professionals to return services to their communities. The NIH suggested that to address these problems, more minority scientists in these fields and more minority and nonminority investigators were needed to turn their attention and research focus to disparities in health.

As a result, each T32 grant proposal must document how it will diversify student and faculty populations and increase the participation of individuals from underrepresented racial and ethnic groups especially those shown by the National Science Foundation to be underrepresented in health-related sciences (see www.nsf.gov/statistics/). The program also must show how it will improve recruitment of individuals with a physical or mental impairment who are limited in one or more major life activities. Additionally, programs should recruit persons from disadvantaged backgrounds, meaning those with an annual income below established low-income thresholds as determined by the government (see aspe.hhs.gov/poverty/indix.shtml). Finally, persons from social, cultural, or educational environments are also encouraged to apply, including persons from certain rural or inner-city environments that have been inhibited from participating. The renewal applications must include details on how to encourage recruitment of minority scholars.

Connections that may increase minority recruitment include the NIH Black Scientists Association (bsa.od.nih.gov/), the National Name Exchange Program, and the Western Name Exchange Program. The latter two involve a consortium of 29 universities that annually collect and exchange names of talented under-

---

✎Tip

At the present time, proposals are not scored on the actual recruitment plans; however, in the future, these plans may be included in the overall evaluation process. Currently, if the recruitment and retention plan to enhance diversity is judged to be unacceptable, there is a bar to funding that cannot be removed until an acceptable plan has been submitted. The determination of acceptable is made by the NIH institute that will eventually fund the proposal. If the proposal is received without a plan, it could be returned without review.

represented ethnic minority students who are in their junior or senior year of their undergraduate education. These efforts exist to identify talented pools of students eligible for recruitment to graduate level programs. An effort called GO-MAP has facilitated access to the database for both programs since the mid-1980s. Additionally, the McNair Scholars Database Directory exists for sharing the names, addresses, majors, and areas of interest for seniors who will graduate in December and May. The names come from the students who have applied for the McNair Postbaccalaureate Program for low-income first-generation college students and students underrepresented in graduate education. The database is distributed to all graduate school deans in the country for use in recruitment.

Other ideas include gathering names from Project 1000, and the NIH-MARC STAR programs. Students' names can be obtained and phone calls can be made to begin the recruitment process. Accomplishments of students in the program should be provided on the Web site, with testimonials about their experiences. The program also can be advertised to targeted populations in colleges and universities that serve underrepresented students to increase the applicant pool. Mailings can be sent to undergraduate departments in your discipline, particularly targeting schools with underrepresented students, especially at historically black colleges and universities, Hispanic-serving institutions, and tribal colleges.

Training in the Responsible Conduct of Research

Since July 1990, the NIH has required that all training grants and mentored K proposals submitted include plans for the instruction in the responsible conduct of research. Applications must include a description of instruction in scientific integrity. Applications without such plans will not be reviewed.

Areas that must be covered are documented in the proposal and include conflict of interest, responsible authorship, policies for handling misconduct, data management, data sharing, and policies regarding the use of human and

---

Tip

Because the NIH encourages institutions to provide instruction in the responsible conduct of research to all graduate students, postdocs, and research staff regardless of their source of support, mentors must make this a priority. Ideas for mentoring might include sitting in on a local human studies committee (institutional review board) to actively participate in the ethical conduct of science or, if allowed, joining the institutional review board. Also, trainees should actively pursue institutional responsible conduct of research (RCR) activities either using the Internet or in person and seek a role model who values this training. The NIDA-K committee that reviews all T32 grant applications actually requires ongoing training and a substantial plan to be documented. That committee would score as inappropriate those applications that specify only using HIPAA training or a prior course in ethics. For more information, see grants1.nih.gov/grants/guide/notice-files/not92-236.html. The Office of Research Integrity also has considerable Web-based resources for use by T32 directors at ori.dhhs.gov/.

animal subjects. Plans must be detailed enough to address the topic, the format, participation of faculty who attends the training, and the frequency of the program.

Review Criteria

The appropriate scientific review groups are convened in accordance with standard peer review procedures from the NIH (see www.csr.nih.gov/refrev .htm). These committees evaluate applications for scientific and technical merit according to the guidelines of the NRSA. Following the NIH review guidelines, generally only the top half is reviewed, and assigned a priority score. The NIH review guidelines are very detailed and must be followed exactly. Tables are now formatted for the applicant; they should be utilized for all submissions in exactly the format given. According to the guidelines, the following issues are pertinent when making funding decisions:

- The scientific merit of the proposed project as determined by peer review
- The relevance of the program priorities
- The availability of funds
- Diversity of the pool of trainees

In many of the NIH institutes, T32 grants are not reviewed by a committee solely dedicated to T32 or training mechanisms. As a result, reviewers may not be aware of the specific nuances regarding review guidelines or the explicit explanation of the tables needed. Therefore, applicants would be advised that they should briefly explain the various tables. Proposals are scored on the following issues (taken directly from the NIH criteria):

Training Program

Are the objectives, design, and direction of the proposed research training program appropriate? Does the proposed program provide suitable training for the levels of trainees being proposed and the area of science to be supported by the program? Is the quality of proposed course contents and training experience appropriate for all levels of trainees to be included in the program? Are inter- and multidisciplinary and interprofessional research training opportunities or novel concepts, approaches, methodologies, or technologies appropriately utilized?

Training Program Director

Questions will arise during review whether the program director has the scientific background, expertise, and experience appropriate to direct,

Training Program

For the training program criterion, the applicant must show the expertise of each faculty member, the courses that are offered specifically for these trainees, and the grants that each faculty member has active or pending.

manage, coordinate, and administer the proposed research training program. Reviewers are concerned with whether the training program director plans to commit adequate time to the program.

Preceptors/Mentors

Is the caliber of preceptors/mentors as researchers, including successful competition for research support in areas directly related to the proposed research training program, appropriate for their role in the training program? Are there a sufficient number of experienced mentors with appropriate expertise and funding available at the applicant institution to support the number of trainees and levels of trainees being proposed in the application?

Training Program Director

The section on the program director should include detailed plans on the organizational structure of the training program, including how the program will be managed, who will help select the trainees, how trainees will be monitored, how they will select their mentor, and so forth. One unique aspect of some training grants is the appointment of an ombudsperson—someone who is appointed by the director to discuss complaints and resolve issues.

Past Training Record

Is the past research training record of the program, the program director, and designated preceptors/mentors appropriate? How successful are former trainees in seeking further career development and in establishing productive scientific careers? Statistically speaking, NRSA graduates are more likely to find employment in faculty and research positions. However, the evaluation of a T32 grant focuses exclusively on whether the pending application shows credibly their training program will fit this mold. Specifically, the review addresses whether there is evidence of successful completion of programs, receipt of subsequent fellowships and/or career awards, further training appointments, and similar accomplishments. Is there evidence of a productive scientific career among trainees who graduate, such as a record of successful competition for research grants, receipt of special honors or award, a record of publications, receipt of patents, promotion to scientific positions, and any other measure of success consistent with the nature and duration of the training received. What is the track record of proposed mentors in similar research training programs? Is there a record in retaining health-professional postdocs (i.e., individuals with the M.D., D.O., D.D.S., D.N.Sc., etc.) for at least two years in research training or other research activities, if appropriate?

Preceptors/Mentors

To review the preceptor/mentor criterion, reviewers will want to see the publications and current or any future (pending) grant support of the faculty as well as a complete discussion canvassing the nature of their collaborative relationships.

Tip

Data on past training records should be available from the required tables. Reviewers are concerned with how successful a program is at filling the training slots. Because slots can be filled any time from July 1 through June 30 of that funding year, it is important for the applicant who is going in for a renewal to state that slot X will be filled by June 30 of that year so that reviewers do not "ding" the applicant for unused slots. However, if a slot has not been filled in a previous year or if a trainee has left before 12 months, there should be adequate justification given.

Institutional Training Environment, Commitment, and Resources

Here, reviewers are concerned with the quality of the research environment for the proposed research training program. Questions arise during review regarding the level of institutional commitment, quality of available facilities, and suitability of courses, research experiences, and research training support. Is the proposed program slotted to be an integral component of the applicant institution's overall research program/mission?

Trainee Recruitment, Selection, and Retention Plan

Reviewers deliberate whether the quality of the applicant pool and plans for the selection and retention of individuals appointed to the training program are appropriate. Specifically, what is the size and quality of the applicant pool? Are the recruiting procedures, trainee selection criteria, and retention strategies appropriate and well defined? Are there advertising plans or other effective strategies in place or anticipated to recruit high-quality trainees? For competing renewal applications reviewers will want to address how successful the program has been regarding efforts to recruit and retain individuals from diverse underrepresented populations?

Institutional Support

Institutional information will be extracted from the letters of support included with the application. Letters should be specific and not generic.

Institutional Diversity

Reviewers like to see that trainees come from institutions other than the sponsoring institution and that they are not all being trained by the same individual.

Evaluation and Tracking Plan

Reviewers want to see there is an adequate evaluation plan and that it is sufficiently detailed to track career outcomes of trainees. This information is highly informative whether the program is successful. Does the evaluation plan include a system for tracking participants following program completion, such as publications, grant proposals, and awards, and is there a systematic means to plot career trajectories of supported trainees? For competing renewal applications reviewers want to know if there are plans to make changes that improve program performance and the assessment of outcomes. Competing renewal applications must describe the program accomplishments to date, following the application instructions, including the evaluation and outcome measures report. In addition to these above stated criteria, applications that request short-term research training positions also are assessed using the following criteria: Is the quality of the proposed short-term research training program appropriate? Are the commitment and availability of the participating faculty, program design, availability of research support, and training environment well suited for short-term training? Does the program have access to candidates for short-term research training and the ability to recruit high quality, short-term trainees from the applicant institution or some other health-professional school? Does the research training program include features that might be expected to persuade short-term trainees to consider careers in health-related research? What is the effect of the short-term training program on the quality of the regular research training program or any existing, stand-alone short-term research training program? Are the number of short-term positions, and the plan to integrate the short-term training program into the regular research training programs appropriate? Is there a plan to follow the careers of short-term trainees and to assess the effect of the training program on subsequent career choices? For competing continuation applications, what is the success in attracting students back for multiple appointments?

Protection of Human Subjects From Research Risk

The applicant must assure that with the involvement of human subjects, participants will be protected from research risk.

Inclusion of Women, Minorities, and Children in Research

The applicant must ensure adequate plans to include type of gender, as well as all racial and ethnic groups (and subgroups), and children as appropriate for the scientific goals of the research. Plans for the recruitment and retention of subjects also will be evaluated.

Care and Use of Vertebrate Animals in Research

If vertebrate animals are to be used in any project, five items are assessed, as outlined in the guidelines.

Biohazards

If materials or procedures are proposed that are potentially hazardous to research personnel and/or the environment, the reviewers must determine if the proposed protection is adequate.

Additional Issues

Budget

Reviewers assess how reasonable the proposed budget is; for a T32, this translates to the stipend level requested and the number of slots.

Leave Policies

Trainees receive vacation and holidays at the same rate as persons in comparable training positions at the

Trainees

If this is a new submission, the applicant must demonstrate that the program will be able to recruit and sustain the number of training slots requested, as well as the level of training proposed. For example, if six slots are requested, all at level 5 (six years or more post-Ph.D.), the applicant must demonstrate that it will be possible to recruit six trainees, all of whom are experienced and well along in their career.

institution. Summers are still considered active research periods. Trainees may receive stipends for up to 15 calendar days of sick leave per year, which can be used for medical conditions including time off for pregnancy and childbirth. A period of terminal leave is not allowable. Guidelines are posted at grants1 .nih.gov/grants/policy/nihgps_2003/NIHGPS_Part11.htm.

FINAL THOUGHTS ON THE MATTER OF T32 GRANTS

In 2003, the scientific research society Sigma Xi launched a survey of postdocs to better understand the full scope of issues regarding graduate training opportunities around the United States. Out of 174 institutions invited, 46 participated, including 18 of 20 top tier employers. Responses were even obtained from persons working inside the NIH. Through email, 22,000 postdocs were invited to participate; 34% did (sampling error was less than 1%; see postdoc.sigmaxi.org for extensive demographics of the sample). Highlights of the survey results indicate that 75% of the institutions had an administrative office for training. About 70% of trainees reported being satisfied overall with their current experience, with unhappiness stemming from low wages, lack of benefits, and a mismatch between expectations and outcomes. In about 25% of the cases, trainees did not consider their advisor to be a mentor. A little less than one-third of the trainees reported receiving no training in research ethics (31%) or proposal writing (37%). Two-thirds reported no training in negotiating skills.

Training directors are going to have to do much better, in this era of multidisciplinary translational research. With organizations becoming much more loosely coupled, institutions are going to need to give more structured oversight and provide more formal training. Postdocs reporting the highest amount of structured oversight and formal training were more likely to be satisfied, to give mentors high ratings, to have low numbers of conflicts, and to publish more papers than are postdocs with less oversight and training.

Recently, substance abuse researchers gathered for a conference titled Reflections on 40 Years of Substance Abuse Research. Many fields of science were represented, including ethnography, pharmacology, epidemiology, treatment, neuroscience, and prevention. Many of those in attendance were training directors currently or previously. The original title of the meeting was going to be the "Gray Beards Conference" to reflect the graying or aging of the field. It estimated that 30% of investigators will retire over the next decade—in all fields of science. This number may be an underestimate for physicians but is alarming nonetheless. As the field moves forward with retirements and job vacancies, training the next generation of scientists is becoming more important than ever. Let's hope the NIH agrees.

FINAL TIPS FOR SUCCESS

- Follow all of the T32 instructions exactly
- Have a good training program director
- Enlist great mentors who love to mentor
- Document all of your and their successes
- Contact the NIH institute for ideas and information

And until e-submission is accepted for T32s, get a big box, because the grant applications are very large!

SBIR Funding

A Unique Opportunity for the Entrepreneurial Researcher

Jeffrey A. Hoffman, Susanna Nemes, & William B. Hansen

The will to brilliance never leads to the greatest insights, only simplicity does that.

—Lou Andreas-Salomé

THE SMALL BUSINESS Innovation Research (SBIR) program represents a unique federal funding program that, as of 2005, has been awarding more than $2 billion of grants and contracts annually. Federal agencies with extramural research budgets of more than $100 million are required to administer SBIR programs using an annual set-aside of 2.5% for small businesses. These monies are intended to stimulate research and development of innovative products or services that have the potential for commercialization and public benefit. Small businesses are defined as for-profit companies with fewer than 500 employees. Currently, 11 federal agencies participate in the SBIR program: the Departments of Health and Human Services (DHHS), Agriculture (USDA), Commerce (DOC), Defense (DOD), Education (DoED), Energy (DOE), Homeland Security (DHS), and Transportation (DOT); the Environmental Protection Agency (EPA); the National Aeronautics and Space Administration (NASA); and the National Science Foundation (NSF).

The Small Business Technology Transfer (STTR) program is a related set-aside program to facilitate cooperative research and development between small businesses and U.S. universities or nonprofit research institutions funded by federal agencies with extramural research and development budgets of more than $1 billion, using 0.3% of their budget. Currently, five federal agencies participate in the STTR program: DOD, DOE, DHHS (NIH), NASA, and NSF. The intent of both the SBIR and STTR programs is to facilitate research and development of innovative products and transfer this technology from the research setting into the commercial marketplace. Small businesses are a pivotal hub for the transfer of research-based technology from the "laboratory to the living room." Although most of the general principals of writing grant applications for the SBIR and STTR are similar, there are some different requirements associated with SBIR and STTR programs that investigators should carefully consider by reading the current solicitation for each funding mechanism prior to any grant preparation. In this chapter, we focus primarily on SBIR grant applications that may or may not include collaboration with research institutions.

SBIR PROGRAM OVERVIEW

Program Background

The SBIR and STTR programs represent different sources of financial support than other grant opportunities that exist in the NIH portfolio of funding mechanisms. The SBIR and STTR funding mechanisms specifically require involvement of small for-profit businesses. This noted difference from other possible funding avenues is small, but not trivial. The goal of the SBIR/STTR program is to build capacity for technology transfer through entrepreneurship and influence the marketplace with new technology that can advance science. This stands in stark contrast to other funding mechanisms that seek to advance knowledge without considering the effect of technological enhancements on the marketplace.

An important consideration in the SBIR process is why the government actively seeks to foster technological development in the marketplace. One of the cardinal responses to this question is based broadly in a philosophy shared by members of Congress and supported by many presidential administrations. The philosophical position suggests that the translation of science and research findings to practical applications, particularly those that benefit directly people, requires a broker, agent, or company to initiate technology transfer. This philosophy includes an unspoken, unwritten assumption that, while knowledge generation should be for the public good, government agencies are not the ideal mechanism for making knowledge functional in solving health and other problems. Indeed, the opposite is quite often true: Government is usually an inefficient mechanism for managing emerging technologies. The private sector simply does a much better job. The SBIR/STTR program recognizes that entrepreneurs are the means by which advances in knowledge are able to find their way into daily life.

A historical case in point helps illustrate the importance of SBIR funding. The SBIR program started with a pilot project funded in 1977 through NSF and under the inspiration of Roland Tibbetts. During the second round of reviews (submitted in 1978), a small firm applied for SBIR funding in order to develop a computational method for alphabetizing lists on a personal computer. It should be recalled that the Apple I was introduced in 1976, the Apple II was introduced to the market a year later, and at this historical juncture in time, few people owned computers. Personal computers were novelties with limited if any application software and only rudimentary (by today's standards) operating systems. So, when the reviewers considered the proposal, they had doubts that software to complete this task could actually be developed. Nonetheless, the project was deemed innovative and funding was awarded. The small business that received funding took the name Symantec and, within the short period of six years, developed Q&A Software, their first product. Today, of course, Symantec is regarded as a giant in the computing industry, having engineered a wide range of highly useful and protective antivirus software applications. In many respects, the company owes its humble beginnings to SBIR funding. Interestingly, the small seed funds provided to the company have been more than repaid to the government in the form of business tax revenues.

Of course, not every small company that receives SBIR startup funds has a similar success story. Running a small business for an SBIR-funded company is much the same as running a small business supported by any other kind of funding. Long-term success is determined by the company's ability to attract capital either through investment or production. Without a flow of capital sufficient to cover expenses, any business will fail. What companies need in addition to funding includes a clearly defined vision of the future, the potential to create products and services that someone wants and can pay for, the ability to manage day-to-day operations, the ability to fulfill orders once they arrive, and the ability to respond to a changing market place. The history of SBIR/STTR has a long list of successes to brag about. However, like any other field, there is a longer list of companies that received one or two SBIR grants and then disappeared off the radar screen, never to be heard from again.

Company Models

Before you apply for an SBIR or STTR, consider why you want to go down this road. Once thought of as low prestige, SBIR/STTR funding has now become as difficult to obtain as funding for an R01 or independent investigator research grants. There are other ways of getting funding that may be better suited to what you want to do. We have seen several different models of pursuing SBIRs/STTRs that you may wish to consider. Below we briefly review these models.

Model 1: The Breakaway Company

This is the model the three authors of this chapter have pursued. All three of us started companies, Danya International, Social Solutions International, and Tanglewood Research, which were intended to be our sole livelihood. In our situations, getting SBIR funding is a part of our make-it or break-it mentality. We left academia behind, or never put our foot in the academic door in the first place, because we started with a vision that did not fit the mold of purely academic responsibilities. Breakaway companies typically cast away from other moorings as quickly as they can. They become the full-time employment of their founders and plan to survive based on hard work and creative thinking. Breakaway companies involve a great deal of risk and little front-end security. However, despite the risk, we view such companies as having the greatest potential for long-term success. Everyone who comes to work for such a company typically adopts the attitude of the leader and begins aggressively developing new products and services. These companies learn very quickly the concept of a customer—a word rarely understood by researchers from an academic background. Successful breakaway companies maintain a clear vision of what they can become that spans the next decade or beyond.

Model 2: The Tethered Company

This model of company is typically created by someone who has a commitment to pursuing academic goals—or has such a lucrative academic position that he or she chooses not to leave. The tethered company becomes a way of marketing products and services for which there exists a viable market on the side and usually outside of academia. The rule that requires the principal investigator (PI) to be more than 50% time with the small business creates a challenge for these people. Because these companies are sideline businesses for usually very talented researchers who are faculty at some prestigious academic learning center, it is often the case that the key person in the company hires someone else to be principal investigator of their SBIR/STTR projects. Our view is that such companies may have limited potential for long-term sustained growth. A company designed along this model approach can survive if there is a ready-made market for the limited numbers of products and services such companies are likely to create. It is also possible that a tethered company will produce a few products that will be bought out by someone else. However, our experience is that the tethered company employees will either soon adopt the less than full commitment and attitude of the part-time leader or, if they are ambitious, will leave to start their own companies. Nonetheless, this type of company is ideal for a researcher who has ideas and research that can be turned into easily marketed products. Also, if the researcher would like to see the company go more in the direction of a breakaway company, she or he may want to partner with someone possessing an advanced business degree (i.e., MBA) or relevant business experience to manage day-to-day operations of the company. Keep in mind, though, that manning the helm of a company designed to harness the energies of several independent researchers provides its own challenges. One overriding challenge arises because of certain demands in the work environment. For instance, workers must maintain a high level of creativity and at the same time instigate a successful research environment based on tried-and-true scientific methods and analytic practices. The end result is a group of independent investigators that tend to be a quirky if not eccentric bunch.

Model 3: The Remora Approach

Remoras (a member of the genus Perciformes and family Echeneidae) are tropical fish 30 to 90 cm long that attach to sharks or other large aquatic creatures, including whales, manta rays, stingrays, and sea turtles. Remoras create a suckerlike motion with their dorsal fins to attach to the skin of larger marine fish. The remora's claim to biologic fame is that it provides small services to the larger transport fish, including cleaning off dead skin and removing parasites in exchange for a place to live. The symbiotic interaction (also called phoresy or commensalism) of the remora and its host also exists in the business world. Often, an investigator not affiliated with a for-profit small business seeks to attach his/her work effort to an existing business entity. The STTR grant mechanism fits this business model quite well. The investigator attaches to a specific company using one of the two business models already mentioned. The company zeitgeist or corporate ethos will maintain similar long-term operating goals and succeed much as we described for the tethered or breakaway company models. For example, several of us have met and worked with academic researchers who have very interesting ideas about new products but do not have the energy or interest to start their own businesses. They are probably wise in deciding not to initiate a breakaway or tethered company, both of which require extensive effort and time commitment. What the academic desires is a cost-effective means to transform their ideas into something they might use to make a little money on the side. Sometimes the ideas are really interesting and are unchallenged in the market place—a new approach that inherently has some market potential.

Remora business endeavors have a reduced chance of long-term success in the SBIR/STTR business for several reasons. They face certain challenges because the leader of the project often lacks one of the key ingredients of success (a clear vision of the future, the potential to create products and services that someone wants and can pay for, the ability to manage day-to-day operations, the ability to fulfill orders once they arrive, or the ability to respond to a changing market place). If a project is funded using a remora business model, the smaller company's success depends largely on the more enterprising company that provides the "ride." In other words, the remora business approach necessitates attaching a smaller company to a larger company with the intention of some service or information "exchange." There is rarely a long-term commitment from the host to carry the project beyond its funded period. Furthermore, executive staff working at the host business and investigators at the remora must conduct extensive negotiations about profit sharing, fulfillment, branding, and so forth, before the product created can survive in the market place. Each of these issues has the potential to sink or seriously put into jeopardy a deal. Success, we are reminded, is hard to achieve even when natural advantages exist in abundance. Having barriers to overcome can severely limit a company's potential for success.

Leaders of breakaway and tethered companies need to carefully consider the benefits and challenges of working with remora researchers. On the plus side, if the remora researcher truly has novel ideas that can turn into marketable products, an SBIR/STTR grant may turn into a stepping stone for personnel recruitment. On the other hand, if extensive babysitting is needed, if you are constantly distracted from your own pursuit to deal with human resource and personality "issues," you may want to avoid the remora. It all depends on the degree to which a symbiotic business relationship can be established and the plusses outweigh the minuses.

Based on the business model descriptions provided above, there are several pieces of advice worth noting. First, before investigators start down the SBIR/STTR road, they should examine not only their ability to write a decent proposal, but also their ability to start, grow, and manage a business. A series of questions may help to clarify our meaning here with regard to suitability. Do others around you—including your partner, spouse, or other support system— have confidence in your abilities? Do you have adequate (if any) resources to survive without continuous funding? Can you describe your vision of your company beyond what the next grant or contract is about? Do you know how to build a strong team and manage a diverse group of people? Can you meet a payroll, pay taxes, and offer an attractive slate of fringe benefits (e.g., medical, dental, and life insurance, 401k or annuity options, and flexible benefits spending plans)? Have you had enough adversity in your life that you have successfully overcome to have confidence that you will deal well with future challenges? Are you someone who can get things done? Are you lucky? (Luck has been described as what happens when preparation meets opportunity.) These are all questions an investigator should ask and answer honestly as they travel a path toward deciding whether they are suitable for SBIR/STTR funding and an SBIR/STTR lifestyle.

Perhaps the best piece of advice, which represents the collection of all our own personal trials with SBIR funding, suggests that if there exists an easier method to accomplish your research goals, you should consider it. Unlike R01 researchers who face their primary challenges getting funded and then getting published, SBIR/STTR researchers must face not only the challenge of getting funded, but also the added challenge of building a successful business operation that can bring their intellectual creations to market. Both challenges go hand in hand and cannot be separated, especially since the intellectual bench science and creative work necessitate a marketing and business mentality.

Small Business Requirements

There are a number of other critical requirements and specific variations to the SBIR program that should be noted. To remain eligible the small business concern applying for an SBIR/STTR grant, must be at least 51% owned and controlled by one or more individuals who are citizens or permanent residents of, or permanent resident aliens in, the United States; or (for SBIR only) it is a for-profit business concern that is at least 51% owned and controlled by another for-profit business concern that is at least 51% owned and controlled by one or more individuals who are citizens of, or permanent resident aliens in, the United States. In addition, generally, all SBIR/STTR research must be performed in its entirety within the United States.

Furthermore, SBIR and STTR grants have strict performance guidelines for. For instance, the PI is the individual, identified in the grant application, responsible for scientific oversight, administrative leadership, and technical direction for the project. At the time of award and during the conduct of the proposed project, the *primary employment* of the PI receiving an SBIR grant must be *with the small business concern* listed as one of the performance sites. Primary employment means that at least 51% of the PI's time is spent in the employ of the small business concern, and this precludes full-time employment at another organization. For STTR grants, the PI must commit a minimum of 10% effort to the project and the PI/project director must have a formal appointment with or commitment to the small business concern listed in the application, and this must be officially documented.

The PI must possess sufficient qualifications to assume a leadership role (scientifically and administratively) or include other investigators who complement the PI's professional qualifications. It is recommended that if the PI does not have a graduate-level degree, preferably a Ph.D. or M.D., another member of the team should have an advanced graduate degree along with considerable research and business expertise in order to oversee the evaluation of the product. The person with the research expertise can be included on the team as a co-investigator or as an expert consultant. There are no restrictions on the co-investigator's affiliation with the small business or the percentage effort that co-investigators needs to spend on the project, but this time commitment should be realistic based on the tasks they will be performing. Although review committees generally have somewhat less rigorous academic standards for the qualifications of the PI for an SBIR grant than for R01 grants, such as not requiring a Ph.D., M.D., or advanced graduate degree or, related to this acumen, a high number of peer-reviewed publications, the PI and co-Investigators should have a track record of success in an area of research and/or product development relevant to the application.

Phases

The SBIR funding program is organized in three performance phases. Phase I is intended to establish the technical merit and feasibility of a proposed product or service. Phase I is generally awarded for a six-month period with a funding ceiling of $100,000. Requests for funds exceeding this amount or a time period longer than six months need to be well justified. During Phase I, some type of prototype is generally developed and evaluated on a pilot basis to determine the feasibility of proceeding to Phase II. Phase II generally entails the full development of a product over a period of up to two years with a budget of up to $750,000. A longer time period and/or additional funds can be requested but will require a clear justification. During Phase II, a more rigorous evaluation of the product is generally conducted. These are general guidelines but the specific requirements are determined by agency and exceptions are also allowed with permission from the agency. In most cases, both the Phase I and Phase II projects can receive no-cost extensions. No-cost extensions generally allow continued research or development activity, which rely on unexpended direct cost dollars from a previous funding cycle (i.e., no more money but more time). Phase III is the commercialization phase and entails the commercial marketing and distribution of the product by the small business. Some agencies provide some minimal support or technical assistance for Phase III. Generally, the small business is responsible for the funding of this phase but may seek other sources of capital or partnerships for this commercialization phase.

Fast-Track Mechanism

Another variation of the application process for some agencies including NIH is the fast-track mechanism. This mechanism allows applicants to submit the Phase I and Phase II applications simultaneously, along with a more detailed commercialization plan. The purpose of the fast-track mechanism is to reduce the period of time between Phase I and Phase II. The time period between the two phases can be at least a year, and possibly longer if reapplication for funding is necessary and especially if the Phase II application is submitted only after Phase I will be completed. Because Phase I captures information regarding feasibility, many SBIR applicants tend to hold off their Phase II application until Phase I is completed. The fast-track mechanism should be considered when a product has high potential for commercialization, an evaluation plan has been fully developed and is poised for implementation, partners have been aligned for both phases, and a long delay between Phase I and II could be detrimental to the project. However, fast-track applications generally receive rigorous attention by reviewers, and we advise potential applicants not to utilize this particular mechanism until the small business has demonstrated some record of success within the SBIR/STTR program. It is important to include a section in the fast-track proposals in which you specifically justify the need for continuous funding through the fast-track mechanism.

Supplemental Funds

In the case of most SBIR grants, supplemental funds can be requested once a grant is awarded. In general, the supplemental funds can be up to 25% of the grant award amount. The availability of supplemental funds is largely determined by how much funding in an agency's set-aside is left unspent at the end of the fiscal year. Supplemental funds can be requested to complete additional related work that would enhance the viability or success of a project. For example, an SBIR awarded to develop program materials for a health promotion program, might require supplemental funds to develop an additional instructional video, construct program or intervention materials in another language, or develop materials that can be used for another age group (and that might require additional focus groups for market testing). All of these avenues of program development are likely to increase the commercial potential of the product line. Funding supplements should be requested as early as possible once a grant is awarded, mainly because the scope of work outlined in the supplement request will need to be completed at the same time as the parent SBIR grant. A supplement will not be awarded if requested during an extension period of the parent grant. Requests for supplements to Phase I grants should be in the first month of the grant or shortly thereafter. This provides sufficient time for the supplement request to be processed and for the proposed work to be completed. For Phase II grants, requests for supplements should be made during the first year of the grant. Earlier submission is always better when requesting an SBIR supplement. It is advised that the PI discuss these issues with the assigned project officer prior to any such requests. The application process is simple, consisting of a letter describing the need for the additional product, the steps that will be taken to complete the product and a budget. The supplement application is in essence, a three- to four-page mini-proposal.

SBIR Versus STTR

When trying to determine whether to submit an SBIR or STTR application, there are several factors to consider. First, there is generally substantially more funding available for SBIR grants than for STTR grants; however, the SBIR mechanism tends to be more competitive because there are so many more applications in any given round (e.g., STTR funding at NIH is roughly 10% of total SBIR/STTR funding). Also, fewer agencies use the STTR program, and Phase II is generally limited to $500,000, as opposed to the dollar limit of $750,000 for SBIR grants. One major advantage of submitting an STTR is that when the relationship with the PI or key personnel is with a university or a nonprofit research institution, the PI is permitted to be employed by the research institution and is only required to commit a minimum of 10% time to the project.

Additionally, when intellectual property is regarded as key to the success of the project and is owned by the university or research institution, it may be preferable to submit an STTR in order to avoid certain legal issues that arise with ownership and distribution of intellectual property. The STTR requires that a contractual agreement be reached with the university regarding the roles of the company versus the university with respect to allocation of rights of ownership and rights to commercialize intellectual property. This agreement extends to revenue or royalty sharing. In legal jargon, these agreements fall under the purview of "Allocation of Rights in Intellectual Property and Rights to Carry Out Follow-on Research, Development, or Commercialization."[1] These types of arrangements often entail very complex legal and organizational issues that require lengthy and sensitive negotiations—and may require multiple levels of approval by the university bureaucracy and can take an extended period of time—possibly beyond planned submission deadlines. A model agreement for STTR grants is available for review at the NIH SBIR/STTR Web site (grants.nih.gov/grants/funding/sbirsttr/sttrmodelagreement.doc). The STTR mechanism may be useful to the university in order to facilitate the introduction of research-based products into the marketplace—as well as to provide more entrepreneurial business experience for faculty and graduate students. If the role of the university is one that is not so integrated or fundamental, it may be preferable to have the university serve in the capacity of a subcontractor on an SBIR application, which does not generally require such extensive negotiation and agreement prior to submission.

SBIR Contracts

Although the focus of this chapter is primarily on writing SBIR and STTR grant applications, NIH and some other agencies also have an SBIR contract program, with annual solicitations for SBIR contract proposals. The contract mechanism has many of the same eligibility requirements as the SBIR grant program but falls under a different set of regulations that are designed for managing contracts rather than grants. Contract solicitations specify in more detail the type of product or service the government wants developed, have a different application format, and are considered under a separate review process from grants. Although we do not cover contracts in any great detail here, the best advice is to consult with the appropriate agency prior to submission. Overall, contracts represent another excellent source of funding for developing product lines, and most of the SBIR/STTR information in this chapter is highly relevant to contract proposals.

The SBIR program represents an incredible opportunity for the research community to use an entrepreneurial approach to advance science and translate science to the practical realm. This funding mechanism does not require re-payment; however, it has become highly competitive, and it is critical to follow the guidelines of the solicitations and to meet the requirements of the evaluation criteria to the fullest extent possible. The individual authors of this chapter have been successful SBIR grant writers, primarily in developing behavioral health products with NIH funding. In the next section, we share some critical and formative lessons learned and provide important guidance that should be helpful toward writing successful SBIR/STTR applications.

STRATEGIES FOR COMMERCIALIZATION

There are many challenges to the commercialization goals of the SBIR program, especially within the public health sector supported by the NIH grants. If a product or service truly possesses significant commercial potential, it is unlikely that you would want to choose the SBIR program as your first source of funding because of the very slow bureaucratic process and long time it takes to obtain the funding and conduct the research. Therefore, most products and services de-veloped under the SBIR program address unique or specialized public health needs where private sector funding is generally not available. This type of niche marketing can be useful to product developers and help them focus exclusively on an identified market. In addition, commercialization schemes for many types of public health products or services target small markets, making it difficult to find sufficient startup capital to market or sell these products. Finally, often the government is also working to address similar public health needs and likewise is developing similar products and services that are offered to the public for free— and it is difficult to compete with free. Nevertheless, there have been break-through products funded by the SBIR program, and there are some useful tips and strategies that should enhance your opportunities for successful commer-cialization or increase societal benefits.

First, it is essential that you gain a good understanding of the potential market for your product or service. Identify end-users who will buy it. Develop a surefire business plan detailing strategies for sales and distribution. Conduct market analyses to find out whether demographics (income) support your mar-keting strategy. A good question that should be addressed right in the beginning is whether the target audience has the resources to purchase the product. Develop a specific marketing plan. Amortize the marketing plan back on the costs of marketing and sales to ensure the product is priced accordingly and will net a positive cash flow. These are only a few of the many essential questions that need to be asked and evaluated as part of the strategic business plan. Once you have an understanding of the market, you have to decide the best way to reach the target audience. Often, the market plan is developed by outside parties. Most companies that have the ability to win an SBIR grant and conduct the research required do not possess the financial resources or skills to market, sell, and distribute a product. It is often best to form strategic partnerships with third-party companies for these purposes, including publishers, distributors, manufacturers, and marketing companies. Another useful tactic involves affiliating with national organizations that address the unique health or social needs of specific target populations. If you are planning to market the product yourself, be prepared to invest substantial resources into marketing, sales, and fulfillment in a competitive market.

A different strategy involves developing products or services that fulfill a requirement of federal or state governments. For example, many states require educational drunk driving programs; thus, developing a curriculum with instructional videos that meet this requirement helps create a niche market with a viable consumer base. It can also be helpful and important to get your product or service approved by a government agency, including receiving accolades for interventions as a "model program." The National Registry of Evidence-Based Effective Programs and Practices (NREPP), funded by the Substance Abuse and Mental Health Services Administration (SAMHSA), recently created a national registry with strict guidelines for admission as evidence-based intervention programs. Rigorously evaluated violence, drug abuse, mental health, reading and achievement, and drunk driving are only a few of the select programs that can make the grade. SAMHSA and NREPP created a Web site for listing the model criteria and also presenting programs that have achieved this merit (www .modelprograms.samhsa.gov).

The research evaluation component conducted through the SBIR can help to establish credibility for this type of recognition. SBIR funding can also be very helpful in obtaining investment capital from angle investors or venture capital firms. Demonstrating the ability to receive SBIR funding from a government agency can add credibility from the perspective of an investment analyst. Using SBIR funding to leverage other investment sources is considered positive and is encouraged by the SBIR program. Third-party partnerships are also an excellent mechanism for marketing SBIR products. For example, Danya International, Inc. where Jeff Hoffman is CEO, has developed a strategic partnership with Hazelden Publishing and Educational Services, Inc., to publish some of Danya's drug and tobacco treatment manuals. Hazelden published Danya's *Living in Balance: Moving From a Life of Addiction to a Life of Recovery* in 2003, and it has been one of their best-selling products for the past couple of years. Hazelden has the resources and capabilities to market a behavioral health product like this, whereas Danya did not. Hazelden published, marketed, and distributed the SBIR product to the public, and Danya receives a royalty payment—resulting in successful commercialization of the product. Another strategy is to adapt and translate products to reach other vulnerable populations, which may not possess sufficient resources compared to mainstream groups. For example, Social Solutions International Inc., where Susanna Nemes is CEO, is building a niche revolving around culturally adapted and translated substance abuse educational products for minority populations. Another successful strategy is to develop a suite of related products to be marketed together. Tanglewood Research, where William Hansen is president, has done this with All Stars educational substance abuse prevention materials, being marketed in conjunction with evaluation support services (Evaluation Lizard—an online tool for conducting prevention program evaluations where surveys match a program's targeted mediating variables) and professional development and training (Prevention ABCs—online and DVD instruction to enhance program providers' skill and understanding of prevention methods). In all three examples, extensive research and development were coupled with existing niche marketing strategies to make highly attractive products available to large commercially appropriate audiences with a notably high demand factor.

Another successful strategy for both winning and commercializing an SBIR grant is to build on a body of successful research already completed for a product and then use the SBIR funding mechanism to make the product more commercially viable and marketable. Dr. Gilbert J. Botvin, founder and president of National Health Promotion Associates, Inc. (NHPA), developed the Life Skills Training drug abuse prevention program and conducted rigorous high-quality evaluation research from an academic setting over a period of many years, demonstrating its effectiveness. NHPA was able to utilize SBIR funding to enhance, refine, expand, and further evaluate this program to develop a more commercially viable product, thereby translating the original research into more widespread practice. Another example of the successful implementation of this strategy is illustrated by Inflexxion, Inc., founded by psychologist and CEO Simon Budman, which took one of the most widely used and validated substance abuse assessment instruments available in the public domain, the Addiction Severity Index (ASI), originally developed by Dr. Tom McLellan and associates at the University of Pennsylvania, and used SBIR funding to develop an interactive CD-ROM multimedia version of this instrument. Inflexxion also has developed versions of the instruments in different languages, including Spanish and Chinese, as well as an innovative Web-based data collection and reporting system that can be utilized by state-funded and large private substance abuse treatment agencies. Inflexxion, with 2006 revenues nearing $10 million, has moved dramatically over the previous five years from having nearly 90% of its funding support coming from SBIR grants to receiving the vast majority of its revenues from commercialization of SBIR-related products. As can be seen from these two brief examples, both NHPA and Inflexxion have invested heavily in the marketing and sales of their products with very successful returns on their investments.

Finally, commercialization can also be attained through building on the capabilities obtained through SBIR funding. For example, Danya International has built on its health communication expertise developed primarily through various NIH-funded SBIR products over a period of 10 years to obtain several large multi-million dollar government contracts that require the company's specific expertise and that have a substantial social impact on HIV and drug use prevention and child and family health. This indirect type of successful commercialization can result in the creation of new jobs and increased public tax revenues, as well as the continued transfer of technology from research to real-life settings.

GETTING STARTED WITH YOUR SBIR APPLICATION

One simple way to look at how to be successful in writing SBIR grant applications is to use the "SBIR" acronym to guide your writing, in this way:

Small: Keep your project small in scope. Don't be overly ambitious. Make sure the project has a reasonable timeframe and appropriate budget. Most important, your application should propose a project that can be completed successfully within the milestones and project aims set forth.

Business: The proposal should include a solid, well-constructed product business plan. The application needs to show evidence there is commercial potential for the product—including product analysis (i.e., competition) and product market information. The application should demonstrate capability to sell or distribute the product utilizing either the small business group's expertise or that of the PI.

Innovation: Make sure the product is unique and innovative—that it offers something new, different from what already exists in the marketplace. Whether the product uses new technology, renders considerable advances in science, or supplies much needed creative development, ensure that the product takes the field a step forward in innovation.

Research: A successful SBIR application has to include a sound research platform—both in the development of the application and in the implementation. Make sure the application has adequately addressed any relevant research already completed and proposes an experimentally rigorous and methodologically sound research design, and that the collective staff from the research or small business end maintains strong, credible research capabilities with a system of accountability.

A question often posed to the chapter authors always seems to resonate around "what is the secret to winning SBIR grants?" The answer, truthfully speaking, is that there really is no secret—keeping the project small, focused, and highly innovative, with a clear business plan and revenue model and a rock solid research design—these are the keys to winning SBIR grants.

Getting started requires obtaining a copy of the solicitation for the federal agency where you plan to submit your application. You can generally find this by searching the Internet for SBIR under your agency of interest, or you can go to www.SBIRworld.com and search by agency. Once you get the appropriate solicitation, make sure that you read the instructions very carefully. This may be overwhelming at first because of the exhaustive number of regulations and guidelines related to government grants in general, and SBIR grants in particular. But it is important to get an overview of the complete set of requirements and instructions before you get started writing. Once you have reviewed the instructions, you will need to select the topic area that best fits your project. For the NIH, the topics listed are generally quite broad and reflect the mission of each of the specific NIH agencies. Some other agencies specify in greater detail what types of projects they will fund (this is also true for NIH SBIR contracts as opposed to grants).

EVALUATION CRITERIA

After you have reviewed the instructions and identified the topic area, the best place to start writing any grant application is to begin with the evaluation criteria. Chapter 3 on the essentials of grant writing makes similar suggestions and is worth reading in conjunction with this chapter. When you first begin to conceptualize your product or project—use the evaluation criteria to carefully lay out your thoughts. Review the solicitation for the agency where you are planning to submit your application and begin with the evaluation criteria. For NIH, the evaluation criteria are stated in the current solicitation and are summarized as follows:

1. Significance:
   - Does the study address an important problem?
   - Is the argument supporting the need for this product/project made clearly/well?
   - Does the proposed project have commercial potential, and/or social benefits and can these be clearly articulated?
   - Will it make a contribution to the field?
   - Is the proposed product an improvement over what is already available? How does the proposed product compare to similar products?
2. Approach:
   - Is the proposed plan a sound approach for establishing technical and commercial feasibility?
   - Is the work plan reasonable in the available amount of time? Is the timeline well structured? Are the project goals realistic or overly ambitious?
   - Does the applicant acknowledge potential problems and consider alternative strategies (is there a limitations section)?

- Are the milestones and evaluation approaches appropriate? Can the aims be accomplished with the proposed plan? At the end of Phase I, will be team be able to show that their product does what they want it to do?
- Will the target audience be reached with the proposed product/ap-approach?

3. Innovation:
   - Are the aims or product original and innovative? Does the project employ novel technologies, approaches, or methodologies? How is the proposed product different from what already exists in the field?
   - Does the propose product challenge current paradigms or overcome current obstacles?
   - Is the proposed innovation appropriate for the target audience?

4. Investigator:
   - Is the PI capable of supervising, coordinating, and managing the proposed project?
   - Is the work proposed appropriate to the experience level of the PI and other researchers? Does the investigative team have experience doing this type of project?
   - Has the PI or other members of the team been successful with other SBIR grants?
   - Is there a description of the consultants—are they appropriate? Do they cover any areas of expertise not covered by the research team? Are there letters of support from the consultants?
   - Can the PI devote sufficient time to this project?

5. Environment:
   - Is there sufficient access to resources (e.g. equipment, facilities, personnel) to complete the project?
   - Does the environment contribute to the probability of success?
   - Are there collaborative arrangements that will increase the likelihood of success? Will the collaborative arrangements assist in areas that the small business needs support (e.g., recruiting, conducting pilot study)? Are there letters of support from the collaborators?
   - Is there a strong commitment of support by all participating organizations?

6. Additional Criteria for Phase II Applications:
   - Did the applicant meet the Phase I goals? Did they demonstrate feasibility? Produce what they said they would produce? If not, did they explain why? Is there a solid foundation for Phase II?
   - Is the commercial potential addressed in detail including plan, competition, market analysis, sales of similar products, partners for mar-

keting, etc.? Letters of support from partners? Is there a high degree of commercial potential?
- Is there a detailed product development plan?
- Is there a data and safety monitoring plan—if necessary (if it is a clinical trial)?

7. Additional Criteria for Fast-Track Applications:
   - Are there clear criteria for meeting Phase I goals before moving to Phase II?
   - Is there a reasonable justification for doing a fast track?
   - Does the team have experience with SBIR grants? Have they been successful in completing them in the past?
   - Has the team done similar projects? Have they included lessons learned that can help with this new project?
   - Is there a detailed Product Development Plan?
   - Is the commercial potential addressed in detail- plan, competition, market analysis, sales of similar products, partners for marketing, etc.? Are there letters of support from partners? Is there a high degree of commercial potential?

8. Additional Criteria for Resubmissions (include previous reviewer comments with the new proposal):
   - Did the applicant address all of the reviewer comments adequately? It is essential to address these concerns in a respectful, erudite manner and tone.
   - Do the changes improve the revised application?
   - Are there any new areas of concern that now need to be addressed?

It is essential that you are confident that you can fully address every one of these evaluation criteria. Keep in mind that the application will be reviewed by a group of independent researchers and experts who will be using these exact criteria to evaluate and score your application. Therefore, carefully addressing each and every one of these evaluation criteria is a sine qua non of constructing a solid, well-written, and meritorious application. Also, after you write your application, it is important to go back and specifically review these designated areas to make sure that you have fully satisfied the review criteria. In fact, we recommend that you have an independent review of the draft application by other researchers in your organization, colleagues, or consultants. Your colleagues can then use these questions as formal guidelines to draft a critique and make recommendations for improving the application. Chapter 18 on revisions and resubmissions makes this same point, and it represents a healthy way to learn from outside sources about any undiscovered glitches prior to submission and formal review.

CONSTRUCTING AND WRITING AN SBIR GRANT APPLICATION

All SBIR and STTR grant applications are now submitted electronically at www .grants.gov. As many of us have discovered recently with this change in submission format, electronic submission can be a time-consuming and a daunting process. Small businesses applying for funds need to register with several federal agencies—Central Contractor Registration (www.CCR.gov), Grants.gov, and the institute where the funding application will be sent—before the submission process can begin. A DUNS number must be obtained from Dun & Bradstreet (smallbusiness.dnb.com). Registration can take several weeks; therefore, careful planning should guide you to obtain your DUNS number early. Make sure that you follow the electronic submission instructions very carefully and give yourself several days before the final deadline to make sure that you are able to submit the application properly. If you do not follow the rules for font size, margins, page limits, and so on, your application may be rejected and not even be reviewed. The main text of the application, referred to as the Research Plan (sections A–D), is limited to only 15 pages for Phase I and 25 pages for Phase II applications. This page restriction does not include NIH biographical sketches, letters of support, or the Human Subjects section. Requirements and the titles of the various sections differ between contracts and grants. Make sure to review the instructions prior to each submission as the rules frequently change.

You have to include a very large amount of information in these few pages, so think this process through very carefully, write clearly and logically, and do not waste any space. You will be able to attach a bibliography of references cited in the Research Plan (and this does not count toward the total page count). Although there is no page limit for the references, it is important to select only those literature references pertinent to the proposed research. Below we review briefly each of the major sections of the grant application. The lettering sequence from A through K in the next section of this chapter corresponds to the sections of the PHS grant application form.

A. Specific Aims

Clearly state the overall goal and specific objectives of the project. General goals can be stated first, followed by specific indications. Number these items sequentially so you can refer back to them in later portions of the application. Indicate how you will demonstrate the feasibility of the project in Phase I. Provide a clear description of the product or service being developed and its potential for innovation and commercialization. It is very easy to be overly ambitious in Phase I—make sure that your objectives can be reasonably accomplished in six months for less than $100,000. That amount of time and money can fly by very quickly—and it is essential that you demonstrate feasibility—so keep it small. At most, one page is recommended for this section. The onus of this section is to show that your company can cobble the resources necessary to streamline your production efforts and ready the product in the suggested timeline. If you cannot deliver what is promised in Phase I sometime during the six-month period, you stand little chance of obtaining additional Phase II funding for larger and more protracted commercialization and field-testing efforts.

B. Background and Significance

Clearly describe the technical or social problem your product or service will address. Demonstrate that you are completely familiar with the current literature and research related to this specific problem. This section entails around two to three pages at most and necessitates brevity and poignancy. Describe any theoretical underpinnings to your approach. If you are making a technical refinement on an existing product (i.e., creating an interactive DVD for a health promotion program), make sure to highlight why this modification is essential and describe the magnitude of its potential impact on end-users. Indicate any research or development work that you or your team has done related to the problem and how it is related to your plans for the project. State the significance of your project for the target population, and/or for society at large, and clearly indicate the commercial potential by describing the market for the product or service. It is always helpful to describe commercial success of similar products, but also indicate what makes your product unique and innovative.

C. Preliminary Studies/Progress Report

Although preliminary data are not required for a Phase I application, reviewers generally prefer to see some initial efforts to test the utility of your proposed project. Therefore, we highly recommend that you include information based on previous published research, a small pilot study, or even qualitative material obtained from focus groups, all of which helps demonstrate the potential success of your proposal. If you have not conducted any preliminary studies, obtained materials based on a needs assessment, or collected pilot data, use this section to highlight other similar projects that the staff or company have done. This will demonstrate that the company/team has experience in performing similar work and is capable of completing the proposed work. For Phase II applications, you will need to complete a Phase I final report in this section following the instructions for presenting your accomplishments in Phase I. It is important to remember that you will need to demonstrate that you accomplished the objectives detailed in the Specific Aims. Therefore, Phase II objectives must be realistic, objective, and clearly definable. For fast-track applications, you will submit the Phase I final progress report after Phase I is completed, and the awarding agency will use this report to determine whether sufficient progress has been made to proceed with Phase II, so it is imperative that you articulate your accomplishments clearly. This is not a time to be modest—continued funding depends on demonstrating realistic accomplishments. For Phase I applications, we advise that you limit this section to two to three pages, whereas for Phase II and fast-track applications, a length of six to eight pages is more suitable and recommended.

D. Research Design and Methods

For both Phase I and Phase II applications, this section will provide a detailed description of the research design, methods, experimental procedures, and study protocols used to evaluate the product or service. You should specify all of the critical details for how the research will be carried out from the inception of the project and construction of any technical materials (software and hardware), including the recruitment of subjects all the way to statistical analysis of the data. This section should follow rigorous academic standards for conducting research relevant to your project. You must indicate how you will conceptualize and measure (reliability and validity) the objectives described under the Specific Aims. When submitting Phase I applications, you must specify the criteria that will be used to demonstrate the feasibility of your product or service. One of the most common problems in preparing SBIR applications is inadequate time and attention paid to the details and requirements of the research plan. Make sure that you give yourself and your team plenty of time to think through all of the various research design issues, potential confounding factors, and how to address them, and even providing the justification for why you selected the proposed design rather than alternative choices. A major design issue that is often over-looked is the estimation of power for your study. Particularly if you suggest a field test, you must have a sufficiently sized sample to ascertain the psychometric properties of any instruments or tests of the technical feasibility of the product. Power is adequately addressed in chapter 4, and we encourage readers to learn from the important insights on sample size estimation and power calculation provided in that chapter. If all else fails, seek expert consultation on this matter before you begin constructing the grant, since being forced to revamp your design after conducting power analyses can thwart your progress.

You should provide a clear description of the sequence of activities and a timetable for the project. Keep in mind that the time frames are generally shorter than would be allowed for any type of long-term research with adequate time to measure changes at follow-up. Therefore, in the discussion of potential diffi-culties and limitations, you should address the rationale for the procedures used keeping in mind the time frame of an SBIR grant and demonstrate that you have considered appropriate alternatives. Describe any new methodologies you plan to use and provide a clear justification and rationale, as well as any new or novel concepts, approaches, tools, or technologies. Depending on the length of the previous sections of the Research Plan (not including the Introduction for revised applications only), you will have between 8 and 10 pages to describe the structure of Phase I and 14–17 pages to describe Phase II.

E. Protection of Human Subjects

According to federal guidelines, the protection of human subjects is considered of paramount importance when federal dollars are used to fund research. In light of this, the section on protection of human subjects must be addressed thoroughly and carefully if human subjects are involved in your proposed research. Chapter 16 provides an intensive and detailed look at some of the necessities and, likewise, some of the pitfalls encountered with human subjects sections. The information in that chapter provides a very useful backdrop for all grants and contracts and can embellish an SBIR application tremendously, but a few brief comments here are still in order.

The Health and Human Service "Protection of Human Subjects" regulations (45 CFR Part 46) define a human subject as a living individual about whom an investigator conducting research obtains data through intervention or interaction with the individual or identifiable private information. *Make sure that you carefully review the guidelines for the protection of human subjects in the application guide* and describe how you will ensure that human subjects be appropriately protected, how informed consent will be obtained, and how specimens and/or private (personal health) information will be protected. Describe the risks and benefits with a clear justification for how any reasonable risks are outweighed by the potential benefits of the proposed product and research. Do not assume there are no "risks" associated with your research because you do not feel your work is intrusive. The mere use of human subjects poses risks. Do not assume that if you utilize survey questions, for instance, to obtain feedback on a product, there are no risks associated with implementation of this approach.

If your research does not involve use of human subjects, then you should clearly state: "No human subject research is proposed in this application." It is of paramount importance that you clarify whether human subjects are involved in your project. Use of an expert panel as part of your research objectives would not be considered human subjects; however, use of participants in a focus group or as part of a small pilot study collecting qualitative data clearly fits the bill for human subjects. A good rule of thumb is to be conservative in this area, so if you are not certain whether your study involves the use of human subjects, consult with your institutional review board or obtain advice from an expert in the field. If you remain uncertain, it is safer to develop a plan for human subjects rather than have your proposal receive a poor score or have funding held up because you did not provide an adequate plan. It is generally assumed that if human subjects are involved, both women and minorities will be included in the study. If your study delimits the sample to males only or excludes children, you must provide a reasonable scientific justification. You must indicate the estimated number and percentage of women and minorities in the study and how they will be recruited in a scientifically acceptable manner. Describe the estimated numbers of women and minorities in a targeted/planned enrollment table. The plan for recruitment of women and minorities should match with materials included in other sections of the proposal.

You may encounter situations where your sampling efforts are proscriptively designed around under sampling a particular age, gender, or race group. For instance, if women are notorious for not attending group meetings or fail to enroll as often as men in studies of a similar ilk, it is not sufficient to say that women are not compliant and therefore will not be recruited. You have to develop aggressive, scientifically valid, and replicable methods of recruitment to reach the hard-to-reach. If, on the other hand, women are disproportionately underrepresented in your population (i.e., a study of anabolic steroid use among collegiate athletes), then it is scientifically valid to state that women do not use a particular substance, health alternative, or commercial product as often as men and thus will not be a formative part of your sampling efforts. The same applies to race and age groups, although you should be careful if you are excluding race groups for any reason whatsoever. You should explain how you obtained sample estimates and whether they are based on enrollment figures from similar treatment programs, city demographics, census indicators, or epidemiological information obtained from a national survey (you need to provide citations for each of these various sampling strategies).

It is also essential to address whether participants under the legal age of 21 will be included in your study. If your study precludes sampling of youth under the age of 21, you should indicate why, providing an explanation along sampling lines, developmental arguments, safety concerns, cognitive ability, or whatever argument fits your sampling and recruitment plan. Age groups can be delimited with regard to sampling if it would be inappropriate to use children for a particular study, given that they are legal minors. However, merely delimiting youth because their base rates are notoriously low for certain behaviors calls the appropriateness of the product for youth into question. Nonetheless, if youth under the age of 21 will be included, you should indicate the proposed number of participants and a recruitment strategy. In the event that your design necessitates inclusion of children (legal minors), indicate how you have ensured that there is adequate expertise in working with children among the team members. If the children are legal minors under the age of 18, parental consent is required in addition to a child assent form. Consent and assent forms must state the study protocols in a language compatible with the reading levels of the target audience. Therefore, be careful to explain the study in great detail when using children and to use simple words familiar to their age level. For example, the term "anonymous" or "confidential" must be clarified using a child's mindset.

A Flesch-Kincaid readability index will indicate the developmental appropriateness of your consent/assent forms.[2,3]

If your project involves a clinical trial (not usually developed for Phase I), include a detailed data and safety monitoring plan and describe the general structure of the monitoring entity and mechanisms for reporting adverse events to the NIH and/or your cognizant institutional review board. The more detail you provide in the data and safety monitoring plan, the more likely you get rave reviews because you demonstrate a sound knowledge of the demanding scientific requirements to conduct research.

F. Vertebrate Animals

If you indicated that vertebrate animals are involved in your research, you must address several points covered in the instructions to ensure the proper treatment and protection of animals in accordance with research standards. If not, just indicate that it is not applicable to your research project.

G. Literature Cited

This section requires documentation of sources used in the application. There is no formal requirement stating the method to list references. Some investigators use the endnote style based on the Council of Science Editors' *Scientific Style and Format* (also called the Vancouver style). This method of endnotes and literature documentation utilizes a numbered system with superscript note numbers inside the text and then lists the sources by number in section G. The Vancouver style will save you space in the text but is harder to manipulate should you need to reduce or modify sections of the grant in an effort to save space (in which case, the text must be renumbered, albeit some newer software packages such as EndNotes handle this with ease). Other methods include the author/date parenthetic style based on the *Publication Manual of the American Psychological Association*. A third method is the Uniform System of Citation. The methods vary on the finest of points, but consistency is the mark of a solid proposal. If possible and appropriate, make sure to include the work of reviewers who are on the review committee for your proposal. You can obtain information regarding reviewers at the NIH Web site for your committee. The most important point to remember is that consistency is a hallmark of well-scored proposals and should be a standard operating procedure in your proposal construction.

H. Consortium/Contractual Arrangements

In this section, you must explain the programmatic, fiscal, and administrative arrangements to be made between the small business and remaining organizations participating in the project. In particular, you need to provide a rationale for including other organizations emphasizing how each organization or consultant augments the project with their expertise and how inclusion of individuals or a business entity will enhance the project's overall success. Like a business plan, the wording of this section should highlight the necessity of the partner, what unique business or research skills they bring to the table, and how they will blend this operationally with the small business entity.

For Phase I SBIR applications, at least two-thirds or 67% of the research must be carried out by the small business concern. The amount budgeted for all consultant and contractual arrangements may not exceed 33% of the total budget (including indirect costs and fees).

For Phase II SBIR applications, at least one-half or 50% of the research must be carried out by the small business concern. The amount budgeted for all consultant and contractual arrangements may not exceed 50% of the total budget (including indirect costs and fees).

For Phase I and Phase II STTR applications, at least 40% of the work must be performed by the small business concern and at least 30% of the work must be performed by the single partnering research institution.

I. Resource Sharing Plan(s)

Projects with $500,000 or more in direct costs in any year must include a brief one-paragraph description of how final research data will be shared, or explain why data sharing is not possible. Also, all applications where the development of model organisms is anticipated must include a description of a specific plan for sharing and distributing unique model organism research resources or explain why it is not possible.

J. Consultants

Letters of support from organizations or consultants that can demonstrate a commitment to the project and that will enhance the probability of success and/or commercial potential of the project can add much value to the application. However, these letters must add real substantive value or they will appear to be adding fluff to the proposal. You must attach appropriate letters from all consultants confirming their roles on the project and rate for consulting services, the latter of which bolsters any budgetary requests. Follow the specific instructions for the required information to be included in consultant letters and then provide a draft sample letter to your consultants that they can complete and put on their letterhead. Also have them provide you with an NIH version of their biographical sketch, a template of which exists on the NIH Web site. If consultants bring vastly different sets of skills to a project, make sure to highlight these differences, honing in on their uniqueness and ability to move the project forward. Letters of support should amplify the consultants' skills and be personalized in the event the PI has a long-standing relationship with the consultant or business entity.

K. Appendix

Phase I SBIR and STTR applications generally do not allow inclusion of appendices. Phase II applications allow appendices that include materials developed in Phase I, related publications, patents, or copies of instruments and consent forms. However, only the primary reviewers are likely to see these appendices. Consistent with NIH regulations regarding appendix materials, it is strongly advised that any information deemed critical to the evaluation of the application be included in the text of the application.

COMMON PITFALLS IN APPLICATIONS

There are numerous pitfalls—if not fatal flaws—associated with certain SBIR grant applications. Noting these weaknesses will give readers some insight into why applications receive low scores and ultimately do not receive consideration for funding. Some of the more common problems encountered include applications that (1) are overly ambitious and unrealistic, (2) lack innovation, (3) contain a poor research design (including problems with sample recruitment, subject retention, follow-up, statistical analyses, and stated research goals), (4) demonstrate inadequate knowledge of the research literature, (5) lack evidence supporting potential for commercialization or social impact, and (6) do not follow the grant application instructions carefully. These weaknesses are highlighted by Jo Anne Goodnight, the NIH SBIR/STTR program coordinator, who listed some of the most common reasons cited by NIH reviewers for an application's failure to gain the study section or reviewers' enthusiasm, including:

- Poorly defined test of feasibility in Phase I application
- Methods unsuited to the objective
- Problem more complex than investigator appears to realize
- Not significant to health-related research
- Too little detail in the research plan to convince reviewers the investigator knows what he or she is doing; that is, no recognition of potential problems and pitfalls
- Direction or sense of priority not clearly defined; that is, experiments do not follow from one another and lack a clear starting or finishing point
- Lack of focus in hypotheses, specific aims, and or research plan
- Investigator too inexperienced with the proposed techniques (and failed to enlist collaborators with complementary expertise)
- Proposal driven by technology, that is, a method in search of a problem
- Rationale for experiments not provided, that is, why the experiments are important as well as how they are relevant to the objective

- Lack of alternative methods in case the primary approach does not work out
- Proposed model system not appropriate to address the proposed questions

These and many other reasons, some of which can be difficult to anticipate, may presage the death knell for an application. This is not necessarily a reflection of the intelligence or competency of the PI or research team—this is a highly complex process with multiple requirements from research, business, regulatory, and governmental perspectives. It often takes all three allowable submissions to get an SBIR application funded, even from some of the best researchers. If your application is not funded, you should carefully analyze the reviewer comments to determine whether or not the weaknesses of the application can be corrected and assess whether or not to resubmit the application. If you are considering resubmitting, it is advisable to get feedback on the application from the government project officer at the agency where you want to submit before you resubmit the application—this can be very helpful. Any advice you glean from the project officer will be helpful to give you a sense of the committee's gut feeling regarding the application (see chapter 18 on revisions and resubmissions). NIH regulations permit only two resubmissions of an application. It goes without saying that one of the keys to success in the SBIR world, as in most other areas of life, is persistence—so don't let a rejection keep you down.

RESUBMISSIONS

When resubmitting an application, you are allowed a specific number of pages to address the previous reviewer comments. This is a brief summary of changes to the application that highlights responses to reviewer comments and key improvements to the application—be clear, concise, and respectful of the reviewers. It is not uncommon for reviewers to say that something was missing in the application that was actually there. For instance, do not say: "if the reviewer had read the application more carefully ... " but rather indicate that you "recognize this concern and would like to elaborate more specifically that ... ." The introduction for Phase I and supplemental applications is limited to one page; Phase II and fast-track applications can be up to three pages—do not exceed these limits. This section is critical, as one of the review criteria for a resubmission is whether or not the previous reviewer comments were adequately addressed.

BUDGET

Make sure that the project is reasonable within the allowable cost limits and that the budget matches your technical proposal (cost accounting is covered in some detail in chapter 15). The percent effort allotted to personnel should be reasonable to accomplish the work to be done. Reviewers often comment if the percent effort of key personnel is too low. It is important to make sure staff is not covered more than 100% on government contracts. In addition, carefully consider who is listed as "key personnel," because the percent effort of the key personnel cannot be changed dramatically. You may also need to get permission to change any of the key personnel. Government budgetary issues are guided by a range of cost principles that can be highly complex in and of themselves, and a full discussion of these is beyond the scope of this chapter. However, we do touch on a few basic points. The budget includes allowable direct costs such as salaries, consultant and subcontracting costs, materials and supplies, rental fees and equipment, travel, and other costs directly associated with carrying out the proposed project; indirect costs such as fringe benefits, overhead, and general and administrative costs that must be negotiated with the federal agency; and fees, with are permitted up to 7% of the total costs of the grant. If your company does not have a negotiated indirect rate, it is generally recommended that you use a rate of 20–25% of total direct costs in your budget planning because for initial Phase I awards, this rate will generally be applied without negotiations.

CONCLUSION

The SBIR program offers an incredible opportunity for entrepreneurial researchers who want to develop products and services that have commercial potential. The SBIR grant mechanisms pose many challenges; however, success in the program can be very rewarding and help to launch a research-based business. We want to emphasize that the SBIR program can be used to advance knowledge in your field of endeavor. We encourage you to try to conduct your research in such a way that you can produce publications and scientific presentations that go beyond the commercial goals of your project. The SBIR program, especially under the NIH, has the potential not only of generating innovative commercial products that can enhance public health, but also of helping creatively address the health and social needs of people suffering from various conditions that impair their ability to live life problem-free. Most of us are not in this business purely for commercial success, but to make a difference in the world—and the SBIR program can be a helpful vehicle in this endeavor.

14 Federal Grants and Contracts Outside of NIH

Karol Kumpfer & Julia Franklin Summerhays

The more mistakes we commit the faster our learning curve slopes skyward. Actually, it is not mistakes but attempts that are the oxygen of success.

—Craig Lambert, *Mind Over Water: Lessons on Life From the Art of Rowing*

Up to this point, many chapters have focused almost exclusively on the NIH grant funding mechanisms. In addition to the full gamut of the NIH research grants and other types of grants discussed in prior chapters (fellowships, R01, R03, R21, K, SBIR/STTR, center grants, training grants, etc.), nonresearch services or demonstration/ evaluation federal grants are also a major source of funding for universities, private nonprofits, and nongovernmental organizations (NGOs). It would be remiss to not include a chapter emphasizing these sources of funding, particularly given the increased number of applications submitted to these funding sources and volume of funding available. This chapter focuses on U.S. federal funding sources that generally fund providers for nonresearch activities such as program development, direct client services, conferences, staff training, equipment, evaluation services, secondary data analysis, and other nonresearch activities. A substantial amount of federal funding is earmarked by Congress each year for these nonresearch activities and should be considered by researchers and nonresearchers alike.

As the NIH funding levels for new grant starts decreases, more university researchers are partnering with community agencies to implement and evaluate the effectiveness of model programs or promising programs. In many cases, however, these "nonresearch" activities involve more complicated research in the form of high-quality implementation and outcome program evaluations than are sometimes conducted in NIH research grants. Hence, the applicant should not underestimate the complexity or level of scientific knowledge needed to successfully compete for these nonresearch grants in today's grant or foundation climate. In many respects, a grant writing team will have to be very familiar with both research and literature reviews of what works for various targeted population. The most successful grants often involve a partnership between community practitioners and university researchers.

This chapter is organized primarily on the phases or steps involved in getting and implementing a grant: locating funding sources, the application process, writing and managing the grant writing process, tips on writing successful grants, the review process, and managing and reporting on a federal grant that is not part of the NIH portfolio. A final section addresses a very important component outlining mechanisms for publishing results (a major component to contracts and deliverables).

FEDERAL FUNDING SOURCES OUTSIDE OF NIH

What Are the Nonresearch Funding Sources/Agencies Besides NIH?

There are many different types of federal agencies that offer nonresearch grants, cooperative agreements, or contracts in the U.S. federal government. The largest federal source of nonresearch funding is the Department of Health and Human Services (DHHS), which has a total FY 2006 to 2007 budget of $698 billion, with $28.6 billion set aside for research grants within the NIH institutes and centers. These numbers indicate that there is at least $500 billion available for nonresearch grants and contracts, which is considerably more than is available for the NIH research portfolio.

Examples of federal agencies within DHHS where the authors of this chapter have submitted nonresearch grants include the Centers for Disease Control and Prevention (CDC), Substance Abuse and Mental Health Services Administration (SAMHSA) and their three centers—the Center for Substance Abuse Prevention (CSAP), the Center for Mental Health Services (CMHS), the Center for Substance Abuse Treatment (CSAT)—the Administration for Children and Families, Agency for Health Care Research and Quality, Health Resources and Services Administration, Indian Health Services, Office of Minority Health, and the Administration on Native Americans. Outside of the Department of Health and

Human Services, additional nonresearch funding sources are the Department of Education (DoED), Department of Defense, National Institute on Justice, Department of Agriculture (USDA), and Department of Transportation, to name a few. Lists of the grants being offered by these agencies are available at Grants.gov (www.grants.gov).

Purpose

The general purpose of most of these nonresearch grants is to fund local service agencies to deliver evidence-based or promising interventions. This also includes creating opportunities for these service agencies to test the effectiveness of various programs as part of methodologically rigorous evaluations with new local populations. Sometimes the demonstration/evaluation funding is to develop a new cultural or age-appropriate service and to evaluate its effectiveness with a new population. These grants are called "knowledge development" grants aimed to create new knowledge about the effectiveness of a new service or an adaptation of an existing evidence-based model with different populations. For services grants, the aim is simply to disseminate useful services for the public good.

Distinction in NIH and Non-NIH Funding: The Unique Niche for Knowledge Development, Dissemination, or Demonstration/Evaluation Grants

In order to be successful in applying for nonfederal grants, readers of this chapter should be familiar with the purpose of these grants and some recent history and trends in funding. In particular, there has been a trend to make funding available for increased numbers of field tests of evidence-based practices (EBs) found effective in NIH-funded research. The federal government funds these nonresearch grants and contracts because of their need to support the dissemination of effective programs to improve health and educational services to the general public.

Over the past two decades, the substantial congressional investment in research has paid off in a large number of evidence-based programs or practices in medicine, public health, agriculture, education, and other social areas. Unfortunately, for many years practitioners have felt comfortable in taking on the difficult task of creating their own health and social services models or services without regard to any demonstrated or proven effectiveness. Clinical research on effectiveness in practice settings has been extremely rare. In many cases, unproven programs were used and rigorous evaluations were absent. For instance, Arthur and Blitz[1] estimated that only about 10% of the substance abuse prevention programs delivered in schools or communities were those found effective through NIH-supported research studies. About 30% were commercially marketed programs, and about 60% were developed by practitioners. In addition, most of these programs were not implemented with fidelity or in name only. In contrast, the USDA and its land-grant state universities have developed sophisticated dissemination systems through cooperative extension divisions nationwide to help farmers implement research-based practices. This has resulted in highly effective and efficient farms across the United States. In the health and social services area, the NIH did not envision a role in dissemination or favor encouraging adoption. As a result, field practitioners (those people in the trenches) had little access to information about evidence-based programs and practices.

Over the past decade or so, considerable concern and frustration was voiced by the NIH research community about the lack of dissemination and adoption by community practitioners of social services and health programs or practices with proven evidence of effectiveness in research studies.[2-5] Most academic researchers did not feel comfortable becoming commercial marketers and also lacked the time and expertise to get their program adopted and used by practitioners. Additionally, many university communities do not reward fellow academicians for developing their own companies and possibly limited the faculty's attention to pure research or teaching. This has led to a noticeable underutilization of NIH research productivity, and much of the body of evidence-based programs has not been disseminated to practitioners. This gap from research to service has recently been recognized by the government[6] as well as by the research community.[7]

To help rectify this problem, in the mid-1990s the CDC developed review systems to create lists of evidence-based clinical treatment programs. As we approached the new millennium, the *Guide to Community Preventive Services* (www .thecommunityguide.org) came online for major areas of health, beginning with tobacco cessation and prevention. The international Cochrane Collaboration (www.cochrane.org), a nonprofit organization dedicated to dissemination of systematic reviews of evidence-based health care interventions, was founded in the United Kingdom in 1993. By 2000, its online reviews were already being used by doctors worldwide. These efforts also reinforce the critical need for thorough literature and research reviews to locate EBs.

The DoED was one of the first federal agencies to begin publishing information on programs that work. These publications were often disseminated to the public for free, but access for practitioners was somehow limited. Beginning in about 2000, many federal agencies began to create Web-based lists of approved evidence-based programs with proven outcomes that could be funded by their agency. Since then, the percentage of effective programs being implemented in the community has increased considerably, particularly those funded through local, state, or county agencies, but many with federal funding. In addition, universities became more favorable toward research parks representing joint collaborations between university professors and commercial enterprise. These collaborative enterprises were funded by contracts or Small Business Innovations Research (SBIR) and Small Business Technology Transfer (STTR) grants (see chapter 13 for more information on these mechanisms).

FROM RESEARCH TO PRACTICE

With this historical picture in mind, it is easy to see that nonresearch or services agencies within the federal government serve a very useful function today. They are not just services agencies funding any type of practitioner-developed program, but represent the "bridge from research to practice." To clarify the distinction between NIH research and non-NIH research, it is essential that readers understand the different phases that transpire from research to practice. Research institutes or centers in NIH as well as the National Science Foundation fund primarily what are called Phase I to III research studies. These begin with Phase I hypothesis development, move onto Phase II methods development, and continue with Phase III randomized control trials, which are also called efficacy trials.[8,9]

The "nonresearch" or services agencies listed above fund studies that focus on testing services. They also fund studies that engage translation of evidence-based models that were determined to be efficacious in Phase III controlled intervention trials. Translation studies then apply evidence-based programs with different populations in more real-world settings in the field. These translation studies help determine whether the results obtained in research settings, which can be quite methodologically rigorous, will hold up in practice settings.

A Phase IV study is an effectiveness trial, or a defined population study, where an EB is tested by a services agency to see if the EB is still effective when there is less oversight by the program developer and less control of program implementation fidelity. Implementation fidelity is critical to the success of any program and is usually artificially boosted in research settings. Thus, translation studies are essential to determine whether program implementation fidelity can be obtained in real-world settings and with less rigorous oversight by the research community. A Phase V dissemination study, sometimes called a demonstration and implementation study, tests the EB in a much larger, multisite study to determine whether wider dissemination activity influences program findings. If the evaluation results still produce large effect sizes and good cost–benefit ratios, then states and county governments can have greater confidence in recommending that local services agencies implement these EBs with their local state, county or federal pass-through funds.

As figure 14.1 shows, these nonresearch funding sources now stress more funding for Phase IV and V effectiveness and dissemination studies. Even with this greater emphasis, there may be some confusion given the Phase IV and V studies are often called replication or evaluation studies. This confusion arises primarily because the agencies supporting these studies are technically not supposed to be engaged in conducting pure research. While there is considerable overlap in the actual activities of the NIH and non-NIH research grants, technically non-NIH grants are not earmarked for supporting research, but rather emphasize services and evaluation. To make this distinction even fuzzier, NIH has also begun funding more Phase IV and V community effectiveness and dissemination studies as part of congressional mandates for more translational research. This flurry of research activity is essentially driven by a need to better understand dissemination practices including principles of adoption and institutionalized that influence uptake of evidence-based programs by communities.

NIH[10] calls this research type II translational research and distinguishes this from type I translational research, which is the application of laboratory and pre-clinical studies (Phase I and II research) into practical efficacy trials (Phase III research). Because many applications to nonresearch agencies will involve a variant of type II translational research, the reader interested in giving their grant a competitive edge is advised to read some of the recent articles[11] outlining tips for successfully conducting replications or adaptations of evidence-based models in community practice. Rohrbach and colleagues[12] recently reviewed a number of different theoretical frameworks (e.g., diffusion of innovations theory[13]), organizational change theories, and individual and group behavioral change theories[14] that provide a backdrop for type II translational research. They also reviewed factors related to successful implementation of the evidence-based model. Factors fueling successful implementation centered on the organizational climate, quality of leadership rather than the quality of the selected evidence-based program, and heightened program implementation fidelity resulting from sufficient training and technical assistance. Fidelity is the degree to which a program is implemented as designed by the developer.[15] This process is measured using fidelity checklists by an evaluator who monitors the number of activities specified in the program manuals that are actually implemented.

Figure 14.1. Continuum of Substance Abuse Prevention Research. Substance Abuse and Mental Health Services Administration: Center for Substance Abuse Prevention. (Jansen, Glynn, & Howard, 1996[16]; Greenwald & Cullen, 1985[17])

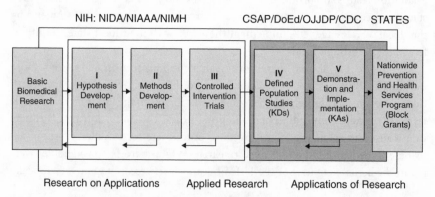

The strong emphasis on finding and implementing (with fidelity) the most effective evidence-based programs has diminished somewhat the earlier emphasis on hiring or training high-quality and effective implementers. This should not be the case because target outcomes are most likely 80% related to the quality of the implementation and 20% related to the actual curriculum used. For instance, several studies have examined the qualities of effective therapists, but fewer studies have extended this premise to prevention activities,[16] where a great deal more needs to be studied concerning qualities of effective implementers. Rohrbach and colleagues[12] also studied the importance of high-quality implementation and point out that "the science related to implementing evidence-based programs and practices with fidelity and positive outcomes lags far behind the science related to developing the programs" (p. 303–304).

UPS AND DOWNS IN FUNDING

Over the past few years, there has been a noticeable decrease in funding for new grants at NIH. This has been most noticeable for high-cost intervention research studies. To offset the loss of these important studies, there has been a rise in partnerships or jointly funded studies linking NIH with non-NIH agencies (e.g., SAMHSA). In these cases, the NIH institute or center funds a university, non-profit institute, or research think tank to conduct program evaluation research, and then SAMHSA funds a community agency to test the actual intervention.

In some cases, funding lines are intended to evaluate promising existing services models developed by local service agencies. If the program is able to obtain promising results using a nonrandomized trial (but includes a comparison group), then evidence from the pilot study can be used to help the community service agency or the evaluators apply for a Phase III efficacy trial at NIH (where there will be greater demands placed on design and methodological rigor). According to this framework, the traffic on the bridge between research and practice needs to be two ways. One flow of information comes from testing promising models developed in the field. A second flow of information comes from testing adaptations with new cultural, age, gender, or local populations. There needs to be feedback between these two processes in order to refine existing evidence-based programs and inform the larger literature of their efficacy. Collaborative grants of this nature are able to involve regular services agencies that are often the primary grant recipients, with university groups serving as the independent evaluators on a subcontract.

Locating Evidence-Based Programs and Policies

Many of the agencies listed above have Web sites where they list evidence-based programs that have been found in research studies to be effective with many different populations. For instance, the first author of this chapter was director of

CSAP at SAMHSA until 2000. As a prevention research scientist with several National Institute for Drug Abuse and National Institute on Alcohol Abuse and Alcoholism grants at the time, she was fully aware that there were many effective substance abuse prevention programs that had proven efficacy in randomized clinical trials that were not being used by practitioners.[17] To help practitioners locate the best programs, the author funded a consortium of universities to compile a registry of effective prevention programs. The result was the National Registry of Evidence-Based Programs and Practices. This online source of evidence-based programs (www.modelprograms.samhsa.gov) is now being expanded from model programs reviewed by SAMHSA (CSAP, CSAT, CMHS) to also contain model programs for the DoED and Office of Juvenile Justice and Delinquency Prevention. What started out as a small seed to nurture a knowledge base has grown into an enormous registry covering much of the NIH and other agency funding for efficacious prevention programs.

We place a great deal of emphasis on field evaluations of evidence-based models in this chapter because local services agencies need to know whether funding from federal (or even state) agencies is primarily earmarked for replication trials of approved programs. One of the major reasons reviewers will score an application poorly is because the applicant proposes to implement a program not considered by the reviewers to be appropriate for the target population. It makes sense, knowing this in advance, to peruse the Web sites of the funding agency in an effort to see if they provide a list of approved "best practices," "model programs," or "evidence-based programs." This effort alone prior to submission will greatly enhance chances of funding and possibly lead to a successful program outcome.

Eligibility Criteria for Who Can Apply

The types of grants we discuss in this chapter differ in several ways from the NIH research grants. First and foremost, eligibility criteria are generally broader and include small private nonprofit service agencies whose mission emphasizes more the delivery of high-quality services to the general public or specialized subpopulations. Individuals cannot apply for these federal funds. Only agencies with nonprofit or profit status recognized by the Internal Revenue Service can apply. Box 14.1 shows the recently published eligibility criteria.

From a logistical point of view, there are some advantages to having the local services agency submit the grant. Less of the funding will be burned up by indirect costs. Universities frequently charge more than 50% above and beyond direct costs to manage grants (see chapter 15 for a more detailed explanation of the differences between direct and indirect costs). On grants from NIH, these cost factors are not much of an issue because NIH will simply pay the indirect cost tariff using a DHHS negotiated rate. However, most of these nonresearch grants

> ### Box **14.1**
>
> Eligible applicants are domestic public and private nonprofit entities. For example, State and local governments; federally recognized tribes; State recognized tribes, urban Indian organizations (as defined in Public Law 94-437, as amended); public or private universities and colleges; community- and faith-based organizations; and tribal organizations may apply. The statutory authority for this program prohibits grants to for-profit organizations. No more than one application may be submitted from one organization.

have a maximum limit for the amount of funding requested that includes both the direct and indirect costs. Fortunately, most local services agencies have indirect or administrative cost rates hovering between 15% and 30%, which is much less that 50–70% charged by universities. If the local services agency does not have a DHHS negotiated indirect cost rate (also called facilities and administration costs or F&A), they can simply charge a 10% provisional indirect rate. A federally approved audit in their first year will then inform them whether to increase the indirect cost rate. The yellow book audit can be performed by a certified public accountant with oversight provided by the regional DHHS offices for negotiating indirect cost rates (phone audits are possible). Information on government auditing standards (2007) can be downloaded from www.gao.gov/govaud/d07162g.pdf.

Examples of Types of Funding Sources

Most non-NIH federal agencies offer grants, cooperative agreements, and contracts on an annual basis. While grants are the most common form of funding vehicles, a number of federal agencies are turning more to cooperative agreements. Cooperative agreements permit a greater element of control by the federal agency using a project officer to monitor closely grant activities. Be sure to check within the proposal announcement to see if you are applying for a grant or a cooperative agreement.

Contracts carry with them a greater degree of agency oversight, usually provided by a project officer working for the federal government. Basically, a contract is a mechanism for a federal agency to seek provision of services that the federal agency staff is unable to perform. Services of this nature usually require specific staff expertise or involve enormous logistical planning that may occur on an infrequent basis. Examples of contract services include national evaluation services, training and dissemination services, technical services, and conferences. Contracts of this nature usually run anywhere between $500,000 and $10 million. Companies competing for these contracts in the Washington, DC area generally go by the moniker "beltway bandits." These companies often have close working relationships with the agency directors or project officers because of their close proximity or based on prior contracts. As a general rule, beltway bandits have many highly qualified staff or consultants because of increased flexibility in hiring and, sometimes, have political clout useful to the agency in getting or maintaining funding. The major exception is when regional training and technical assistance centers are being bid out on a contract basis. Some of these are won by consulting agencies or universities that are outside of Washington, DC. The incumbent contractors are the most likely to win these bids unless there is some discontent on the part of the federal agency project officer regarding past performance. Some contracts can only be awarded to a small business, a minority or woman-owned 8(a) business, or a 501(c) nonprofit company.

SBIR/STTR Grants or Contracts

Many federal research agencies also participate in research grants and contracts that have as their major purpose the translation of the research into commercial products or services that can benefit the public. The federal government does not envision for itself a role disseminating the results of the research it funds or in developing commercial products that can be better marketed by the private sector. However, it does see for itself a role in research or evaluation of commercial products that can be used in technology transfer or effective dissemination of research findings. Eleven federal research agencies have a 2.5% set-aside in their budgets for SBIR grants. Five federal agencies also have a 0.3% set-aside for STTR grants. The STTR grants involve collaboration between a university and a small business, but the award goes to the small business with a subcontract to the university (see chapter 13 for details on STTR and SBIR grants). Regulations permit that either grant mechanism can only be awarded to American-owned, independently operated businesses with no more than 500 employees.

Locating These Funding Opportunities

In the last few years, all branches of the federal government have consolidated their announcements of funding into a single Web site at Grants.gov (see appendix 1). This is one of the most comprehensive online resources for grant opportunities. Managed by the DHHS, this Web site provides access to more than 1,000 federal grant programs. Previously, hard copies of announcements were published in a number of different sources such as *Federal Grants and Contracts Weekly* and *Commerce Business Daily* or on each federal agency Web site.

Another source that is useful for universities is the Community of Science. By registering with its Web site (www.cos.com), researchers can create a personal profile that includes specific research interests and receive weekly email alerts with current funding opportunities. Networking with colleagues who have current funding is a good way to get familiar with specific agencies and what types of projects they might fund. It is also a good idea to contact project officers at federal agencies to be sure your research idea fits in with their funding strategies.

Funding for Discretionary Grants

The type and number of grants available each year change based on the new congressional appropriations budget. The Senate Appropriations Committee passed S 370 on July 20, 2006, that included $142.8 billion for discretionary spending, an increase of less than 1% over FY 2006 levels and $4.5 billion over President Bush's request.

The full Senate and House approvals should happen normally before the end of the federal funding year on October 1, but in many years, because of politics or an election year, these deliberations can be shelved until after November. If this case, Congress can pass temporary spending bills, which are called continuing resolutions. These measures allow the government to operate at the prior year's levels in the event that it misses the fiscal deadline. If these continuation funding bills are not passed, then the government shuts down and employees go home, which has happened in the past, making clearer to citizens why government services are important.

EXAMPLES OF CURRENT GRANTS OFFERED

Because the first author is a former CSAP director, and primarily owing to familiarity with certain government agencies, this section provides examples emphasizing SAMHSA grants. The easiest way to determine what the horizons hold for new grant funds is to track the congressional appropriations process and language. A good Web site to obtain funding information is appropriations.senate.gov, which is maintained by the Senate Appropriations Committee, a group of legislators who are generally favorable to health and human services grants. In 2006, the Senate recommended $3.3 billion in funding for the SAMHSA for fiscal year 2007. This amount is $12.7 million above the comparable fiscal year 2006 level and $77.3 million above the administration request. If funded this could mean some additional discretionary grants.

Center for Substance Abuse Prevention

The House and the Senate both recommended a small increase for CSAP in 2006, with the Senate recommending a total of $197.6 million and an increase of $3.9 million from last year for Programs of Regional and National Significance (PRNS). Many of the discretionary grants given to small agencies that CSAP funded directly for the past 15 years have ended. Sample programs included the High-Risk Youth programs, Pregnant Women and Infant grant program, the Adolescent Female grants, and the Family Strengthening programs (140 per year). However, a few grant programs still exist, including the new Prevention of Methamphetamine Abuse grants, which appropriated $3.3 million for 11 grants last year.

Most of the discretionary grant funds for CSAP (about $106 million) have been moved into Strategic Prevention Framework State Incentive Grants for the states to award to grantees. The other major funding source for small services agencies is the large Drug-Free Communities Support Program. This community coalition grant program is provided with funds from the White House Office of National Drug Control Policy to SAMHSA for CSAP to award and administer community grants. This antidrug program provides grants of up to $100,000 to about 750 community coalitions that mobilize their communities to prevent youth alcohol, tobacco, illicit drug, and inhalant abuse. This year, 107 new grants were funded, so it should be understood that high-quality applications to this funding source have a high likelihood of funding. In addition, since 2004 CSAP has funded HIV grants in an effort to develop local capacity to provide mental health and substance abuse treatment and prevention services for individuals living with and affected by HIV/AIDS. These funds will assist states with out-reach and training, addressing the special needs of racial and ethnic minorities and studying the costs associated with delivering integrated care. SAMHSA an-ticipates funding the discretionary grant programs in FY 2007, based on the president's FY 2007 budget request.

Center for Substance Abuse Treatment

This agency received $2.15 billion in FY 2006, with about $1.7 billion dedicated to state block grants that it distributed to the states on a formula for allocation to local treatment agencies. About 20% of this amount is supposed to be dedicated to prevention. This program funds the backbone of our nation's alcohol and drug treatment agencies. About $398.6 million was dedicated to discretionary grants for PRNS. The administration recommended a Methamphetamine Treatment Initiative of $24 million, but Congress may not approve this expenditure and include it within the Targeted Capacities Expansion grant program. The Senate also recommended $15 million for treatment programs targeting pregnant, post-partum, and residential women and their children. This amount is $4.1 million above the comparable level for fiscal year 2006, so there could be extra funding for these grants. Also, $31.1 million was recommended for the Screening, Brief Intervention, Referral, and Treatment program to identify and treat early drug users.

Center for Mental Health Services

The Senate Appropriations Committee recommended $911.8 million for mental health services, or $28.1 million above FY 2005. The same committee recom-mended $290.9 million for programs of regional and national significance or

$27.9 million more that could increase the number of new grant starts. CMHS funds youth suicide prevention and early intervention programs for about $30 million. The CMHS also fund grants to prevent youth violence through the Safe Schools/Healthy Students interdepartmental program and about $25.7 million for the State Incentive Grants for Transformation program, and also funds the Statewide Consumer Network Grants and Statewide Family Network Grants. The National Child Traumatic Stress Network is also funded by CMHS for about $30 million, and $12 million is used for grants to fund mental health services to the homeless as well as funds for an Elderly Treatment and Outreach Program.

Typical Timelines

Unlike the NIH grant application receipt dates for new grants (chapter 1 reviews the newly revised NIH timelines), federal nonresearch agencies generally have only a single receipt date each year. Moreover, these receipt dates may vary for different announcements within a single agency. To make grant receipt dates even more unpredictable, there is considerable variability for an ongoing agency request for proposal (RFP) or funding initiative. The reason for this variability is because funding announcements depend on congressional approval of agency funding. Furthermore, once approved, a project officer overseeing a particular grant portfolio has to turn this appropriation around, write the grant announcement, and match the congressional line-item appropriations.

For this reason, many agencies do not write their grant announcements until after the final appropriations occur. This means that they may not post the announcement until sometime between February and April, with deadlines for submission in late spring or even early summer. If this happens, the agency will be pressed for time to get the grants reviewed and award the funds by September 30 each year (the new federal fiscal years begin in October). Federal agencies have to spend their current year appropriation or have them obligated in completely negotiated grantee contracts by September 30 at the end of the federal fiscal year or they will loose these funds. Grants will be awarded only one year at a time with continuation funding dependent on congressional approval each year and up to the total number of additional years that the agency specified in the grant announcement.

While there are a number of grants listed on Grants.gov by various agencies in the fall each year, many of these may not be funded yet. The agency project officers have published the grant announcements, but generally there is caveat in the wording of each announcement specifying that funding and funding levels will depend on the final congressional appropriations for that year. It is a good idea to check on the likelihood of funding for some announcements, if there are proposed cuts in the new budget in this area. For instance, this year the Senate agreed with the president in proposing to eliminate several line items for funding, including the $94 million dollar DoED Smaller Learning Communities grants popular with grant seekers and the $4.9 million dollar Dropout Prevention program. In their bill, the Senate further proposed to eliminate the $99 million for the Innovative Education Program Strategies and $36 million for the Credit Enhancement/Charter School Facilities. Many programs were flat-funded, meaning no increase over last year.

Nonresearch grants are shorter in planned duration than the typical five-year research grant. They are generally awarded for three years, but some for as little as one year. Often these one-year grants are called planning grants or pilot studies. Technically, your grant, if funded, will generally be contracted to have a start date of October 1 and end date of September 30. However, new grantees are likely to not get their awarded funds until several months later. So if you actually begin on time on October 1, up-front funding by the agency may be necessary to begin hiring staff and beginning project activities. If not possible, then the project is likely to not spend all of its first-year funds and you may have to ask for carryover funds. In some years, carryover funding has been denied because of government overexpenditures.

THE APPLICATION PROCESS

Paper Submissions

In submitting these grants, follow carefully the directions in the full announcement. Do not confuse the short description of the funding announcement on Web sites or Grants.gov for the actual RFPs, or other funding announcements. These federal agencies have you download a longer description of what they want, which should include a short literature review on why this grant initiative is needed, promising approaches and research, eligibility, amount of funding and number of grants expected to be funded, due dates, sections of the grant and what should go into each, review criteria and points for each section, and reporting requirements, as well as where to get an application kit with the required title or face page, budget forms, and certifications, and references. You must also get this application kit as well as the RFP. The application kit that is generally used takes the form of a PHS 5161 or PHS 398 form, so be sure to note which type of forms the agency wants the proposals submitted on. Which application kit you order is specified in the grant announcement. Be sure you have both the RFP or RFA (request for applications) printed out, and a copy of the application kit, which can also be downloaded from Grants.gov.

Electronic Submissions

The online application process through Grants.gov should be quick and easy; however, until you are used to this method of submission, there is a steep learning curve, which can cause frustration if you have not allowed enough time. The first step is to register in the system. To do so, you must have a DUNS number, which you receive from Dun & Bradstreet if your agency does not have one. Allow enough time for this—registration can take several weeks. Next, get the funding opportunity number and/or Catalogue of Federal Domestic Assistance (CFDA) number of the desired grant. Next, you should download and install the PureEdge Viewer, a free program that is necessary to access the grant applications. Once you have the viewer installed, you should download the grant application package and instructions. All of the required forms and documents are now at your fingertips. You can work on the forms offline, uploading them as you complete them. The system is designed to alert you if there is any missing information on each form. Grants.gov provides a training demonstration, "How to Complete an Application Package", at www.grants.gov/images/Application_Package.swf. Once again, be sure to begin the final submission several days ahead of the deadline, because if there are mistakes anywhere within the application forms, the computer finds them and will ask you to go back to make those corrections before it can be submitted.

TYPICAL SECTIONS OF A NON-NIH GRANT

Non-NIH grants typically have the following sections. Be sure to notice the pages limitations for your narrative, which are 25 single-spaced pages (sections A–D). Box 14.2 provides examples of the different sections: Need, Proposed Approach, Staff and Organizational Experience, and Evaluation. These are the sections rated for your total points in the review criteria. Note that this is only a *typical* example of the types of sections and content wanted. Other formats or outlines are used by other funders. Be sure to follow guidelines for the desired sections of the grant as specified in the application instructions in the announcement.

One tip on writing the narrative is that the length of each section should mirror the number of points assigned to that section. Therefore, in the example used, the proposed approach section should be the longest section, and the next longest is the evaluation, and shortest is staffing and organizational capability. A frequent error by beginning grant writers is to not include enough detail or clarity on how the funds will be used in terms to address reviewers' questions about the program activities. The grant should detail (a) what program will be implemented, length, dosage, content, and adaptations process; (b) number and type of staff who will implement; (c) when and where implemented; and (d) with which types of clients (number, demographic characteristics, and needs). Be sure to clearly specify recruiting and retention procedures for clients and numbers expected to complete the program, rather than supplying only numbers beginning the program. Hence, the anticipated attrition rate and ways to reduce attrition through incentives should be specified.

A professional evaluator who is proposed for the grant should write the evaluation section. The evaluator frequently writes not only this section but also

---

Box **14.2**
_____

Project Narrative (no more than 25 pages for sections A–D)

Section A: Statement of Need (20 points)

Section B: Proposed Approach (35 points) (purpose, goals, objectives, evidence-based intervention, adaptations needed, logic model, diversity issues, timeline, advisory group, collaborating organizations and groundwork done, potential barriers and methods to overcome them, and project sustainability plan)

Section C: Staff and Organizational Experience (15 points) (organization and staff capability, list of staff and evaluator, cultural characteristics of key staff and whether bilingual and bicultural, available resources [e.g., facilities, equipment], location and compliant with the Americans with Disabilities Act [ADA])

Section D: Evaluation and Data (30 points) (required Government Performance Reporting Act [GPRA] or bNOMs performance outcome measures and any additional measures, reliability and validity of measures, process and fidelity measures, and data collection, and data management, analysis, interpretation and reporting with measures in an appendix)

Supporting Documentation

Section E: Literature Citations

Section F: Budget Justification, Existing Resources, Other Support (narrative justification of each line item)

Section G: Biographical Sketches and Job Descriptions (two pages or less for each, one-page job descriptions for key personnel following examples PHS 5161-1 instructions at available at www.hhs.gov/forms/PHS-5161-1.doc.

Section H: Confidentiality and Participant Protection/Human Subjects (procedures assuring confidentiality, participant protection and the protection of human subject regulations following information about Protection of Human Subjects Regulations at www.hhs.gov/ohrp.

---

much of the grant for no cost in exchange for being awarded the final evaluation subcontract if the grant is funded. This section should include a process and an outcome evaluation, questions to be addressed, hypotheses, client or community change objectives, and long-terms goals as specified in your logic model. The type of evaluation research design used should be mentioned—a true experimental randomized control design, or a quasi-experimental design and type, or a nonexperimental design. See Cook and Campbell's seminal book, *Quasi-Experimentation: Design and Analysis Issues in Field Settings*,[18] for a complete description of different types of evaluation designs. An additional piece of this required prose in a grant application regards computation and consideration of power in terms of the number of subjects and expected effect sizes (see chapter 4 for detailed computations and examples).

The measurement instruments should each be described in a short paragraph or a table with number of items per scale, reliability and validity, and which participants complete the survey (e.g., child, adolescent, parent, or adult data are triangulated). The data collection methodology should be clear including who collects the data, whether the data is self-report and the method of data collection (e.g., individual or phone interviews, group surveys, mail-out surveys, computer Web-based surveys, or direct laptop surveys), implementer report, mechanical measures, archival data, and so forth. How confidentiality is will be maintained should be briefly mentioned here and in more detail in the Human Subjects section. Data analysis should match the evaluation design. End this narrative with a discussion of how the results will be disseminated using either conference presentations in combination with scientific reports and publications, and make mention of any credits to the funding agency.

TIPS ON WRITING SUCCESSFUL FEDERAL NON-NIH GRANTS

Grant Activities and Evaluation

One of the major differences between the research-based NIH grants and non-NIH grants is that technically non-NIH or service and evaluation grants are not considered research grants. The ramifications are minor in terms of the quality of the science in many cases. High-quality program evaluations are frequently required that can involve more complicated process evaluations than are often required on research grants that have better control of the interventions. Outcome results are also generally required, but not as complicated and frequently not employing randomized control trials, but only matched comparison groups. Hence, while the process evaluations can be more complex, the outcome evaluations can be less complex but no less difficult to negotiate with the community services providers. Deciding on the best comparison groups can be difficult. Some federal agencies will require a wait treatment comparison group; others, a dosage equivalent credible treatment comparison group. Each quasi-experimental design has its own strengths and also difficulties in terms of demonstrating positive effects. Some agencies want longitudinal designs with measured follow-up.

One nonresearch grant we have some familiarity with was funded through CSAP and required a four-year follow-up posttesting period and standardized measures agreed upon by 12 different cross-site grantees from different universities. In other words, the "nonresearch" requirements were more stringent than independent research grants funded through NIH. Another CSAT grant just completed for adolescent residential treatment also was quite complex from a design standpoint and required a two-year follow-up with all outcome measures determined by a private research firm for all grantees. The data were collected and entered directly into the cross-site evaluator's national Web site database. Hence, the research requirements were very stringent and demanding, including data-sharing agreements. The required data collection form was about 50 pages long and took about two to three hours for a client to complete. It is highly unlikely that this private contractor had approval from the office of management and budget for this long evaluation instrument, yet all grantees were told they had to use this form to be funded. A full-time "tracker" for the quarterly longitudinal follow-up was hired by the evaluator at our local university. This individual had the primary task of locating prior drug treatment clients and was set with the task of obtaining a benchmark standard for percent completion rate at each follow-up period. This high water mark for follow-up rates was used as a benchmark to determine continued funding.

Who Is the Primary Recipient of the Grant?

Another major difference between research-based NIH grants and non-NIH grants is that the university researchers or evaluators are often subcontractors and not the primary investigators. Hence, the recipients of these federal services grants are generally limited to community services agencies. Even if not specified in the list of eligible agencies, recipients are more often nonprofit agencies, faith communities, schools, or state or tribal governments, rather than universities. One reason this occurs is because the reviewers of these grants are often from NGOs, and they regard the NIH grants as appropriate for universities and the service grants better suited for NGOs.

SPECIFIC KEYS TO SUCCESS

In order to be a successful applicant, an NGO generally has to partner with a university or private evaluation company or consultant. A prominent feature of this collaboration is that the consultant group usually writes the grant or at least the evaluation section. Some of these grants are written on a fee-for-service basis; however, federal funding agencies look down on this practice because the person who wrote the grant will not be involved in actual implementation. According to the federal agencies' mindset, the grant writer may have little concern for whether what is promised in the text will actually come to fruition. To safeguard against these practices, some federal agencies now require the NGO to provide information at the end of the grant application detailing who wrote the grant and clarifying their implementation role. If the grant writer is a hired professional and not committed to implementing the project, the grant has a lower chance of being funded.

Importance of Community Collaboration

Because non-NIH grants are considered services grants with an evaluation component, a collaborative relationship is often needed. Community agencies should seek out university faculty and students who can help design, construct, and staff a high-quality evaluation. The budget amount earmarked for the evaluation is sometimes specified in the grant guidelines as between 10% and 20%. While it appears that this will detract from the amount of funding to be devoted to direct services, collaboration with a university professor or faculty can be very advantageous in helping write a winning grant. Moreover, the professor can help meet staffing needs using undergraduate and graduate students who need internship or elective credits in their specialties. This provides a tremendous cost savings to the grant. For instance, work-study students can be hired for as little as $2.50 per hour out of pocket, with the federal government grant to the university paying the balance of the $7.50 per hour. Hence, collaboration with a university can pay off in delivery of more direct services because of the very low staffing cost by employing university work-study students.

Implementing Evidence-Based Interventions

An additional advantage of the university and community agency collaboration is knowledge of the selection of the most effective research-based interventions to offer in the grant. University faculty members are often experts who can readily access the research literature regarding EBs, and they have extensive knowledge regarding program evaluation methodology. The agency staff can offer the knowledge of the clients and work with the researchers on how to make the EB interventions more locally and culturally relevant and effective. A winning grant often proposes to take an existing EB with strong support in the research literature and make it more locally, age, gender, or culturally appropriate. This increases adoption with minor adaptation. The grant should specify a process for this adaptation and include a table of specifications to show how each intervention strategy is modified.

Concept Papers or Letters of Intent

A formal letter of intent (LOI) is more frequently requested by federal agencies about one month in advance of the final submission. An LOI should include a one- to five-page summary of your proposed research. The major reason for the LOI is to determine about how many grants will be submitted, but it is also an additional chance to ask for feedback on how to improve your grant. One tip about these LOIs is that if you don't even see the announcement until after the deadline for the LOI submission, you can still submit a grant because LOIs are not mandatory. However, submitting an LOI in a timely manner helps you to obtain feedback from the project officer. This activity then helps you to shape your application and construct a winning idea. The project officer also can give you tips on writing the grant and activities that the review committee generally does not like to fund, as well as what type of application is likely to get funded.

Keys to Preparing a Budget for a Winning Grant

One major consideration in a winning grant is getting the most services to the most clients for the least amount of money—the proverbial "biggest bang for the buck." One good tip is to begin with the budget before even writing the concept paper or LOI to send to the project officer. We recommend starting with a budget because then you really know how much money you will have for various parts of the grant such as client services, evaluation, indirect costs, and total costs. Unlike the NIH grants, non-NIH or service grants specify a funding limit that includes both the direct and indirect costs. If the grant announcement does specify a range or an upper limit on funding, you can divide the total amount of funding available that is generally stated in the announcement by the number of grants they will fund, to get the average amount of funding for each grant. Be sure to stay within these budget limits for both your direct and indirect costs. Do not try to be much below that amount, because reviewers are likely to not see the grant as competitive in scope. Also, project officers will not want to have a large number of smaller grants to manage. If the announcement says they want to fund 10 grants, then that is the number of grants they want to fund for the average amount of funding. In the words of the Red Queen in *Alice in Wonderland*: "When I use a word it means exactly what I intend it to mean—no more and no less."

To get down to calculating the amount of funding you will have for your budget for direct service costs (personnel, training, equipment, materials, etc.), you need to subtract your indirect costs. Hence, if the limit you can apply for is $100,000 per year, you have to subtract from that your indirect costs (sometimes called overhead costs or facilities and administration costs). If your agency has a federally negotiated indirect rate (overhead rate) of 25% of your direct costs, then you only have about $80,000 for direct services. This can be derived by dividing $100,000 by the factor of 1.25 to get $80,000. You can double check this amount by multiplying $80,000 by .25 or 25%, which totals $20,000, and then adding that to $80,000 to result in the total direct and indirect grant total of $100,000. Once you have the total direct cost amount of $80,000, you have to subtract from that the amount of your university evaluation subcontractor's direct costs and also its indirect F&A costs. These indirect cost rates can be pretty high at universities and up to 50% or 75% of direct costs. So if your university researchers want $10,000 for their evaluation services, and the university indirect rate is 50%, then the total cost of the subcontract will be $15,000 (direct $10,000 + $5,000 indirect cost F&A = $15,000). This now becomes $15,000 in direct costs in your budget. This leaves you only $65,000 for direct services at your agency ($80,000 direct costs − $15,000 for the university evaluation subcontract).

However, this is less expensive than having the university as the primary grant recipient. In this case, with an indirect rate of twice as much as the NGO (50% vs. 25%), there is less funding for the direct services ($66,667 vs. $80,000). This is another reason that universities are often not as competitive in getting non-NIH grants because they cannot deliver as many direct services to clients because of their high indirect rates. Sometimes the university researcher can get a special waiver by the university office of sponsored project or research to cut the indirect rate in half for special circumstances. Keep in mind that universities survive to a great deal on their grant indirect costs. These monies help them control their overhead costs, which include building construction and maintenance, faculty lines, library expenses, administration (institutional review boards), and ancillary costs not covered directly in their budgets. For instance, most health sciences centers at state universities have only about 10% of their funds as line items directly tied to the budget and covered by state. The balance of their budget costs comes from research grants and clinical services. Therefore, if they believe that they can benefit from a lucrative grant, but their rate for indirect costs is not competitive, they may be willing to negotiate a lower rate. Also, there are different indirect cost rates for different types of grants services. For nonresearch grants that are primarily being delivered off campus, there may be a rate that is considerably lower (about half) because university facilities and equipment are not being used. Some federal agencies such as the DoED simply limit the indirect rate a university can charge to 8%.

STEPS IN DEVELOPING A WINNING GRANT: WORKING WITH PROJECT OFFICERS

As chapter 2 of this volume outlines in considerable detail, it is very helpful to have the support of the funding agency project officer before submitting a grant. Even if an LOI is not required a month in advance, which is becoming more common, it is a very good idea to contact the project officer specified on the grant application by email and arrange a phone call. Use this opportunity to describe your specific idea, ask for any suggestions on improvements, and offer to send by e-mail a one- or two-page concept paper. Getting the interest and support of the project officer can make the difference in getting funded or not. They know the special quirks of the reviewers and the emerging priorities of their agency. With the fluctuation in reviewers from grant cycle to grant cycle, non-NIH service grants may suffer from a lack of reviewer continuity. NIH project officers have an advantage in predicting how a review committee will stand on a grant because the committee members are often "standing" committees with members who serve for several years.

In the case of non-NIH grant, the review committees are often "special" review committees with new members each year drawn from a large pool of potential reviewers, generally practitioners in the field and a few junior university researchers. Also, the reviews are generally conducted only once a year, so if you are not funded, you do not go back to the same committee members. This can be a disadvantage because even if you improve the grant based on suggestions from a prior review, you will most likely not have the same reviewers the next year even if there is a release in the next year for the specific grant announcement. For tips on how to respond to reviews and resubmission, see chapter 18 this volume, which stresses the importance of contacting your project officers at the agency to see if they have any additional guidance on how to improve your grant based on the reviewers' comments. Sometimes program officers attend the reviews in Washington, DC and may have additional comments about the discussion of your grant by the reviewers that was not captured by the written reviews. The reviews are written prior to the committee meeting. If the reviews are done by phone or just sent back to the federal agency using email, the project officer will have less information to share. However, the project officer may be able to provide some insight when the comments are written and there has been sufficient time to mull them over. In general, what you want is to have this project officer really excited about getting your concept funded. Most agency staff members are very committed professionals whose job it is to see that the highest quality programs and services are funded by their agency.

REVIEW PROCESS

This section discusses review criteria and typical reasons that funding may be denied.

Review Criteria

Unlike the NIH grants that have standard review criteria (see chapter 1 covering peer review and chapter 3 examining review criteria)—significance, approach, innovation, investigators, and environment—the non-NIH grant review criteria are tailored to the specific announcement. The general format contains quality ratings for the different sections of the grant based on the total points assigned to each section. Box 14.3 shows the typical evaluation criteria for non-NIH federal agency grants.

Why Do Grants Fail?

As mentioned above, a disadvantage of non-NIH grants is that often there is no second chance to get funded. Committees are created for a special announcement and sometimes the agency does not offer the same funding the next year or the agency changes its funding priorities. This places the onus on the applicant to write a successful winning grant the first time it is reviewed. NIH has conducted some investigations examining why many grants are not given better

---

Box 14.3   Sample of Evaluation Criteria

Your application will be reviewed and scored according to the quality of your response to the requirements listed below for developing the project narrative (sections A–D). These sections describe what you intend to do with your project and replace the narrative instructions in the PHS 5161-1 application forms. The number of points after each grant section heading is the maximum number of points a review committee may assign to that section of your project narrative. Note that, although the budget for the proposed project is not a review criterion, the review group will be asked to comment on the appropriateness of the budget after the merits of the application have been considered.

---

priority scores. Surveying across numerous internal review group sections, the single most stated reason for grants not being funded is because the data analysis section was not clear or was of poor quality. Hence, even with these nonresearch grants, it is important to have an evaluator who really knows the most sophisticated design and analysis issues. These are called research methodologists, not just statisticians. Their expertise includes psychometrics (measurement concerns), survey design, sampling, power estimation, laboratory protocols, consenting of subjects, subject recruitment and follow-up methods, epidemiology, research strategies, interviewing, and data management (collection, collation, and computerization), to name just a few skills. Most of these highly trained individuals will work on grants as consultants for a daily rate.

Failure to Be Reviewed

The reasons for failure of many grants to do well in review are even more complex for federal services grants. First, there a several reasons your grant may not even make it to review. Consider the events listed in box 14.4 that can transpire prior to review.

Box 14.4   Reasons for Failure to Be Reviewed

Grant was received past the deadline.
Grant was not complete—missing required forms or information.
Grant is over the page limit or margins are smaller than specified in the
    announcement.
The font size is smaller than allowed in the announcement, which is generally
    12-point font.
The budget is too large for the size of grants funded as specified in the
    announcement.

Failure to Get a High Enough Review Score

In a non-NIH grant review, generally about two to four members of a special review committee are asked to be the primary reviewers and to write a summary of a particular grants strengths and weaknesses. These individual reviewers often have to score the grant based on a range of possible scores for each section of the grant. Thus, it is imperative that applicants carefully follow the required sections of a grant, because these match the sections in the reviewers' scoring templates. Section headings should be worded precisely as the application dictates, for easy identification. Applicants should carefully read the grant announcement and obtain a clear picture of what is required in each section and what components are scored by reviewers. Reviewers need to be able to identify components of the application; find information; have no trouble making headway of charts, tables, figures, and diagrams; and feel comfortable with the grant writing style.

What Are the Key Components of a Review?

First and foremost, reviewers want to be excited about the ideas embedded in a grant application. The grant should contain innovative ideas that are couched in reasonable fiscal prudence. In reality, grants should offer the biggest bang for the buck but at the same time be thoughtful. Reviewers need to quickly capture how the grant outlines the service agency's organizational strengths, service delivery options, and penchant for meeting deadlines. There is also the possibility that luck is operating in your favor. For instance, your grant may offer a specific line of services or include a target population that overlaps quite heavily with the specific interests of the reviewer. When this happens, you may have greater luck during the review, since there is a voice in the room speaking on your behalf.

General Tips for Funding

A federal nonresearch grant, like any NIH grant, has to be well written and easy to follow. It also has to look nice, with appropriate formatting (font, paragraph layout, text effects, and font size), inserts (charts or diagrams), and graphics (pictures are worth a 1,000 words!). It is imperative that your literature review be thorough, documented, and current. A grant with old citations does not suggest careful schol-

---

Know Your Reviewer

Find out who sits on the review committee prior to your submission deadline. This information is available on various government Web sites (see appendix 1). Finding out who sits on standing review committees for NIH peer review is somewhat easier than for nonresearch grants, given that the NIH peer review committee sits for three years. Reviewers for federal nonresearch grants are often ad hoc reviewers; thus, they are likely to attend one or two reviews and contribute based on their expertise. Applicants should also use the most popular evidence-based practices to look current in their own intervention practices.

arship or knowledge of the field (chapter 3 covers this issue for NIH grants, as well). Reviewers are usually well published in the field. In the event your grant is reviewed by an individual who has published extensively in the field, and you do not cite this individual's work, this could be the death knell for your application. It is not uncommon for reviewers to search the reference section of a grant first, seeking to identify whether the application is both current and fair (judicious) in the citations (and the application cites the reviewer or their colleagues).

In terms of where to devote the most attention (and therefore text) in the grant, the activity section is where you describe the actual performance and delivery of services. As an example, an activity section should include at the very minimum the various bullet points outlined in box 14.5.

New grant writers, particularly those who have are recent graduate students, tend to confuse the art of grant writing with developing a comprehensive literature review or needs assessments. These individuals often focus too heavily on building a case from the literature, documenting studies, and describing these studies and their relevance to the present topic. The same can be said of spending too much time hammering home certain points. What happens in these applications is a general neglect of the specifics of what services will be delivered and how they can alter the lives of the constituent population. It is good to remember that the agency staff requesting the new activities is already convinced of the need or they would not have written the specific funding announcement. Mostly, they want to know specifically what the applicant's agency can do to reduce the problem through feasible and cost-effective activities. In this regard, it is important to develop a concerted answer to the question: "Specifically, who will do what, when, where, how, and why?"

Box 14.5   **Specific Activities**

This section should include specific detail regarding the nature of services provided:

Populations that will be serviced

Numbers of clients per year

Demographics of the clients (e.g., ethnicity, gender, age)

Recruitment methods

Methods to reduce sample attrition

Prior experience with clients

Feasibility of recruiting the target numbers of clients

Delivery of services

Training of staff

Quality assurance in service delivery (program fidelity)

Implementation evaluation documenting numbers of hours of services

Outcome evaluation (pre- and posttest using standardized measures)

Logic Models

To assure the activities are closely linked to the funding announcement's stated needs and objectives, it is very helpful to create a logic model appropriate for the grant. Logic models are constructed different ways, but generally they look somewhat like the graphic schematic portrayed in figure 14.2.

It is easiest to create a logic model from the right side of figure 14.2, or at least beginning with a list of goals. Generally, you should have no more than three goals (this keeps your project focused on deliverables). For instance, the first author developed a logic model for family-based substance abuse programs that included a primary goal to "reduce 30 day alcohol and drug use." Two additional and measurable subgoals included increasing quality of life and reducing health care costs.

The objectives are written next and should revolve around anticipated changes in the designated risk and protective factors or mediators (i.e., intervening measures). These factors are identified based on the research literature as proximal predictors of the problem. Examples of mediators (which happen to be risk factors for drug use) include knowledge, attitudes, beliefs, or behaviors that will likely lead to a reduction in the problem and that are malleable through the proposed activities. The next step includes listing the activities that will be implemented including recruiting clients, hiring staff, training staff, implementing the program (number of sessions, length of sessions, type of sessions), and evaluating services. Last is the list of resources needed to implement the different activities, such as the facilities, materials, and personnel required right down to the name of the evaluator who will conduct the evaluation. Once you have created a logic model that everyone agrees with in terms of clearly specifying the goals, objectives, activities, and resources needed, you are ready to write your grant.

Tip

It is advisable to begin the grant construction process with the budget. Calculating your budget prior to writing the grant helps because you need to be sure you have enough funds to implement all of the services promised in the grant. The budget should include all of the proposed personnel, regular salary, and fringe benefits. All proposed staff positions should have people named to those positions, so that the reviewers believe that the project is feasible because you have excellent staff for the project. Be sure you get commitments from all proposed staff including letters of commitment included in the grant for all positions with people listed as well as their PHS biographical sketches. Be sure that the bio-sketches are updated and that they are in the current PHS format, which gets revised frequently. Check your grant application kit from Grants. gov for the proper forms. The final budget should be put on the proper PHS forms. Web sites for the bio-sketch and budget forms are listed in appendix 1.

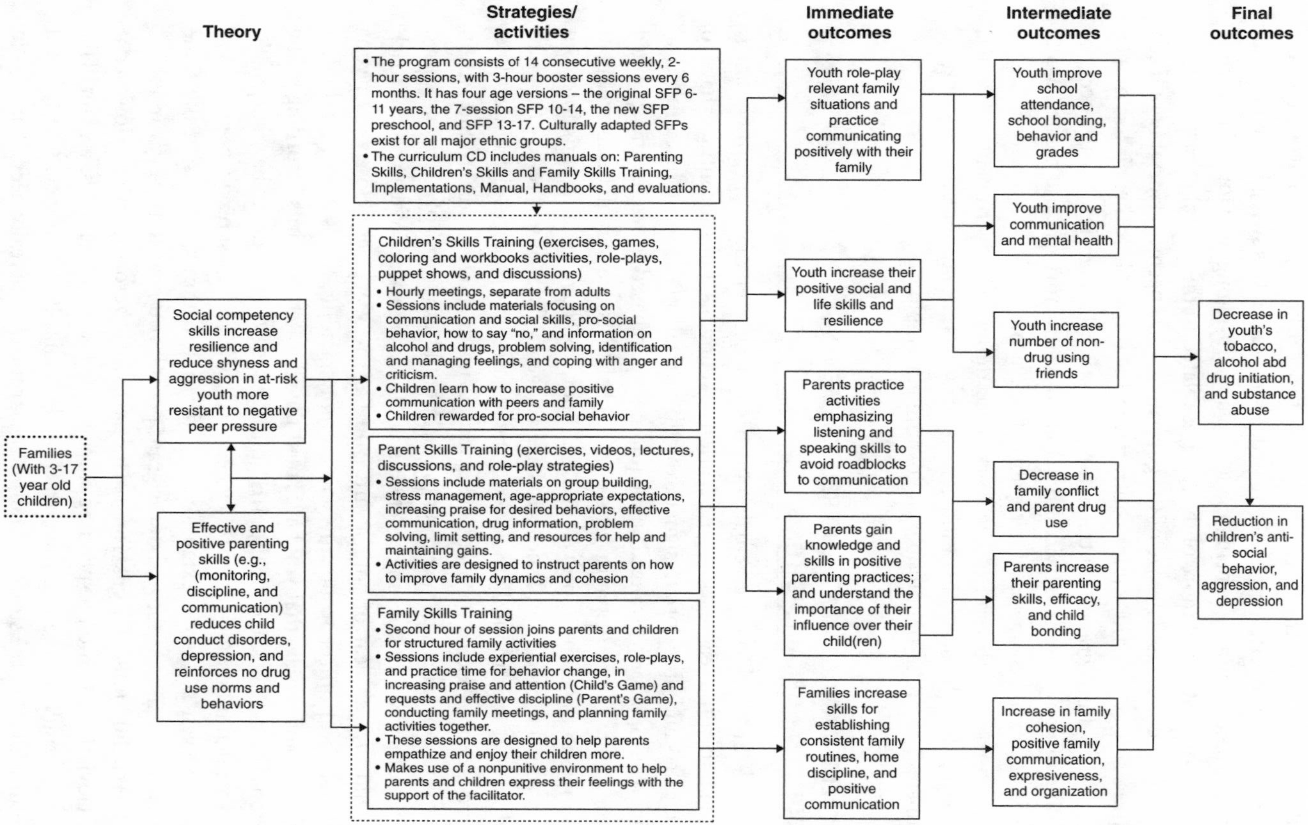

Theory
Strategies/ activities
Immediate outcomes
Intermediate outcomes
Final outcomes
Families (With 3-17 year old children)
Social competency skills increase resilience and reduce shyness and aggression in at-risk youth more resistant to negative peer pressure
Effective and positive parenting skills (e.g., (monitoring, discipline, and communication) reduces child conduct disorders, depression, and reinforces no drug use norms and behaviors
• The program consists of 14 consecutive weekly, 2-hour sessions, with 3-hour booster sessions every 6 months. It has four age versions – the original SFP 6-11 years, the 7-session SFP 10-14, the new SFP preschool, and SFP 13-17. Culturally adapted SFPs exist for all major ethnic groups.
• The curriculum CD includes manuals on: Parenting Skills, Children's Skills and Family Skills Training, Implementations, Manual, Handbooks, and evaluations.
Children's Skills Training (exercises, games, coloring and workbooks activities, role-plays, puppet shows, and discussions)
• Hourly meetings, separate from adults
• Sessions include materials focusing on communication and social skills, pro-social behavior, how to say "no," and information on alcohol and drugs, problem solving, identification and managing feelings, and coping with anger and criticism.
• Children learn how to increase positive communication with peers and family
• Children rewarded for pro-social behavior
Parent Skills Training (exercises, videos, lectures, discussions, and role-play strategies)
• Sessions include materials on group building, stress management, age-appropriate expectations, increasing praise for desired behaviors, effective communication, drug information, problem solving, limit setting, and resources for help and maintaining gains.
• Activities are designed to instruct parents on how to improve family dynamics and cohesion
Family Skills Training
• Second hour of session joins parents and children for structured family activities
• Sessions include experiential exercises, role-plays, and practice time for behavior change, in increasing praise and attention (Child's Game) and requests and effective discipline (Parent's Game), conducting family meetings, and planning family activities together.
• These sessions are designed to help parents empathize and enjoy their children more.
• Makes use of a nonpunitive environment to help parents and children express their feelings with the support of the facilitator.
Youth role-play relevant family situations and practice communicating positively with their family
Youth increase their positive social and life skills and resilience
Parents practice activities emphasizing listening and speaking skills to avoid roadblocks to communication
Parents gain knowledge and skills in positive parenting practices; and understand the importance of their influence over their child(ren)
Families increase skills for establishing consistent family routines, home discipline, and positive communication
Youth improve school attendance, school bonding, behavior and grades
Youth improve communication and mental health
Youth increase number of non-drug using friends
Decrease in family conflict and parent drug use
Parents increase their parenting skills, efficacy, and child bonding
Increase in family cohesion, positive family communication, expresiveness, and organization
Decrease in youth's tobacco, alcohol abd drug initiation, and substance abuse
Reduction in children's anti-social behavior, aggression, and depression

Figure 14.2. Sample Logic Plan for Nonresearch Services Grant

Trends—What Is Being Funded

In the last few years, the federal budget for services has decreased, while the cost of running the government has increased. As a result of this swing in the financial pendulum, less funding is being made available through grants for small services agencies or NGOs and more of the services related to the federal government are bid out on contracts. The size of the government has been considerably reduced as these services get bid out for contract, but the downside is there is less money available to fund grants/contracts for small services agencies. This process of bidding out government services to preferred contractors has also created a cottage industry of beltway bandits capable of delivering services to the government. Hence, in reality the size of the work force doing the governments work has increased, but the administration can say they technically "cut the size of government," meaning the number of government employees.

PROJECT MANAGEMENT AND REQUIREMENTS
IF FUNDED—GPRA REPORTING

As if all this work on the actual grant has not been enough, once the grant is funded, then the real work begins. Various documents and subcontracts have to be created and appropriate signatures affixed. Staff needs to be hired, physical space developed or rearranged, and equipment purchased as needed and specified in the grant. The principal investigator (PI) has to assure that all funds are spent as shown in the grant-approved budget. If not, you have to get permission from your federal fiscal officer. It helps to have an agency fiscal officer review the grant and meet at least monthly to review expenditures and balances per budget line. There is some "executive" latitude or authority to move funds around within your personnel and other expenses totals, but only about 10% of each can be used on the other without getting federal fiscal officer approval. When you approach the end of each year of your award, you have to work very closely with your internal fiscal officer to be sure you are not spending funds over your budget limits or, conversely, that you have spent the allocated amounts according to the various budget lines. Unlike the NIH grants, it is getting harder to have surplus or unexpended funds and request they be made available in a subsequent grant next year (or even a no-cost extension to add years to the budget using the same allocated dollars). At the end of the grant period, you have to be very careful not to overspend funds. The goal is to balance as close to zero as possible. However, it is inadvisable to go on a spending spree in the last two months of a grant. This usually results in a red flag and attracts auditors like bees to honey. Auditors will question whether the supplies, equipment, or travel were really needed or used in a timely manner for the grant.

Most non-NIH grants require you to collect specific outcome data required for congressional reporting regarding agency success. These data fall under the purview of the Government Performance Results Act (GPRA). As a means of increasing accountability for line item funding amounts to the various federal agencies, Congress now mandates that each federal agency determines an appropriate definition of success for their specific grant funding. To exemplify this accounting system, CSAP has its grantees collect data from clients on 30-day use of alcohol and illegal drugs. Special 30-day frequency-of-use questions, called standardized GPRA measures, are designed by the agency's evaluation contractors, and all grantees collect these data directly from clients.

THE QUINTESSENTIAL NATURE OF A GRANT WRITER

It goes without saying that successful grant writing requires a multitude of talents. One way to characterize these individuals suggests that grant writers are "dreamers and schemers" epitomized by hard work and a penchant for organization and time management skills. Above all, grant writers need to write in a clear, consistent, and convincing manner. A professor teaching a course on grant writing once said to her graduate students, you should be "able to sell refrigerators to Eskimos." If that is not enough, grant writers need to have a head full of winning and creative ideas. These ideas need to match the funding announcement goals and objectives, and they need to be considered innovative and exciting by the review committee.

The Big Picture

When all is said and done, the grant proposal must be cost-effective and convince the reviewers that it is feasible. Grant production, in its entirety, requires participation by a team of experts rather than a single grant writer. Once a grant has been awarded, be sure to maintain good relationships with the grant's project officer and fiscal officer by completing all reporting requirements.

PUBLICATIONS AND PRESENTATIONS

Completion of the grant is not signified by finalization of implementation. That is only the real first step after all of the logistical issues have been resolved (e.g., subject recruitment). Now that implementation is done, there must be a reservoir of data that have been collected and need to be organized into reports. A major component of grant production regards publications and presentations at conferences, scientific meetings, and even congressional or senate hearings. Despite having an orientation toward services, the types of grants that are the focus of this chapter also entail an element of research. This means collating the data, analyzing the data statistically, and summarizing the data and statistical findings in reports. It is essential that all publications (including PowerPoint presentations at meetings) credit the funding agency. Footnotes and acknowledgments are the industry standard for doing this in scientific publications. Be sure to send the project officer a copy of any publications. A number of these nonfederal agencies also have required conferences where program implementers and evaluators are expected to attend and present on their grants. Be sure to carefully read the grant instructions because they frequently mention that you should include in your application budget funding for the PI, program coordinator, and evaluator to attend these conferences, which are generally held in Washington, DC.

One other point worth noting is that positive findings following implementation can auger well for your agency. In other words, some federal agencies have what they call mentoring grants. These grants are used to help past grantees that ran successful evaluations to mentor other agencies and assist them in the process of learning more about implementation and evaluation.

SUMMARY AND CONCLUSIONS

This chapter has covered funding opportunities outside of NIH with a focus on nonresearch activities such as program evaluations of evidence-based programs and practices. There are a number of federal nonresearch grants, cooperative agreements, or contracts available from federal agencies. The best source for locating the announcements for these grants is through the universal portal Grants.gov. These grants can be as difficult to write as federal research grants. Some are longer than the NIH standard 25-page single-spaced narrative because they include required tables and matrices, such as Administration on Native Americans grants, where the narrative can be more than 60 pages long. Some are very short and relatively easier to construct, including DoED grants. The amount of funding for nonresearch grants is considerably larger than the approximate $28.6 billion in funding available for all NIH research funds. Because of decreasing levels of funding for new grants at NIH, researchers and practitioners should consider partnering to apply for the nonresearch grants, which have a larger pool of money available.

In addition to these pointers, this chapter has briefly attended to the different phases of research and pointed out the growing need for and emphasis on applied research. The demand for successful programs and cost-effective expenditures of government federal dollars on programs that work requires greater emphasis on developing evidence-based programs. Once developed in the context of randomized controlled field trials, a second stage involves determining whether treatment, intervention, or service programs produce similar outcomes with new and different populations than those that they were originally tested on. Funding trends currently stress practice agencies selecting the best evidence-based program for their population's unique needs and then conducting as high a quality process and outcome evaluation as can be managed within the limitations of the budget.

On the face of things, the types of grants described in this chapter are not easy to implement, nor are they easy to evaluate. In fact, nonresearch grants can be equally or more challenging than NIH research grants to implement with high quality and fidelity. Based on a lengthy career in the service sector as well as holding an agency director's position inside the government, we offer the following "sage" advice: Do not be fooled into thinking that just because these are nonresearch grants, they are any easier to obtain or implement. Because the requests for proposals are often a one-shot affair, you do not get a second or third chance to improve your grant as you do with NIH grants that can be revised and resubmitted. These nonresearch grants can be very challenging and take a committed leader or PI and staff to implement effectively as planned in the grant.

However, the rewards are many in improved services and staff moral when they can say with confidence that what they are doing really works. In addition, a successful grant can lead to increased funding from other local county or state funding sources. In addition, it can lead to a successful NIH grant because your agency has demonstrated capability and capacity to implement evidence-based programs with fidelity and high quality. If you have made some unique adaptations based on cultural, developmental, gender, or special population appropriateness of an evidence-based model, you could also develop a training and dissemination system to help other agencies adopt this effective service. So there are many benefits to a successful grant to balance the hard work that it does take. Be resilient, and if your first attempt does not produce funding, continue to look for similar grant announcements where you can use your "boiler plate" materials to produce a more successful grant. That is the most important tip within this chapter: The more grants you submit, the more likely you are to be successful. Even the best-funded researchers who have obtained their monies from NIH have had to resubmit their grants multiple times to get funded. Therefore, don't be discouraged, and move forward. This is the only way to success in this grant writing field.

The Financing and Cost Accounting of Science

Budgets and Budget Administration

MICHELLE A. LEWIS

Biomedical research is an essential enterprise for our society, pursued to a very great extent in laboratories scattered throughout academic health centers by dedicated, expert scientists driven by a quest to help improve quality of life. ... Our nation and others in the "developed world" have both the opportunity and the obligation to meet the challenges of improving the health of our society as well as that of those less fortunate.

—ANDREW R. MARKS, *"The Economy of Science"*

THIS CHAPTER EXAMINES one of the most essential components of grant construction: developing a budget to finance science. All grants submitted to the NIH require a budget, regardless of size or scope of the project. The budget can be modular and contain relatively little detail, only a few numbers placed in neat little boxes at the top of a form. These numbers address the direct costs for different grant years, and the form is followed by a brief narrative for personnel and consortium costs. Larger, more intensive projects entailing data collection, fieldwork, subject contact, or laboratory costs entail a more detailed budget and narrative that cannot be modular in format if they exceed $250,000 of direct costs per year. In contrast, center grants require reams of budget pages detailing cost structures for research or administrative functions performed by the various cores. Likewise, grants that involve consortium agreements and subcontracts also require pages of explanation and detailed financial accounting. In either case, big or small, R03 or

P50, financing scientific inquiry and the execution of a grant requires extensive deliberation about money.

The best approach to constructing budget's for grant applications submitted to the NIH and other Public Health Service (PHS) agencies involves the technique of "cost accounting the science," an approach that emulates or parallels the methods and experimental procedures outlined in the grant proposal. As depicted in figure 15.1, a synergistic relationship between the science and the budget is important to cost account a grant during its basic construction and various stages or phases of grant development.

Any expenditure(s) proposed in the budget, that is not fully supported by the scope of work proposed in the aforementioned sections will raise a red flag to reviewers. Red flags over budgetary issues are less common during review; however, they can be as damaging as human subject concerns. In other words, these types of comments during review raise the specter that the principal investigator (PI) does not fully grasp the project design or is unaware (e.g., junior faculty) of the resources needed to achieve the stated goals of the study. If it becomes evident to a review committee that a possible disconnect exists between the budget and the project design, reviewers may lose enthusiasm even for the very best studies. This type of activity can adversely influence the final priority score. Budgetary concerns raised during review are duly noted during the review by the scientific review administrator (SRA) and program staff and are further addressed internally by the parent-funding institute or center before funding considerations can be made.

The budget needs to measure costs accurately so that decision makers can compare the cost of a program with its benefit, the cost of one program with another, and the cost of alternative methods of reaching a specified goal.[1]

Figure 15.1. Synergistic Components of a Grant Budget

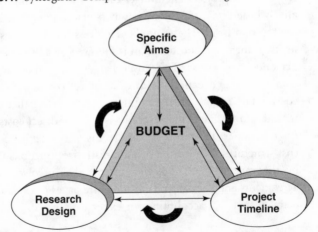

Therefore, any calculation or formula utilized to arrive at a total requested dollar amount for personnel and/or nonpersonnel expenditures should be explained and not left up to the interpretation of the reviewers. NIH reviewers are in the position of making budget recommendations for grants scored within a fundable range. There are two ways in which a comment or recommendation from a reviewer can trickle down into the summary statement. Summary statements are prepared by the SRA staff and used by program staff, council, and grants management to guide them in making funding decisions. On the one hand, a reviewer acting alone can initiate this activity by inserting a section in his/her review detailing budget concerns and submit this to the SRA after a vote on the grant is taken. A second method involves the consensus section of a summary statement that considers the tenor of the entire review committee based on their discussion of the grant at review. If the basic tenor of the committee supports a budget concern, this will also trickle down into the summary statement. This shows that the entire review committee agreed with the budget concern, and this is harder for program staff to ignore when it comes to making funding decisions. Trimming budgets is always stated in terms of percentage cuts. The standard approach is to recommend 10% or 20% reductions as budget modifications. Perhaps the most frequent reasons recommended budget cuts will be made include:

- Inadequate justification of costs
- Insufficient detail on calculations
- Exorbitant costs in comparison to the activities proposed
- Costs too low to adequately achieve the stated objectives of the project
- Costs not economically efficient
- Costs not comparable to other proposals with similar objectives
- Costs that are not reasonable, allocable, or consistent or do not conform to budget restrictions set forth by the funding agency and/or the applicable Office of Management and Budget (OMB) cost principles[2] (information on the precise language for the OMB circulars mentioned can be found by linking to the appropriate Web sites; see appendix 1)

Currently, no page limitations are set on the budget sections of the NIH grant applications (unless the funding announcement specifies otherwise). Therefore, investigators would be smart to provide as much detailed information as possible by justifying *all* personnel and nonpersonnel costs required to develop and implement the proposed research program.

THE ART OF BUDGET PREPARATION

Consistent with the points raised in chapter 3, there is as much "art" as there is science in preparing grants. Budget preparation and grants management also has an element of "art," albeit this activity can be daunting to many new investigators and/or administrative personnel unfamiliar with the process. Even seasoned professionals are often times frustrated by the process of having to refine their budgets to justify the research proposed. While the art of budget preparation and grants management has a significant learning curve, the process is seemingly straightforward. This section contains a good deal of pertinent information that applies to many different grant funding mechanisms to help investigators develop a plan of attack for devising budgets.

A good piece of advice at the outset is that it is very important to carefully follow the budget guidelines provided by the funding agency, coordinate the grant application process as early as possible to overcome unforeseen obstacles, and examine the entire proposal for consistency. By consistency, I mean if your grant proposal relies on urine analysis to detect cocaine abuse in an experiment testing different behavioral treatment modalities with addicts, make sure you provide budget details on the cost of urine analysis. Leaving this item out can have serious adverse consequences when the reviewers get their hands on the grant. Another way to think about consistency is to remember that the budget is part of the grant and the two most important pieces, science and money, are inseparable.

Additionally, all proposed budget costs should conform to the sponsor's published guidelines on "allowable costs" pertinent to the research program or funding mechanism. For example, while the purchase of food may be allowable and justifiable on an R13/U13 (support for conferences and scientific meetings) grant, it is not an allowable direct expense to budget food on an R03 (research project grant program) proposal containing secondary analyses of existing data sets. Referring to the agency funding announcement regarding budget limitations or restrictions prior to preparing the application will save a lot of time and aggravation during the budget and overall grant preparation process. This point is even more important to new investigators who have not yet established their own administrative support team to assist with the initial phases of preparing the application. Regardless of the level of experience of the submitting investigator(s), however, the following questions should necessarily come to mind while drafting a grant budget:

1. *Why is the proposed budget expenditure important to the project, and how does it contribute to the overall goals of the study?* One way to word this section is to include a brief statement regarding the goals of the project and showcase how the investigative team is poised and ready to examine the research questions. The wording would go as follows:

   A goal of this project is to determine whether treatment X is a successful means to eradicate the ever-growing population of the Japanese beetles, which are responsible for destroying the nation's farms and forests. The proposal includes an experienced multidisciplinary team of investigators who recognize the need to combat the problem of the Japanese beetle infestation in support of our nation's Healthy Forest & Crops Initiative.

2. *Who are the individuals that make up the investigative team, and how do their functions and roles on the project influence the budget?* You would list all the key personnel individually and accentuate their backgrounds and suitability for the project. The text to address investigative roles reads as follows:

> Dr. Carlson is an internationally recognized expert in the field of bio-chemistry, and he will devote 40% effort to the proposed research project in all years of requested support. He will be responsible for chemically for-mulating batches of treatment X and reporting his findings to the investi-gative team.

3. *What is the population being evaluated in this project (if any), and how will their participation influence the budget?* Defining the population or sample that will participate in the study is a major issue when resolving costs. The text could read as follows:

> The top 20 producing farmers in the United States with crops affected by the Japanese beetle infestation problem will participate in focus groups and one-on-one interviews to ascertain the impact of the Japanese beetles on their crops and exported vegetation. Ten randomly selected farmers in the control group will receive a placebo treatment, while the other 10 farmers (experimental group) will receive treatment X. One-on-one structured in-terviews will take place twice per year in project years 2, and 4 and the focus groups will occur in years 3 and 5. Monetary incentives will be provided to all farmers who agree to participate in the focus groups and one-on-one interviews. At the conclusion of the study, all farmers will receive a sample batch of treatment X for beetle eradication.

4. *Where does the project take place, and are the facilities available sufficient to carry out the study? If not, does the grant allow a budget line for renovations or alterations to existing space?* Clarifying the participating facilities and outlining their physical and logistic requirements also factor heavily into the budget. The text for this portion could read as follows:

> Dr. Anderson's laboratory and accompanying office space are sufficient to conduct the study without a need to renovate or alter the existing space. One-on-one interviews will be conducted on-site at the farm locations of the study participants.

5. *What other logistics required to conduct the study will influence the budget?* This issue concerns whether outside companies are involved in the pro-

ject, for instance, conducting focus groups, helping recruit study sites, preparing experimental treatment serum, or conducting laboratory assays. Investigators have to resolve the limits of their own expertise and decide how much work will be farmed out. Other issues address the frequency of conducting experimental trials, the number of focus groups, quantifying costs for laboratory assays, and putting a dollar value on the actual treatment regimen. When interventions involve human subject contact, monetary incentives become an issue and drive up the cost of the budget. Likewise, in some studies administration of survey instruments or neuropsychological assessments is a major cost factor. Costs associated with printing, keypunching (or optically scanning), and coding surveys factor into budgets (as does actual data collection). Studies that involve treatments to human subjects involve the treatment itself, plus additional administrative costs for consenting patients; developing patient records; adding nurses, social workers, and researchers responsible for the additional data collection; and conducting laboratory procedures. In many instances, investigators do not properly cost-account these portions of the research study and get hammered during review. In the present example, mass production of treatment X is a major cost factor, as is distribution of the treatment to the farmers. Furthermore, when the study is completed, and treatment X turns out to be efficacious in its eradication of Japanese beetles, study protocols dictate that treatment X will be distributed to all farmers participating in the study regardless of their study condition assignment.

These types of concerns (and others not mentioned here) and their financial considerations should come to mind as you write your proposal. The answers to these questions represent the core issues that will be part of the first draft (of many drafts) of your budget. The first draft of the budget should always reflect the "worse case scenario." This initial phase is used to outline the full direct costs required to conduct the study without any modifications. Continually scaling back the budget after devising this first draft will help shape the research design and the budget into a coherent package.

The remainder of this chapter:

- Offers recommendations to investigators seeking solutions to better manage their growing grants administration needs
- Suggests the use of a multistep, cost-accounting method to prepare budgets for research applications
- Recommends the use of everyday technological aids to prepare research budgets

- Highlights the importance of designing and creating a comprehensive budget package template
- Provides a detailed breakdown of all budget categories on the PHS 398 Form page 4 and suggest several techniques to construct the NIH budget from start to finish

Appendix 15.1 at the end of this chapter includes a sample nonmodular budget and budget justification. Where appropriate, I provide helpful Web site addresses. These Web sites are described in greater detail in appendix 1 at the end of this volume. The sample budget and accompanying budget narrative in appendix 15.1 are modeled from an actual funded research budget submitted to the NIH (the Japanese beetle research topic is happily fictitious). I highly recommend that investigators consult with their institution's sponsored programs office to ascertain whether the techniques suggested in this chapter are consistent with their expectations and that of the funding agency. If your organization is small and does not employ a staffed grants and contracts office, then the NIH Office of Extramural Research (OER) Web site, located at grants1.nih.gov/grants/oer.htm, is an excellent resource for obtaining up-to-date information on funding opportunities, applications and forms, grant policies and guidelines, and information on electronic research submission procedures.

GRANTS MANAGEMENT PERSONNEL

As a bit of personal background, for the past five years I have held the position of research administrator with the Division of Prevention and Health Behavior and the Institute of Prevention Research at the Weill Medical College of Cornell University. The institute director and division chief, Dr. Gilbert Botvin, is an internationally known expert on tobacco, alcohol, and drug abuse prevention. He, along with several faculty members and colleagues, has received millions of federal grant dollars during the past 25 years from various institutes within the NIH in support of research focusing on school-based drug abuse prevention. The remaining portions of this chapter share with the reader the business and financial accounting model that helps funnel grants through the laboratory at Cornell and the professional expertise required in order that we may perform this important work. This financial accounting model has enabled the division faculty to focus its efforts on writing grants while shifting the grants administration and fiscal management responsibilities to the research administrator. If an investigator is in the position to hire administrative personnel to conduct and/or oversee the administrative aspects of grants management, it is highly recommended, but not necessary. If your institution does not have the resources available to hire an administrator (or grants manager) to conduct these functions, however, the work can be done by the investigator. Keep in mind that advanced planning is vital to successfully preparation of the application and timely submission to the funding agency. Most research institutions' grants and contracts offices have personnel to assist faculty with these matters. If your institution (or department) hires a grants manager or a research administrator, that individual should possess the following technical and interpersonal skills:

- Grant-related work experience in either a clinical or academic setting
- Strong knowledge of managing and devising budgets for research
- Advanced computer literacy utilizing Microsoft Excel and Word
- Working knowledge of the internal (institutionwide) and external (funding agency) grant routing and preparation process
- Exceptional level of patience and the ability to display grace under pressure while striving to meet deadlines

THE INSTITUTE FOR PREVENTION GRANT (BUDGET) PREP PARADIGM

Several months prior to the submission deadline, one or more of the faculty will announce their plans to submit a grant application. This usually occurs at weekly research meetings or informally with the institute director. If the application is in response to a program announcement (PA) or a request for applications (RFA), I review the PA or RFA to determine if there are any funding restrictions that may influence budget decisions. For example, some RFAs indicate that the funding agency is willing to fund an application up to a specified number of years with a direct cost cap per year. It is very important to read the funding announcement thoroughly to ascertain whether the final proposal and the accompanying budget are consistent with the expectations and rules set by the funding agency.

Approximately four to six weeks prior to the submission deadline, I schedule a meeting with the PI to determine what should be included in the budget. During this time, we discuss the different ways the experimental or research design can influence the budget. Often I find this exchange can be very helpful to the PI because I might think of certain design features in terms of specific costs that the PI may not have considered. This is where the "cost accounting the science" technique comes into action. The first draft of the budget is the full-cost budget, which includes all costs necessary to operate the project. The budget will undergo several revisions as the PI is now faced with having to make budget cuts and revisions to the project design, in an effort to make the budget proposal more reasonable, allocable, consistent, and allowable per the guidance offered in the OMB circular applicable to the awardee's institution.[2] The last step in this process entails furnishing the PI with a complete draft budget package (including the budget justification) for review. Figure 15.2 summarizes this four-step process.

**STEP ONE:
REVIEW RFA &
DESIGN THE STUDY**

PI & collaborating investigators:
• Identify funding source.
• Review funding announcement.
• Devise specific aims of study.
• Write narrative for study design.
• Create project timeline.
• Evaluate all resources needed.

STEP FOUR:

Finalize the budget:
• Draft budget justification.
• Show all entries in whole
  dollars.
• Submit budget and justification
  to PI for final edits.
• Route application and final
  budget to grants and contracts
  office for signatures.

STEP TWO:

**PI meets with Research
Administrator:**
• Discuss at length resources
  required to conduct study.
• Cost account the science by
  linking expenditures to project.
• RA presents budget to PI.
• PI reworks design to scale
  back budget (if excessive)

STEP THREE:

Review the draft budget:
• Check for calculation errors in
  the formula(s).
• Meet with the PI and discuss
  any inconsistencies.
• If budget is still over the cap,
  present PI with several scenario
  budgets.

Figure 15.2. Detailed Process of Devising a Budget for Grant Applications

TECHNICAL TOOLS OF THE TRADE

Currently, the NIH has two electronic versions of the PHS 398 forms used for its grant applications (located at grants1.nih.gov/grants/forms.htm). All of the forms provided are in Microsoft Word or Adobe Acrobat PDF format, which is excellent for completing a document requiring typewritten text. But what about the forms that require computations, such as the face page, form pages 4 and 5, and the checklist form page? The Microsoft Excel version of the PHS 398 budget pages (including the face page and the checklist form page) are available online from the research administration offices of Columbia University (www.columbia .edu/cu/opg/projadm/project.html [scroll to bottom of screen]) and North-western University (www.northwestern.edu/orsp/forms.html#NIH).

The most important things to keep in mind if you decide to use these or any other PHS 398 form pages downloaded from the Internet is to be certain that you:

• Double-check that the forms *match exactly* the forms provided on the
  NIH grants and application form Web site.
• Periodically check the NIH Web site for updates and/or changes made to
  the forms.
• Delete and/or replace any prepopulated fields that appear on the downloaded forms (if any) with the information pertinent to your institution
  (e.g., applicant information presented on the face page).

- Update the formulas to reflect your institution's fringe benefit rate and the facilities and administrative costs (F&A; also referred to as the indirect costs).

Your time is better utilized working with a spreadsheet program to create and complete the financial information that appears on budget pages, rather than using the Microsoft Word or Adobe PDF versions of the budget pages. Although it is perfectly acceptable to use the Word or PDF version of the budget pages, it leaves open the door for making errors, particularly if you are pressed for time and need to quickly compute the necessary figures.

For the purposes of explaining the examples provided in this chapter, all of the spreadsheets and formulas used here were created and formulated using the Microsoft Excel spreadsheet program. I have no prior knowledge of whether the formulas, commands, or features of Excel are compatible in other spreadsheet software programs. Understanding how to use your spreadsheet program to its full potential will substantially reduce frustrations and drastically reduce the need for manual computations (which is unavoidable if you are using a word-processing program to complete your budget). Below I include some suggestions for organizing a spreadsheet package to facilitate the process of budget preparation for a nonmodular and modular PHS 398 grant application.

THE BUDGET PACKAGE

Nonmodular Format

The nonmodular budget format provides the funding agency with a complete and detailed itemization of the total direct costs the investigator proposes is necessary to conduct the research project. For all new, competing continuation, revised, and supplemental applications requesting *more than* $250,000 direct costs per year, the following PHS 398 budget package is required:

- Form page 1: face page
- Form page 4: detailed budget for initial budget period
- Form page 5: budget for entire proposed period of support
- Checklist form page

In addition to the PHS 398 forms previously listed, I recommend that the user create an "overall budget detail" worksheet (see figure 15.3). This worksheet will function as a comprehensive summary of the entire project budget, which provides explicit details on all expenditures required to carry out the objectives of the research protocol. The overall budget detail worksheet should not be submitted to the funding agency with the grant application. The purpose of creating the overall budget detail worksheet is to streamline the budget preparation process (pre- and postaward). Additionally, the worksheet functions as a supplement to the project timeline provided in the research proposal. If you decide to use PHS 398 budget form pages 4 and 5 (in Excel format), any information entered into the overall budget detail worksheet can be designed to automatically transfer its information into its respective place on the accompanying PHS 398 budget form pages. Figure 15.3 illustrates a suggested format of an overall budget detail (summary budget) for a five-year, nonmodular NIH grant budget. I recommend that you use whatever format works best when designing your overall budget detail spreadsheet and tailor it to meet the specific needs of your project. The time invested in creating an all-inclusive overall budget detail worksheet will drastically improve your productivity in grant preparation.

Modular Format

A modular application is a type of application in which financial support is requested in specified increments without the need for detailed information related to separate budget categories.[3] Since a detailed categorical budget (i.e., the format used for the nonmodular grant application) is not required for modular applications, form pages 4 and 5 are not used with modular budget packages. The modular budget package consists of the modular budget format page and

Figure 15.3a. (Nonmodular) Overall Budget Detail (page 1 of 2)

Excel File Edit View Insert Format Tools Data Window Help — Mon 10:23 AM

Personnel

	Role	YR1 % effort	YR1 cal mths	YR1 Salary requested	YR2 % effort	YR2 cal mths	YR2 Salary requested	YR3 % effort	YR3 cal mths	YR3 Salary requested	YR4 % effort	YR4 cal mths	YR4 Salary requested	YR5 % effort	YR5 cal mths	YR5 Salary requested	TOTAL
Dr. A	PI	40%	4.80	$73,400	40%	4.80	$73,400	40%	4.80	$73,400	40%	4.80	$73,400	40%	4.80	$73,400	
Dr. B	Entomologist	30%	3.60	$22,700	40%	4.80	$31,175	40%	4.80	$32,110	40%	4.80	$33,073	40%	4.80	$34,066	
Dr. C	Biochemist	40%	4.80	$34,766	40%	4.80	$35,809	40%	4.80	$36,883	40%	4.80	$37,990	40%	4.80	$39,129	
Dr. D	Argronomist	20%	2.40	$24,541	35%	4.20	$44,235	35%	4.20	$45,562	35%	4.20	$46,928	45%	5.40	$62,147	
Ms. E	Research Administrator	40%	4.80	$32,721	40%	4.80	$33,703	40%	4.80	$34,714	40%	4.80	$35,755	40%	4.80	$36,828	
Mr. F	Field Coordinator	0%	0.00	$0	100%	12.00	$50,027	50%	6.00	$25,764	100%	12.00	$53,074	50%	6.00	$27,333	
TBA	Research Assistant	100%	12.00	$35,400	100%	12.00	$35,862	100%	12.00	$37,968	100%	12.00	$39,107	100%	12.00	$40,280	
TOTAL FACULTY & STAFF SALARY		$223,917			$305,211			$286,401			$319,327			$313,183			
FRINGE @ 29%		$64,936			$88,511			$83,056			$92,605			$90,823			
TOTAL PERSONNEL COST		$288,853			$393,722			$369,457			$411,932			$404,006			$1,367,970

INSTITUTIONAL BASE SALARY

	BASE YR 1 (4/1/08-3/31/09)		BASE YR 2 (4/1/09-3/31/10)		BASE YR 3 (4/1/10-3/31/11)		BASE YR 3 (4/1/11-3/31/12)		BASE YR 3 (4/1/12-3/31/13)	
	day as of ...4/1/08	...7/1/08	day as of ...4/1/09	...7/1/09	day as of ...4/1/10	...7/1/10	day as of ...4/1/11	...7/1/11	day as of ...4/1/12	...7/1/13
	8 of pp 8.5	19.6	8 of pp 8.5	19.6	8 of pp 8.5	19.6	8 of pp 8.5	19.6	8 of pp 8.5	19.6
	Dr. A $183,500	$183,500	Dr. A $183,500	$183,500	Dr. A $183,500	$183,500	Dr. A $183,500	$183,500	Dr. A $183,500	$183,500
	Dr. B $74,000	$76,220	Dr. B $76,220	$78,507	Dr. B $78,507	$80,862	Dr. B $80,862	$83,288	Dr. B $83,288	$85,786
	Dr. C $85,000	$87,550	Dr. C $87,550	$90,177	Dr. C $90,177	$92,882	Dr. C $92,882	$95,668	Dr. C $95,668	$98,538
	Dr. D $120,000	$123,600	Dr. D $123,600	$127,308	Dr. D $127,308	$131,127	Dr. D $131,127	$135,061	Dr. D $135,061	$139,113
	Ms.E $80,000	$82,400	Ms.E $82,400	$94,872	Ms.E $84,872	$97,418	Ms.E $87,418	$90,041	Ms.E $90,041	$92,742
	Mr.F $47,500	$48,925	Mr.F $48,925	$50,393	Mr.F $50,393	$51,905	Mr.F $51,905	$53,462	Mr.F $53,462	$55,066
	TBA $35,000	$36,050	TBA $35,050	$37,132	TBA $37,132	$38,245	TBA $38,245	$39,393	TBA $39,393	$40,575

CONSULTANTS

	YR1	YR2	YR3	YR4	YR5	TOTAL
Dr. X. Miller	$1,500	$1,500	$1,500	$1,500	$1,500	
TOTAL CONSULTANTS	$1,500	$1,500	$1,500	$1,500	$1,500	$7,500

EQUIPMENT

	YR1	YR2	YR3	YR4	YR5	TOTAL
Super XYZ Machine	$8,000	$0	$0	$0	$0	
	$0	$0	$0	$0	$0	
TOTAL EQUIPMENT	$8,000	$0	$0	$0	$0	$8,000

	YEAR 1	YEAR 2	YEAR 3	YEAR 4	YEAR 5	TOTAL
SUPPLIES						
Super XYZ supplies	$278	$0	$0	$0	$0	
Treatment X concentrate	$0	$300	$0	$300	$600	
Food Coloring	$0	$35	$0	$0	$0	
Evaluation Surveys	$0	$80	$40	$80	$40	
Soil pH Test Meter	$250	$0	$0	$0	$0	
Research Supplies	$280	$288	$297	$306	$315	
TOTAL SUPPLIES	$808	$703	$337	$686	$955	$3,489
TRAVEL						
To farm locations	$0	$2,000	$0	$2,000	$0	
To focus grp			$500		$500	
TOTAL TRAVEL	$0	$2,000	$500	$2,000	$500	$5,000
PATIENT CARE COST						
Inpatient	$0	$0	$0	$0	$0	
Outpatient	$0	$0	$0	$0	$0	
PATIENT CARE COST	$0	$0	$0	$0	$0	$0
ALTER. & RENOV.						
	$0	$0	$0	$0	$0	
ALTERATIONS & REN	$0	$0	$0	$0	$0	$0
OTHER EXPENSES						
Express ship vials	$0	$0	$0	$0	$300	
Focus group company	$0	$0	$10,000	$0	$10,000	
Keypunching Scanning	$0	$70	$35	$70	$35	
Incentives	$0	$1,500	$1,000	$1,500	$1,000	
Computer	$2,000	$0	$0	$0	$0	
OTHER EXPENSES	$2,000	$1,570	$11,035	$1,570	$11,335	$27,510
CONSORTIUM						
Consortium (Direct)	$71,160	$73,205	$75,311	$77,481	$79,714	$376,871
Consortium (IDC) 25%	$17,790	$18,301	$18,828	$19,370	$19,929	$94,218
CONSORTIUM	$88,950	$91,507	$94,139	$96,851	$99,643	$471,089
TOTAL DIRECT COST	$372,321	$472,701	$453,140	$495,169	$498,010	$2,296,340
F&A COST RATE 1	68.00%	68.00%	68.00%	68.00%	68.00%	
MTDC Base	$318,161	$399,495	$382,829	$417,688	$418,296	
F&A COST	$216,349	$271,657	$260,324	$284,028	$284,441	$1,316,799
TOTAL COST	$606,460	$762,659	$737,292	$798,567	$802,380	$3,707,357

Figure 15.3b. (Nonmodular) Overall Budget Detail (page 2 of 2)

the checklist form page, both of can be accessed from grants1.nih.gov/grants/funding/phs398/phs398.html. For all new, competing continuation, revised, and supplemental R01, R03, R15, R21, R41, and R43 grant applications requesting $250,000 *or less* annually in direct costs per year, with direct costs being requested in modules of $25,000 each, use the modular budget format. The overall budget detail worksheet will also be a helpful tool while constructing a budget for a modular application (an example of which is provided in figure 15.4). The major difference between the nonmodular overall budget detail (figure 15.3) and the modular overall budget detail (figure 15.4) is that in figure 15.3, the nonmodular total direct cost (line 78) is the amount carried on to box 7a of the form face page and the modified total direct cost of that amount (line 81) is used to determine the indirect cost of the project (described in further detail below under "Facilities and Administrative Costs"), whereas in figure 15.4, the "modular direct requested" amount (line 62) is carried onto box 7a of the face page. The modular budget presented in figure 15.4 shows that the total direct cost (line 61) calculated in year 1 is $122,955. However, since this is a modular application, the direct cost amount requested for each project year will be in modules of $25,000 (up to $250,000 per year). That being the case, $122,955 rounded to the nearest $25,000 is $125,000. Just a reminder: The overall budget detail should not be submitted to the funding agency.

For the purpose of explaining the techniques and tools required to prepare a comprehensive detailed budget for a research grant, the modular application format is not discussed further in this chapter. The NIH has provided extensive instructions on the requirements for preparing a budget for modular grant

Figure 15.4. Modular Overall Budget Detail

		YEAR 1			YEAR 2			TOTAL
PERSONNEL		X effort	person month	SALARY	X effort	person month	SALARY	
C. CHARLES		50%	6.00	$47,583	50%	6.00	$49,482	
J. JACOBS		20%	2.40	$21,117	20%	2.40	$21,960	
L. LYONS		5%	0.60	$9,175	5%	0.60	$9,175	
S. SIMMONS		10%	1.20	$8,989	10%	1.20	$9,348	
TOTAL SALARY				$86,864			$89,964	$176,828
FRINGE (29%)				$25,191			$26,090	$51,280
TOTAL PERSONNEL				$112,055			$116,054	$228,109
		BASE YR 1 (12/1/08-11/30/09)						
		SALARY AS OF _	12/08-6/09	7/09-11/09	SALARY AS OF _	12/09-6/10	7/10-11/09	
		CHARLES	$93,589	$97,332	CHARLES	$97,332	$101,225	
		JACOBS	$103,834	$107,987	JACOBS	$107,987	$112,306	
		LYONS	$183,500	$183,500	LYONS	$183,500	$183,500	
		SIMMONS	$88,400	$91,936	SIMMONS	$91,936	$95,613	
CONSULTANTS								
	Janite Johnson, M.D.			$1,000			$1,000	
	Michelle Lawry, Ph.D.			$3,000			$1,000	
TOTAL CONSULTANTS				$4,000			$2,000	$6,000
SUPPLIES								
	Research Supplies			$2,200			$2,200	
TOTAL SUPPLIES				$2,200			$2,200	$4,400
TRAVEL								
P1 Travel to conferences				$3,200			$3,200	
TOTAL TRAVEL				$3,200			$3,200	$6,400
OTHER EXPENSES								
	Postage & Fedex			$500			$500	
	Duplicating			$300			$300	
	Books			$700			$700	
TOTAL OTHER EXPENSES				$1,500			$1,500	$3,000
TOTAL DIRECT COST:				$122,955			$124,954	$247,909
MODULAR DIRECT REQUESTED:				$125,000			$125,000	$250,000
F&A COST RATE 1				68.00%			68.00%	
MTDC Base				$125,000			$125,000	
F&A COST				$85,000			$85,000	$170,000
TOTAL COST				$210,000			$210,000	$420,000

applications and, in addition, has provided examples of modular budgets (with same or variable modules and with or without consortium costs). The modular budget samples for budgets with same or variable modules are located, respectively, at grants.nih.gov/grants/funding/phs398/modbudgetsample_same.pdf and grants.nih.gov/grants/funding/phs398/modbudgetsample_variation.pdf. The level of detail provided in an itemized, nonmodular budget package is substantially more than what is required should an investigator choose to submit a modular grant application. Therefore, the remainder of this chapter is devoted to explaining the nonmodular (categorical) budget format.

COMPREHENSIVE BREAKDOWN OF NONMODULAR CATEGORICAL BUDGET

The example study above involving the eradication of the Japanese beetles is also used for illustration in this section. Information provided in figure 15.3 is referenced frequently to illustrate the process by which a nonmodular NIH budget is constructed. This section also details what an investigator should consider during the budget construction process. Box 15.1 provides a sample study design for the Japanese beetle example.

In order to calculate the *actual* personnel expenses for your budget, you will need to have determined facts 1 through 7 for your institution. Personnel costs (i.e., salaries, wages, and fringe) are almost always the most expensive direct cost category of the entire budget. Therefore, more time will be spent in the upcoming chapter section, explaining the proper way to calculate and depict personnel costs on a research budget.

DETAILED BUDGET

Personnel

According to the PHS 398 instructions, this section of the budget should list all personnel (including "to-be-appointed" positions), including their names, role on the project, months devoted to the project, institutional base salary (IBS), salary requested for the project, fringe benefits, and the academic/nonacademic appointment type (e.g., 9-month or 12-month appointment) for each position.[4] In addition, all persons employed by the applicant organization and devoting effort to the project should be listed regardless of whether a salary is requested. If the project involves personnel who are not employed by the applicant organization, depending on their role on the project they can be listed either as a consultant or as having a subcontract (also termed "consortium") with the applicant organization (which is discussed below under "Consortium and Contractual Costs"). The budget justification should identify the role of each individual,

Study Facts

The applicant organization, WCMC, a not-for-profit, university hospital, will be submitting the R01 proposal to the NIH for the June 1, 2007, submission deadline.

The proposed project dates run from April 1, 2008, through March 31, 2013, and involves one subcontract.

1. All WCMC personnel work a 12-month appointment.
2. There are a total of 26.1 pay periods per project year.
3. The WCMC fiscal year runs from July 1 through June 30.
4. A 3% cost-of-living increase is budgeted for all personnel on every July 1.
5. The fringe benefit rate is 29% of total personnel compensation.
6. 1 Most nonpersonnel budget categories assume a 3% inflationary increase per project year.
7. The F&A rate is 68% on the modified total direct cost (MTDC) base.

Study Design

The objective of this five-year project is to determine whether treatment X is a successful solution to rid of the Japanese beetle infestation, which plagues our nation's farms and forests. This project involves recruiting 20 farmers (10 in the control group and 10 in the experimental group) to participate in four in-depth one-on-one interviews (twice per year in project years 2 and 4) and one focus group per year (project years 3 and 5) to learn about current eradication strategies to and ascertain the fiscal impact that the infestation problem has on their crops and exported vegetation.

---

describe his or her specific functions on the project, and provide information on the individual's expertise.

The NIH (and other PHS agencies) has recently eliminated the use of "percent effort" to describe the level of commitment a person devotes to a project. In place of this term, the NIH requires that personnel time be measured in terms of "person-months" defined as a "metric for expressing the effort (amount of time) PIs, faculty and other senior personnel devote to a specific project. The effort is based on the type of appointment of the individual with the organization; e.g., calendar year (CY), academic year (AY), and/or summer term (SM); and the organization's definition of such."[5] The OER has posted an "interactive conversion table" at grants.nih.gov/grants/policy/person_months_conversion_chart .xls that converts an individual's percent effort into what is now referred to as "person-months." PHS 398 form page 4 (detailed budget page) and the new electronic version of form page 4 (i.e., SF424 sections A and B) have been updated to reflect this new business practice.

Figure 15.5 illustrates the *personnel* section of the overall budget detail from figure 15.3. Personnel and their respective roles are listed in columns A and B (this information will be carried over to PHS 398 form page 4). In addition, the detailed layout of the personnel section enables the user to assign different levels of effort per year to each individual to be consistent with their roles and function to the research project. For example, the study design does not include any fieldwork in year 1; therefore, the field coordinator, "Mr. F," will not commit any time to the project in year 1; however, he will commit 100% effort to the project in years 2 and 4 (to coordinate in the one-on-one interviews) and 50% effort in years 3 and 5 (to assist in the coordination of the focus groups). These variations in level of effort from one year to another demonstrate that the PI is cognizant of the needs of his project from one year to another and has carefully thought out what resources are necessary to carry out the project. The budget justification should explain any change in level of effort from one year to the next, and the changes should be consistent with the needs of the project. In order to capture these annual work scope variations, the overall budget detail worksheet (figure 15.3) is organized so that each project year is composed of its own "% effort" column. Upon entering the percent effort for each personnel listed, the figures in the columns labeled "calendar months" and "salary requested" is automatically computed in the respective project year.

All of these computations are dependent upon creating a section on the worksheet to enter each individual's IBS (as is illustrated on the bottom half of figure 15.5).

Figure 15.5. Personnel Expense Budget

Excel File Edit View Insert Format Tools Data Window Help Mon 10:23 AM

	A	B	C	D	E	F	G	H	I	J	K	L	M	N	O	P	Q	R
1																		
2			YEAR 1			YEAR 2			YEAR 3			YEAR 4			YEAR 5			TOTAL
3	PERSONNEL																	
4		Role	% effort	cal mths	Salary requested	% effort	cal mths	Salary requested	% effort	cal mths	Salary requested	% effort	cal mths	Salary requested	% effort	cal mths	Salary requested	
5	Dr. A	PI	40%	4.80	$73,400	40%	4.80	$73,400	40%	4.80	$73,400	40%	4.80	$73,400	40%	4.80	$73,400	
6	Dr. B	Entomologist	30%	3.60	$22,700	40%	4.80	$31,175	40%	4.80	$32,110	40%	4.80	$33,073	40%	4.80	$34,066	
7	Dr. C	Biochemist	40%	4.80	$34,766	40%	4.80	$35,809	40%	4.80	$36,888	40%	4.80	$37,990	40%	4.80	$39,129	
8	Dr. D	Agronomist	20%	2.40	$24,541	35%	4.20	$44,235	35%	4.20	$45,562	35%	4.20	$46,928	45%	5.40	$62,147	
9	Ms. E	Research Administrator	40%	4.80	$32,721	40%	4.80	$33,703	40%	4.80	$34,714	40%	4.80	$35,755	40%	4.80	$36,828	
10	Mr. F	Field Coordinator	0%	0.00	$0	100%	12.00	$50,027	50%	6.00	$25,764	100%	12.00	$53,074	50%	6.00	$27,333	
11	TBA	Research Assistant	100%	12.00	$35,789	100%	12.00	$35,862	100%	12.00	$37,968	100%	12.00	$39,107	100%	12.00	$40,280	
13	TOTAL FACULTY & STAFF SALARY		$223,917			$305,211			$286,401			$319,327			$313,183			
14	FRINGE @ 29%		$64,936			$88,511			$83,056			$92,605			$90,823			
15	TOTAL PERSONNEL COST		$288,853			$393,722			$369,457			$411,932			$404,006			$1,867,970
17			BASE YR 1 (4/1/08-3/31/09)			BASE YR 2 (4/1/09-3/31/10)			BASE YR 3 (4/1/10-3/31/11)			BASE YR 3 (4/1/11-3/31/12)			BASE YR 3 (4/1/12-3/31/13)			
18			day as of	...4/1/08	...7/1/08	day as of	...4/1/09	...7/1/09	day as of	...4/1/10	...7/1/10	day as of	...4/1/11	...7/1/11	day as of	...4/1/12	...7/1/13	
19			8 of pp	8.5	19.6	8 of pp	8.5	19.6	8 of pp	8.5	19.6	8 of pp	8.5	19.6	8 of pp	8.5	19.6	
20			Dr. A	$183,500	$183,500	Dr. A	$183,500	$183,500	Dr. A	$183,500	$183,500	Dr. A	$183,500	$183,500	Dr. A	$183,500	$183,500	
21	INSTITUTIONAL		Dr. B	$74,000	$76,220	Dr. B	$76,220	$78,507	Dr. B	$78,507	$80,862	Dr. B	$80,862	$83,288	Dr. B	$83,288	$85,786	
22	BASE SALARY		Dr. C	$85,000	$87,550	Dr. C	$87,550	$90,177	Dr. C	$90,177	$92,882	Dr. C	$92,882	$95,668	Dr. C	$95,668	$98,538	
23			Dr. D	$120,000	$123,600	Dr. D	$123,600	$127,308	Dr. D	$127,308	$131,127	Dr. D	$131,127	$135,061	Dr. D	$135,061	$139,113	
24			Ms.E	$80,000	$82,400	Ms.E	$82,400	$94,872	Ms.E	$84,872	$97,418	Ms.E	$87,418	$90,041	Ms.E	$90,041	$92,742	
25			Mr.F	$47,500	$48,925	Mr.F	$48,925	$50,393	Mr.F	$50,393	$51,905	Mr.F	$51,905	$53,462	Mr.F	$53,462	$55,066	
26			TBA	$35,000	$36,050	TBA	$35,050	$37,132	TBA	$37,132	$38,245	TBA	$38,245	$39,393	TBA	$39,393	$40,575	

Figure 15.6 provides a detailed explanation on how the "salary requested" amount for Dr. D was computed in year 1 (see figure 15.5, cell E8). According to the information contained in figure 15.5, Dr. D will devote 2.40 person-months (20%) to the project in year 1. That is 20% multiplied by 12 (number of months in appointment). The project is proposed to begin on April 1, 2008, at which time Dr. D's IBS is $120,000 (figure 15.5, cell D23). However, as of July 1, 2008, Dr. D (and all other personnel of WCMC) is slated to receive a 3% cost-of-living increase above his current IBS, at which time his new salary will be $123,600 (figure 15.5, cell E23). In order to determine the total amount of Dr. D's salary to budget on the grant for the grant period in question, his salary and that of the entire project staff must be prorated. In order to prorate Dr. D's salary at 20% effort in year 1, first we must determine what his compensation would be at 20% effort from April 1 to June 30, 2008, at a salary of $120,000 and *add* to that 20% of his effort from July 1, 2008, through March 31, 2009, at a salary of $123,600. The formula used to prorate Dr. D's salary and to calculate his total compensation for devoting 20% effort in year 1 is provided in detail in figure 15.6.

It is essential to keep in mind that if the grant budget years coincided with the applicant institution fiscal year, there would be no need to prorate the salaries, and the computation for determining the "salary requested" would be a matter of simply multiplying IBS by the proposed percent effort on the project. An inexperienced budget person or new investigator might ask, "Why is so much detail so important?" "Why can't I just ballpark the personnel figures?" First, it is rare that the project years for any research project coincide with the applicant institutions' fiscal year. For this reason, prorating the salary is important in order

Figure 15.6. Detailed Calculation of Dr. D's Salary (Prorated)

Formula in **Cell E8:**	=ROUND (((D23/26.1*6.5) + (E23/26.1*19.6))*C8,0)
Translation of formula in lay terms:	=ROUND $\left[\left(\dfrac{\$120,600}{26.1} \times 6.5 \right) + \left(\dfrac{\$123,600}{26.1} \times 19.6 \right) \right] \times 20\%$, 0
Computation:	=ROUND $29,885 + $92,818 × 0.20 , 0
	This section of the formula represents Dr. D's salary from period 4/1/08 - 6/30/08 divided by the number of pay periods in the entire project year (26.1) multiplied by the number of pay periods from 4/1/08 - 6/30/08.	This section of the formula represents Dr. D's salary from 7/1/08 - 3/31/09 divided by the number of pay periods in the entire project year (26.1) multiplied by the number of pay periods from 7/1/08 - 3/31/09.	Dr. D's % effort committed to the project in year 1.

to determine the exact amount of money it will cost to compensate the project or investigative staff for their time. Generally, most institutions budget for cost-of-living and merit increases for their staff at the beginning of each new fiscal year. These increases must be accounted for when projecting personnel costs for a research budget. Therefore, it is necessary to prorate salaries in order to take into consideration any inflationary factors (i.e., cost-of-living increases or project merit increases) that may be timely with respect to the budget.

If you do not choose to prorate the personnel salaries and wages in accordance with your institutions compensation practices, and if the grant gets funded, there will be a dollar shortfall and the funded budget will not meet *actual* personnel costs. For example, let's suppose for year 1 you did not want to prorate Dr. D's salary because it takes too much time to calculate and you would rather ballpark his personnel expenses. In this scenario, the budget proposed to compensate Dr. D $24,000 (i.e., 20% of $120,000 salary), which does not take into account any inflationary factors. However, when we prorated Dr. D's salary (figure 15.5, cell E8), we determined that $24,541 is the actual amount that would need to be charged to the grant. In this instance, you would have actually spent $541 *more* (not including fringe) than what you had budgeted in the proposal to spend! Imagine you used this "ballpark" technique for every individual with committed effort on the project for all years of requested support; you would have overspent on the budget by thousands of dollars.

Approximating personnel expenses for a research budget can prove to be very costly and can be devastating to a funded project. Imagine if we took the previous example one step further. Suppose you had proposed Dr. D's salary to be 3% more than what his actual salary would have been on the grant start date (i.e., $123,600 in year 1). This oversight would result in creating a budget allocating more money (about $179 additional dollars not including fringe) than what you would have actually spent for salary compensation. While that amount might seem nominal to you, if you constantly find yourself seeking ways to scale back your budget because the total direct cost far exceeds the budget ceiling, one solution is to prorate personnel expenses to accurately reflect what you anticipate happening should the grant get funded. The bottom line resonating around these examples is that it is not a good practice to use ballpark figures to represent personnel costs, and padding the budget is also highly inadvisable.

Figure 15.7 provides a snapshot of the year 1 personnel expenses taken from figure 15.5 (accompanied by a detailed explanation of each entry). Each subsequent project year (as outlined in figure 15.5) demonstrates the same core information outlined in figure 15.7 with a 3% cost-of-living increase proposed to take effect every July 1. For the purposes of preparing the PHS 398 form page 4 using the personnel costs derived in figure 15.7, however, the IBS dollar amount is required. To calculate the IBS, simply divide the salary requested amount by the percent effort committed to the project in a given year and the result is the IBS.

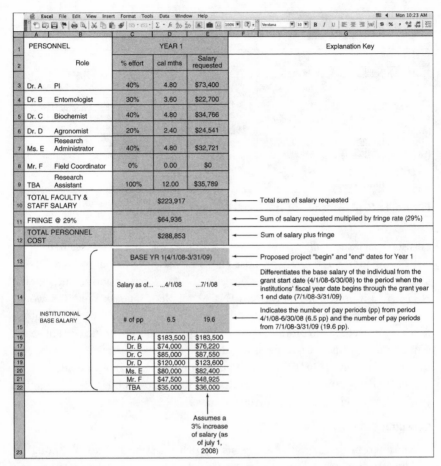

Figure 15.7. Closer Snapshot of Year 1 Personnel Expenses, with Explanations

Figure 15.8 illustrates the method used to calculate the IBS for all project staff of the research proposal. For example, in order to determine IBS to input onto the PHS 398 form page 4 for Dr. D, simply divide $24,541 (figure 15.8, cell E8) by 0.20 (20% effort in decimal form; figure 15.8, cell C8) and the result, $122,705, is the IBS amount to enter on the PHS 398 form page 4 for Dr. D's position.

One additional factor pertains to budgeting personnel costs. The U.S. federal government generates legislatively imposed salary limitations that are updated every January 1 and posted at grants.nih.gov/grants/policy/salcap_summa-salcap_summary.htm. The federal government restricts the amount of direct salary dollars that an individual can charge to a federal grant. As of January 1, 2006, the most an individual can charge to a federal grant is $183,500. For example, Dr. A's IBS is $275,000. However, in the case of determining his base salary for the Japanese beetle proposal, he can charge only $73,400 (i.e., 40% of

			YEAR 1		INSTITUTIONAL BASE SALARY (for form page 4)	Key
PERSONNEL						
	Role	% effort	cal mths	Salary requested		
Dr. A	PI	40%	4.80	$73,400	$183,500	Cell E5 divided by Cell C5 = IBS
Dr. B	Entomologist	30%	3.60	$22,700	$75,667	Cell E6 divided by Cell C6 = IBS
Dr. C	Biochemist	40%	4.80	$34,766	$86,915	Cell E7 divided by Cell C7 = IBS
Dr. D	Agronomist	20%	2.40	$24,541	$122,705	Cell E8 divided by Cell C8 = IBS
Ms. E	Research Administrator	40%	4.80	$32,721	$81,803	Cell E9 divided by Cell C9 = IBS
Mr. F	Field Coordinator	0%	0.00	$0	$0	Cell E10 divided by Cell C10 = IBS
TBA	Research Assistant	100%	12.00	$35,788	$35,789	Cell E11 divided by Cell C11 = IBS

Figure 15.8. Calculation of IBS for PHS 398 Form Page 4

$183,500) per year to *all* years of requested support for the project (see figure 15.5, cell E5). In addition, if Dr. A proposed a 3% increase per year above the current salary cap (i.e., $183,500 year 1, $189,005 year 2, $194,675 year 3, and so on), and the NIH issued a notice of grant award (NGA) for the proposal, the NGA would reflect adjustments to the current and all future years of the project so that no funds were awarded or committed for any of Dr. A's salary over the current year's limitation. The rules regarding salary limitations are very straightforward, and the OER posts annual notices (e.g., Notice Number NOT-OD-06-031 located at grants.nih.gov/grants/guide/notice-files/NOT-OD-06-031.html) to explain that year's salary cap legislation in significant detail.

Consultant Costs

A sponsored project consultant is generally defined as an individual (though it can be a group) providing highly specialized expertise directly related to the science and scope of the sponsored project and whose fees are charged to the sponsored project or to a cost-sharing account.[6] Proper characterization of an individual working as a consultant/independent contractor on a sponsored research project must be based on the federal guidelines provided by the Internal Revenue Service (IRS) and not on cost-saving measures to the research project or as a means of convenience.[6] The service provider cannot be an employee of the applicant institution and is generally hired in a professional capacity to provide specific services under a sponsored agreement (i.e., grant, contract, or a cooperative agreement). To comport with IRS regulations, consultants are responsible for the means and methods for completing the job based on specifications in the contract and must determine how they will accomplish the work, determine their service fees, have significant investment in their business, and have a broad customer base. Misclassifying an employee as an independent consultant subjects the applicant institution to penalties from the IRS and other regulatory agencies.

The IRS has established 20 factors and three categories of control to determine if a service provided by an individual classifies that person as an employee or as an independent contractor of the applicant institution. A copy of this list is located at www.ncarts.edu/formsprocedures/IRS.htm. Awardees of federal grant funding are required to have written policies governing their use of consultants, and these policies should be referenced when considering adding consultants or subcontracts to a project.

Once it has been determined that a service provider classifies as an independent contractor for your research project, the NIH requires that the budget justification identify the individual(s) by name and organization affiliation, specialty, description of service(s) to be performed, their relevance to the grant-supported activities, number of days of anticipated consultation, expected rate of compensation and basis for calculating the fee (i.e., hourly/daily rate or rate per unit of service rendered), terms of reimbursement for travel and meal per diem, and other related costs.[7] Some federal agencies cap the daily rate for consulting services; therefore, the specific agency guidelines should be consulted. As figure 15.3 illustrates, Dr. X. Miller will serve as a consultant on the Japanese beetle project working at a rate of $500/day for three consulting days per year for all years of the proposed project. Refer to appendix 15.1 at the end of this chapter for an example of how the narrative in the budget justification will read for Dr. Miller.

Equipment

The NIH Grants Policy Statement defines equipment as an article of tangible nonexpendable personal property that has a useful life of more than one year and an acquisition cost per unit that equals or exceeds $5,000 or the capitalization threshold established by the organization, whichever is less.[3] All items purchased under this category should be listed, and the budget justification should provide vendor information, a description of the equipment, current prices (including shipping, maintenance costs and agreements), necessity and suitability of the equipment, and any other supporting documentation should be provided in an appendix to the application. Funds budgeted to purchase equipment must be used toward the purchase of new, used, or replacement equipment either figured into the direct costs of the proposal budget or factored into the F&A costs of the institution (which depends on the intended use of the equipment). The type of institution or type of grant determines whether equipment can be purchased; therefore, the funding agency guidelines and those of the applicant institution should be consulted. While project-specific equipment is considered a part of the direct cost to the applicant institution, the total amount for equipment is to be excluded from the grantee's F&A cost base calculation (which is discussed further below under "Facilities and Administrative Costs").

Supplies

Supplies are categorized as items actually used in the course of performing the scope of work, and all tangible property other than equipment.[8] On federally funded projects routine office supplies should be treated as F&A costs and are only appropriate to budget as direct costs if the purpose is for the sole direct benefit of the project.[8] All other supply costs budgeted to the project (e.g., laboratory and/or other research supplies) are routinely considered a direct cost to the project. If the applicant organization is submitting a budget proposal with an inflation factor built in for future years, these estimated costs should be justified and can be based on historical costs determined by previous or ongoing research projects with similar costs.

Travel

Travel costs budgeted onto a federal grant must provide a direct benefit to the research project, must be consistent with the applicant organization's established travel policy, and is subject to the guidance set forth in the OMB Circular A-21, Section 48, under Travel Costs.[2] The travel budget line should include costs for traveling to present a lecture or poster, participate in a panel or symposium, and attend conferences for educational purposes. Travel also can be budgeted for consultation with experts at remote sites, attending meetings required by the sponsor (funding agency), and costs to transport research patients/subjects participating in the research protocol to the site where services are being provided (including public transportation). Most policies allow reimbursement for necessary and reasonable travel and nontravel expenses (i.e., airfare, train fare, car rental, food per diems or subsistence allowances, lodging, and other miscellaneous costs) incurred in the conduct of the business stemming from the research proposal. For domestic and foreign travel, the budget justification should include the purpose and destination of each trip, dates of travel (if known), the mode and cost of transportation, and estimated length of trip and identify the estimated cost per trip per year multiplied by the number of individuals from the project staff traveling.[4]

Patient Care Costs

According to the NIH instructions, if inpatient and/or outpatient costs are requested, the names of the hospitals and/or clinics and the amounts requested for each should be provided in the budget justification. Other anticipated sources of support for the patients' care costs should be disclosed (e.g., health insurance programs or pharmaceutical companies) or expected use of the institution's general clinical research centers.[4]

Alterations and Renovations

The NIH Grants Policy Statement definition of an alteration or renovation (A&R) is work that changes the interior arrangements or other physical characteristics of an existing facility or of installed equipment so that it can be used more effectively for its currently designated purpose or adapted to an alternative use to meet a programmatic requirement. Major A&R (including modernization, remodeling, or improvement) of an existing building is permitted under an NIH grant only when the authorizing statute for the program specifically allows that activity. A&R expenses are not allowable under grants to individuals, foreign grants, and conference grants. A&R must be specifically authorized in the NGA. Otherwise the costs are allowable unless specifically detailed in the terms and conditions of the award. The budget justification should itemize each A&R project by category and justify the costs of repairs, painting, removal or installation of partitions, and so forth. If applicable, square footage and costs should be provided in the narrative, as well.[3]

Other Expenses

The "other" expense category should include an itemization of all other direct costs that are not suitable to place in the existing budget categories (i.e., telecommunication charges, software upgrades, maintenance contracts, postal services, overnight express shipment services, tuition for graduate research assistants, duplicating expenses, data communication costs, patient/research subject incentives, donor fees, publication costs, etc.). The budget narrative should provide detail on the reason why these *other expenses* are needed to meet the objectives of the research proposed.

Consortium and Contractual Costs

The NIH Grants Policy Statement defines a consortium agreement (also referred to as a subcontract, subaward, subprime institution/organization, or subgrant) as a formalized agreement whereby a research project is carried out by the grantee and one or more other organizations that are separate legal entities. Under the agreement, the grantee must perform a substantive role in the conduct of the planned research and not merely serve as a conduit of funds to another party or parties.[3] The prime institution for a research project can have an undisclosed number of subcontracts associated with its proposal as long the subcontractor(s) provides a substantive level effort and brings a level of expertise (otherwise not available at the applicant institution). The collaboration should not duplicate resources already available at the applicant's organization or institution. An example of duplication might be a grant application that requires the expertise of a biostatistician and, instead of using a biostatician at your organization, you seek to collaborate with an outside organization that will render the same services as your internal biostatistics department has available.

In the Japanese beetle proposal, the applicant organization (WCMC) has incorporated the services of Dr. J. J. Hewitt, Director of Biometrics Consulting, LLC, who will devote 30% effort (3.60 person months) during the 12-month academic year to the project. Dr. Hewitt is a nationally recognized biometrician who will be responsible for the collection and interpretation of qualitative data acquired from the farm sites during the one-on-one interviews conducted in years 2 and 4 of the proposed research project. In addition, his company will analyze the data looking for trends and examining underlying relationships between climate, fertilization methods, possible eradication treatments, and the influence of treatment X on these factors. Biometrics Consulting will also examine the influence of numerous agricultural concerns on Japanese beetle survival before and after administering treatment X to the crops. Dr. Hewitt furnished WCMC with a budget proposal (figure 15.9) showing the costs associated with hiring Biometrics Consulting to collaborate on the Japanese beetle project. Since the collaboration requires that a substantive amount of work be conducted in order to achieve the stated objectives of the research, a consortium was more appropriate than compensating Dr. Hewitt as an individual consultant.

If an investigator chooses to submit a competing application containing consortium(s), the following information must be provided to the NIH when submitting the application: (1) a list of all proposed performance sites, including those of the applicant organization and for each consortium Organization; and

Figure 15.9. Biometrics Consulting, LLC Subcontract Proposal

	Role	Base Salary	Effort	Person Months	04/01/08-03/31/09	04/01/09-03/31/10	04/01/10-03/31/11	04/01/11-03/31/12	04/01/12-03/31/13	TOTAL
				Biometrics Consulting, LLC Subcontract Proposal						
JJ Hewitt, Ph.D.	PI	$155,000	30%	3.60	$46,500	$47,895	$49,332	$50,812	$52,336	
Shellie Mack, M.S.	Research Assistant	$45,000	15%	1.80	$6,750	$6,953	$7,161	$7,376	$7,597	
	Total Salaries & Wages				$53,250	$54,848	$56,493	$58,188	$59,933	
	Total Fringe (28%)				14,910	15,357	15,818	16,293	16,781	
	Total Personnel				68,160	70,205	72,311	74,481	76,714	$361,871
Travel					$3,000	$3,000	$3,000	$3,000	$3,000	
Total Direct Costs					71,160	73,205	75,311	77,481	79,714	$376,871
F&A cost (25%)					17,790	18,301	18,828	19,370	19,929	$94,218
Total					$88,950	$91,507	$94,139	$96,851	$99,643	$471,089

(2) complete application budget pages for the first year (form page 4) and each future year of support requested (form page 5) for *each* consortium organization (except for modular applications and awards).[4] Therefore, if the Japanese beetle project involves a collaboration with four subcontractors (which is typical with most P50/P30 Center grant applications), the budget section of the application would begin with the WCMC (the applicant organizations) budget pages, followed by separate form pages 4 and 5 for *each* subcontract (including their own respective budget justifications). The applicant institution will generally require a signed face page and scope of work (which does not accompany the grant proposal) from each consortium institution. However, a statement of intent to participate in a subcontract agreement can be drawn up by the consortium institution(s) and provided as part of the application (placed immediately after the "consortium/contractual arrangement section of the NIH grant application").[4] A signed face page or statement of intent can serve as a provisional contract. In effect, this document commits the consortium institution to conduct the work as outlined in the research plan per the proposed costs outlined in the consortium budget proposal. It is a good rule of thumb to consult the funding agency guidelines and that of your institution regarding their specific requirements for subcontracts. The checklist page for the applicant organization and each consortium should be placed at the end of the grant application, with the applicant organization checklist page first, immediately followed by the checklist page(s) for each consortium.

Consortium budget proposals may include many of the direct and indirect costs allowed by the applicant organization (e.g., personnel, travel, supplies, equipment, and other direct costs relevant to achieving the stated objectives of the research project). The accompanying budget justification for each subcontract should provide the same level of detail as the applicant organization narrative provides (see appendix 15.1).

In November 2004, the NIH published a revised policy on applications that include consortium/contractual F&A costs. This new policy eliminates the incorporation of the consortiums' F&A costs into the applicants direct cost regardless of the budget or budget format used with the application (modular or nonmodular). This notice can be found at grants.nih.gov/grants/guide/notice-files/NOT-OD-05-004.html. A detailed explanation of the calculation utilized to determine F&A costs for a research project is given under "Facilities and Administrative Costs."

Facilities and Administrative Costs

A good deal of this chapter emphasizes financial accounting for direct costs. Salary is a direct cost, as is equipment when the equipment is identified solely for a select research proposal. For instance, a high-pressure gas-liquid chromatography spectrometer that is used to conduct an assay that is part of a single research proposal can be identified as a direct expense. If the equipment is used across several different studies (i.e., a copy machine) with different sources of funding, it cannot be a direct expense charged to one grant. A broad catchall for direct cost expenditures includes personnel, supplies specific to the project, travel, consortiums, and subject compensation or incentives, as well as other expenses that help the investigator execute the research for the identified project. However, every public or private entity (including government agencies) is entitled to collect on a percentage of federal direct cost dollars awarded to their institutions to recover real support costs that benefit sponsored projects (but cannot be exclusively associated with any specific research project or contract).[2] Most research grants are not designed to cover the total cost of the research proposed. The grantee institution in collaboration with any consortium institutions (if applicable) is expected to provide the required physical facilities and administrative services normally available at an institution (services primarily made available through the collection of federal indirect cost dollars). These support infrastructures are essential to operating, and maintaining the institution and the costs associated with operating these programs are "incurred by the grantee for common or joint objectives."[3] Another term used by many institutions is "indirect costs" because they are incurred "indirectly" in the execution of funded research. Circular A-21 defines the *facilities* cost portion of F&A as (1) costs for building and equipment depreciation, (2) interest on debt associated with buildings and equipment, (3) operation and maintenance expenses (e.g., custodial services, repairs, security, and environmental safety), and (4) library expenses (library operations and materials). Circular A-21 defines the *administrative* cost portion of F&A costs as (1) general administration and general expenses (e.g., office of the president, accounting, institutional review boards, and human resources), (2) departmental administration (e.g., academic deans, secretaries, and office supplies), (3) sponsored projects administration, and (4) student administration and services.[2]

The ability for an institution to recover these costs is facilitated by charging the F&A cost *rate* (which is determined through negotiation with the U.S. Department of Health and Human Services [DHHS] Division of Cost Allocation) to the direct cost *base* agreed upon in the negotiations. In the case of for-profit organizations, the F&A rate is then determined through negotiations with the NIH Division of Financial Advisory Services (DFAS). Depending on the structure of the institution and the terms of negotiation with DHHS or DFAS, the F&A cost rate can be charged to the "modified total direct cost" (MTDC) base, or the salary and wage base, or to some other special rate in accordance with the terms of the negotiations. Most commonly, however, the F&A cost rate is applied to the MTDC of the project. MTDC, rather than total direct costs, forms the base for calculating F&A costs to projects. The term "base" is used as a synonym for MTDC because MTDC is the base for distributing F&A costs.[9]

	YEAR 1	YEAR 2	YEAR 3	YEAR 4	YEAR 5	TOTAL
79 TOTAL DIRECT COST	$372,321	$472,701	$458,140	$495,169	$493,010	$2,296,340
80						
81 F&A COST RATE 1	68.00%	68.00%	68.00%	68.00%	68.00%	
82 MTDC Base	$318,161	$399,495	$382,829	$417,688	$418,296	
83 F&A COST	$216,349	$271,657	$260,324	$284,028	$284,441	$1,316,799
84						
85 TOTAL COST	$606,460	$762,659	$737,292	$798,567	$802,380	$3,707,357
86						
87						
88	carry to box 7a of face page				carry to box 8a	
89		carry to box 7b of face page			of face page	
90						carry to box 8b
91						of face page
92						

Figure 15.10. Snapshot of F&A Cost Calculation

Figure 15.10 provides a snapshot of the overall budget detail worksheet in figure 15.3. This snapshot exhibits the final calculations of the budget. At the beginning of this section, the "facts" list disclosed that WCMC's F&A cost is calculated from the MTDC base. The MTDC base (figure 15.10, line 82) is determined for year 1 by using the formula in figure 15.11. The MTDC base excludes any costs budgeted for equipment, patient care costs, A&R, and the consortium's costs and includes all of the other direct costs of the project: personnel costs, consultants, supplies, travel, other expenses, and the first $25,000 of each consortium's direct cost to cover the applicant organization's administrative expenses. Thus, if the consortium's direct cost in year 1 totaled $17,000, the MTDC base calculation would only include $17,000 of the consortium's direct cost (not $25,000). However, in order to collect on the other $8,000 (i.e., $25,000 − $17,000 = $8,000), the applicant institution can collect F&A on the difference ($8,000) in the subsequent project years until the entire $25,000 is collected.

The "total direct cost" (figure 15.10, line 79) is a total sum of *all* direct costs associated with the project (i.e., personnel + consultants + equipment + supplies + travel + patient care costs + alterations and renovations + other expenses + consortium *direct* cost); this sum is what is carried to box 7a of the

Figure 15.11. Modified Total Direct Cost Calculation

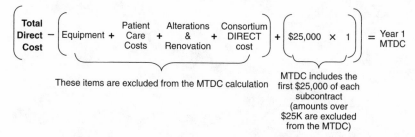

$$\text{Total Direct Cost} - \left(\left(\text{Equipment} + \text{Patient Care Costs} + \text{Alterations \& Renovation} + \text{Consortium DIRECT cost}\right) + \left(\$25{,}000 \times 1\right)\right) = \text{Year 1 MTDC}$$

These items are excluded from the MTDC calculation

MTDC includes the first $25,000 of each subcontract (amounts over $25K are excluded from the MTDC)

PHS 398 face page. The F&A cost (figure 15.10, line 83) is determined by simply multiplying the F&A cost *rate* (figure 15.10, line 81) by the MTDC base (figure 15.10, line 82). The total cost of the project is the sum of the total direct cost (line 79) + consortium's F&A cost (line 75 in figure 15.3b) + the applicant F&A cost (line 83), this sum is entered into box 7b of the face page. Finally, the sum of line 79 (sum of "Total Direct Cost" calculated for all project years) is carried to box 8a of the face page and the sum of line 85 (sum of "Total Cost" calculated for all project years) is carried to box 8b of the face page. The checklist page can be completed by carrying the MTDC base (line 82) amounts to the appropriate section of the checklist form. The next step would involve transcribing all of the computed figures into the respective sections of the PHS 398 budget pages.

Appendix 15.1   Comprehensive Sample Budget and
                   Budget Justification

To further illustrate the main points about budget preparation and computation, this appendix presents a full budget based on the Japanese beetle study example.

Please note that the Japanese beetle topic does not correspond with any proposal submitted by investigators at the Weill Medical College of Cornell University. I have no prior knowledge whether the subject matter is similar to any present, past, or future proposals that are sponsored by federal and/or nonfederal agencies or organizations. The sole reason for using this fictitious study design is to further illustrate important budget concepts described in this chapter and to provide readers with a sample grant budget format used by investigators working in the Institute for Prevention Research at the Weill Medical College of Cornell University.

The budget is prepared using the PHS 398 budget package. The names, addresses, telephone numbers, and other general information provided are fictitious, and if any of the information contained in this section of the application bears resemblance to an actual person, place, or entity, it is purely by coincidence.

SAMPLE NONMODULAR BUDGET AND JUSTIFICATION

Form Approved Through 09/30/2007

OMB No. 0925-0001

Department of Health and Human Services Public Health Services ***Grant Application*** *Do not exceed character length restrictions indicated.*	LEAVE BLANK—FOR PHS USE ONLY.		
	Type	Activity	Number
	Review Group		Formerly
	Council/Board (Month, Year)		Date Received

1. TITLE OF PROJECT *(Do not exceed 81 characters, including spaces and punctuation.)*
Environmentally Safe Application of Treatment X To Eradicate Japanese Beetle

2. RESPONSE TO SPECIFIC REQUEST FOR APPLICATIONS OR PROGRAM ANNOUNCEMENT OR SOLICITATION ☒ NO ☐ YES
(If "Yes," state number and title)
Number: _____ Title: _____

3. PRINCIPAL INVESTIGATOR/PROGRAM DIRECTOR	New Investigator ☒ No ☐ Yes	
3a. NAME (Last, first, middle) Anderson, Jacob, P.	**3b. DEGREE(S)** BS, MS, PhD, MPH	**3h. eRA Commons User Name** janderson
3c. POSITION TITLE Professor	**3d. MAILING ADDRESS** *(Street, city, state, zip code)* 411 East 69th Street New York, NY 10021	
3e. DEPARTMENT, SERVICE, LABORATORY, OR EQUIVALENT Environmental Sciences		
3f. MAJOR SUBDIVISION Weill Medical College		
3g. TELEPHONE AND FAX *(Area code, number and extension)* TEL: (212) 746-1270 FAX: (212) 746-8390	E-MAIL ADDRESS: Jander8640@med.cornell.edu	

4. HUMAN SUBJECTS RESEARCH	**4b. Human Subjects Assurance No.** FWA00000093		**5. VERTEBRATE ANIMALS** ☒ No ☐ Yes	
☐ No ☒ Yes	**4c. Clinical Trial** ☒ No ☐ Yes	**4d. NIH-defined Phase III** Clinical Trial ☒ No ☐ Yes	**5a.** If "Yes," IACUC approval Date	**5b.** Animal welfare assurance no.
4a. Research Exempt ☒ No ☐ Yes	If "Yes," Exemption No.			A2930-01

6. DATES OF PROPOSED PERIOD OF SUPPORT *(month, day, year—MM/DD/YY)*		**7. COSTS REQUESTED FOR INITIAL BUDGET PERIOD**		**8. COSTS REQUESTED FOR PROPOSED PERIOD OF SUPPORT**	
From	Through	**7a.** Direct Costs ($)	**7b.** Total Costs ($)	**8a.** Direct Costs ($)	**8b.** Total Costs ($)
04/01/08	03/31/13	$372,321	$606,460	$2,296,340	$3,707,357

9. APPLICANT ORGANIZATION	**10. TYPE OF ORGANIZATION**	
Name Joan & Sanford I. Weill Medical College of Cornell University Address 1300 York Avenue New York, NY 10021	Public: → ☐ Federal ☐ State ☐ Local Private: → ☒ Private Nonprofit For-profit: → ☐ General ☐ Small Business ☐ Woman-owned ☐ Socially and Economically Disadvantaged	
	11. ENTITY IDENTIFICATION NUMBER 113-162-3978A1 DUNS NO. 060217502 Cong. District 14	

12. ADMINISTRATIVE OFFICIAL TO BE NOTIFIED IF AWARD IS MADE	**13. OFFICIAL SIGNING FOR APPLICANT ORGANIZATION**
Name Randall H. Phillips	Name Barbara Pifel, JD, MBA, RN
Title Manager Grant Accounting	Title Senior Director, Grants & Contracts 1300 York Avenue
Address 100 Broadway, 8th Floor New York, NY 10005-1983	Address WMC Box 89 New York, NY 10021
Tel: (212) 680-7131 FAX: (212) 680-6704	Tel: (212) 821-0959 FAX: (212) 821-0799
E-Mail: rhphilli@med.cornell.edu	E-Mail: blp2001@med.cornell.edu

14. APPLICANT ORGANIZATION CERTIFICATION AND ACCEPTANCE: I certify that the statements herein are true, complete and accurate to the best of my knowledge, and accept the obligation to comply with Public Health Services terms and conditions if a grant is awarded as a result of this application. I am aware that any false, fictitious, or fraudulent statements or claims may subject me to criminal, civil, or administrative penalties.	SIGNATURE OF OFFICIAL NAMED IN 13. *(In ink. "Per" signature not acceptable.)*	DATE

Principal Investigator/Program Director (Last, First, Middle): Anderson, Jacob P., Ph.D.

WCMC (Applicant Organization) Composite Budget

| DETAILED BUDGET FOR INITIAL BUDGET PERIOD DIRECT COSTS ONLY | | FROM 4/1/08 | | THROUGH 3/31/09 | | | | |

PERSONNEL (Applicant organization only)		Months Devoted to Project				DOLLAR AMOUNT REQUESTED (omit cents)		
NAME	ROLE ON PROJECT	Cal. Mnths	Acad. Mnths	Sum. Mnths	INST.BASE SALARY	SALARY REQUESTED	FRINGE BENEFITS	TOTAL
Jacob P. Anderson, Ph.D.	Principal Investigator	4.80			$183,500	$73,400	$21,286	$94,686
Barbara Blocks, Ph.D.	Entomologist	3.60			$75,667	$22,700	$6,583	$29,283
Carl Carlson, Ph.D.	Biochemist	4.80			$86,915	$34,766	$10,082	$44,848
Derrick Dillon, Ph.D.	Agronomist	2.40			$122,703	$24,541	$7,117	$31,658
Evelyn Eves, M.S.	Research Administrator	4.80			$81,802	$32,721	$9,489	$42,210
TBA	Research Assistant	12.00			$35,789	$35,789	$10,379	$46,168
SUBTOTALS						$223,917	$64,936	$288,853

CONSULTANT COSTS **Xavier Miller, Ph.D., 3 consulting days at a rate of $500/day**		$1,500
EQUIPMENT (Itemize) **Super XYZ Machine $8,000**		$8,000
SUPPLIES (Itemize by category) **Super XYZ Supplies $278** **Soil pH Test Meter $250** **Research Supplies $280**		$808
TRAVEL		
PATIENT CARE COSTS	INPATIENT	
	OUTPATIENT	
ALTERATIONS AND RENOVATIONS (Itemize by category)		
OTHER EXPENSES (Itemize by category) **Computer $2,000**		$2,000
CONSORTIUM/CONTRACTUAL COSTS	DIRECT COSTS	$71,160
SUBTOTAL DIRECT COSTS FOR INITIAL BUDGET PERIOD (Item 7a, Face Page)		$ $372,321
CONSORTIUM/CONTRACTUAL COSTS	FACILITIES AND ADMINISTRATIVE COSTS	$17,790
TOTAL DIRECT COSTS FOR INITIAL BUDGET PERIOD		$ $390,111

PHS 398/2590 (Rev. 09/04, Reissued 4/2006)　　　Page [2]　　　Form Page 2

Principal Investigator/Program Director (Last, First, Middle):   Anderson, Jacob P., Ph.D.

WCMC (Applicant Organization) Composite Budget

BUDGET FOR ENTIRE PROPOSED PROJECT PERIOD
DIRECT COSTS ONLY

BUDGET CATEGORY TOTALS		INITIAL BUDGET PERIOD *(from Form Page 4)*	ADDITIONAL YEARS OF SUPPORT REQUESTED			
			2nd	3rd	4th	5th
PERSONNEL: *Salary and fringe benefits. Applicant organization only.*		$288,853	$393,722	$369,457	$411,932	$404,006
CONSULTANT COSTS		$1,500	$1,500	$1,500	$1,500	$1,500
EQUIPMENT		$8,000				
SUPPLIES		$808	$703	$337	$686	$955
TRAVEL			$2,000	$500	$2,000	$500
PATIENT CARE COSTS	INPATIENT					
	OUTPATIENT					
ALTERATIONS AND RENOVATIONS						
OTHER EXPENSES		$2,000	$1,570	$11,035	$1,570	$11,335
CONSORTIUM/ CONTRACTUAL COSTS	DIRECT	$71,160	$73,205	$75,311	$77,481	$79,714
SUBTOTAL DIRECT COSTS *(Sum = Item 8a, Face Page)*		$372,321	$472,701	$458,140	$495,169	$498,010
CONSORTIUM/ CONTRACTUAL COSTS	F&A	$17,790	$18,301	$18,828	$19,370	$19,929
TOTAL DIRECT COSTS		$390,111	$491,002	$476,968	$514,539	$517,939

TOTAL DIRECT COSTS FOR ENTIRE PROPOSED PROJECT PERIOD — $ 2,390,558

JUSTIFICATION. Follow the budget justification instructions exactly. Use continuation pages as needed.

See attached continuation page for budget justification.

WEILL MEDICAL COLLEGE OF CORNELL UNIVERSITY SAMPLE
BUDGET JUSTIFICATION

*Disclaimer

This sample budget justification is for instructional purposes only. If any names or entities referenced, bears resemblance to the name and/or function of an actual person or entity, it is purely by coincidence.

Personnel

All personnel are listed in alphabetical order, with Principal Investigator listed first.

Principal Investigator

Jacob P. Anderson, Ph.D., will serve as the Principal Investigator and his responsibilities will include providing scientific leadership to the proposed research project. Dr. Anderson is an internationally known expert on environmental protection and the sustainability of natural resources. He holds a Ph.D. from the University of Wisconsin-Madison with training and experience in both environmental science and biotechnology.

Dr. Anderson is a senior (tenured) faculty member of the Weill Medical College of Cornell University, where he holds a joint appointment as a Professor of Botany in the Department of Environmental Sciences and the Department of Ecology. Dr. Anderson is also Director of Cornell's Natural Defense of Trees and Plant Life Institute and Chief of the Department of Environmental Sciences, Division of Ecophysiology Research and Vegetation Science.

Dr. Anderson has been a productive researcher, publishing more than 300 scientific papers and book chapters, and has presented more than 175 scientific papers and invited addresses at national and international professional conferences. Dr. Anderson has been a Principal Investigator on 15 major federally funded environmental-protection based prevention projects involving more than 500 farms, national parks, and arboretums. He has served as a member or consultant to numerous governmental and professional advisory committees, including several grant review committees of the Environmental Protection Agency and the U.S. Department of Agriculture.

Dr. Anderson will devote **4.80 person-months** to the proposed research project in all years of requested support. Dr. Anderson will be responsible for providing scientific leadership to the project while overseeing the planning and execution of the research support infrastructure as proposed in the research application. In addition, Dr. Anderson will support the integration of research topics and will set the research agenda and develop new research ideas for future proposals. He will also be responsible for disseminating research findings to the scientific community, overseeing data analyses, and collaborating with key personnel on manuscript preparation and publications. Lastly, Dr. Anderson will exercise oversight of the financial transactions and financial status of the project, to ensure that all charges are reasonable, necessary, and allowable under the terms and conditions of the award.

Entomologist

Barbara Blocks, Ph.D., will serve as the Entomologist, and her responsibilities will include assisting with the instrument development and performing toxicological screenings of the Japanese beetle insects. Dr. Blocks received her B.S. in Entomology from Michigan State University, her M.S. in Entomology with a specialization in Ecology, Evolutionary Biology and Behavior from Michigan State University, and her Ph.D. in Entomology with a concentration in Environmental Toxicology from Michigan State University. Dr. Blocks is currently Professor of Entomology at the Weill Medical College of Cornell University with the Department of Entomology and Director of the Pest Management Center at WCMC. She is a national expert on insect toxicology, molecular entomology, and pesticide education and policy.

In year 1, Dr. Blocks will devote **3.60 person-months** to the project, where she will collaborate with the project staff on developing the survey instrument and visiting the farm sites to collect live samples of the Japanese beetles for further examination at her laboratory. In years 2–5, Dr. Blocks will devote **4.80 person-months** to the project, where will she continue to disseminate her research findings to the project staff and evaluate the toxicology effects of treatment X on the Japanese beetles. Lastly, Dr. Blocks will collaborate with the project staff on manuscript preparation, publications, and presentations.

Plant Biochemist

Carl Carlson, Ph.D., will serve as the Plant Biochemist, and his responsibilities will include formulating and packaging treatment X for distribution to the farm sites. Dr. Carlson received his B.S. in Biology from Columbia University and his M.S. and Ph.D. from the University of Illinois in Plant Biochemistry. Dr. Carlson is currently a Plant Biochemist at Weill Medical College of Cornell University, where for the past 15 years his research has focused on developing new strategies to produce environmentally safe approaches to protect trees and plants from pathogens and insects. Dr. Carlson is currently PI of a five-year NIH study evaluating plant and tree response to climatic and environmental factors and the impact of these stressors on plant and tree health sustainability.

Dr. Carlson will devote **4.80 person-months** to the proposed research project in all years of requested support. His responsibilities will include chemically formulating and packaging treatment X for distribution to the farmers, conducting data analyses, dissemination of scientific findings to the project staff, collaborating with the consultants, and manuscript preparation for the proposed study.

Agronomist

Derrick Dillon, Ph.D., will serve as the Agronomist, and his responsibilities will include conducting the crop variety testing. Dr. Dillon received his B.S. in Agriculture from SUNY Brockport and his M.S. and Ph.D. from Iowa State University. Dr. Dillon is currently Chairman of the Department of Agronomy at WCMC, and his research areas include root and soil interrelationships and the effects of fertilizer and pesticide use on cropping systems in the Midwest. He is a nationally known expert in economic and performance analysis of alternative grazing and pasture renovation systems.

In year 1, Dr. Dillon will devote **2.40 person-months** to the project, where he will collaborate with the project staff on developing the survey instrument and devising diagnostic tests for the farmers to evaluate crop performance on the treatment X program. In years 2–4, Dr. Dillon will commit **4.20 person-months** to the project to administer the crop variety tests. In year 5, Dr. Dillon will commit **5.40 person-months** to the project to evaluate and disseminate the results of the crop variety tests, to evaluate the economic impact of using the treatment X program over other eradication methods, and to collaborate with the project staff on manuscript preparation, publications, and presentations.

Research Administrator

Ms. Evelyn Eves, M.S., will serve as the Research Administrator, and her responsibilities will include managing the daily operations of all grants management activities such as ensuring that project-related activities occur per the timeline provided in the research plan. Ms. Eves received her B.A. in Business from the State University of New York at Albany in 1998 and her M.B.A. from Pace University in May 2003. Ms. Eves served as a research coordinator for the Department of Pediatrics at the Weill Medical College of Cornell University for eight years and has extensive experience in financial and administrative management. She currently manages the daily operations of all administrative activities, including the oversight of financial, personnel, and grant management activities at WCMC.

Ms. Eves will devote **4.80 person-months** to the proposed research in all project years. Ms. Eves will facilitate the business and financial transactions of the project while overseeing the research account(s) associated with the proposed project. She will design databases using Microsoft Access to effectively manage and record daily project expenditures, she will track monetary incentives distributed to the farmers, will set up purchase orders for all equipment and supplies, and will ensure that the consortium is executed. In addition, she will work with research accounting to prepare financial reports as required by the NIH, and furnish the funding agency with requested budgetary and end-of-year fiscal and project-related documentation.

Field Coordinator

Mr. Franklin Fins, M.P.H., will serve as the Field Coordinator, and his responsibilities will include managing the field data collection activities per the timeline proposed in the research plan. Mr. Fins received his Bachelor of Science degree in Biology from State University of New York at Buffalo in 1999 and his M.P.H. in Health Behavior and Health Education from the University of North Carolina at Chapel Hill in 2003. Mr. Fins has held the position of Field Coordinator since December of 1999 under the direction of the PI, Dr. Jacob P. Anderson. Mr. Fins has effectively coordinated the tracking of field activities for previous studies. In addition, Mr. Fins has effectively organized and coordinated data collection activities with more than 5,600 study participants and has supervised more than 30 research/field assistants and more than 20 per diem field staff simultaneously. In addition, he has suggested and implemented methods to improve data collection procedures to the PI on past studies.

In years 2 and 4, Mr. Fins will devote **12.00 person-months** to the proposed research project, where he will supervise all field activities and related personnel on the research projects. Specifically in years 2 and 4, Mr. Fins will schedule and conduct the two one-on-one interviews at the farm sites and, in addition, conduct the soil pH tests at each farm site during these scheduled interviews. In years 3 and 5, Mr. Fins will devote **6.00 person-months** to the proposed research project, where he will assist in moderating the focus groups, monitor and evaluate the firm hired to conduct the focus group to assess intervention fidelity, provide feedback and problem-solving assistance to the focus group moderators and investigators, and supervise, schedule, and coordinate all data collection activities. Mr. Fins has no effort devoted to year 1; therefore, the initial budget page does not list his name or function on the research project.

TBA, Research Assistant

We are proposing to hire **one** research assistant to devote **12.00 calendar months** to the proposed research project in all years of requested support. The TBA Research Assistant will be a hired employee of WCMC. His/her responsibilities will be to assist with finalizing the survey design and recruitment of the farmers for participation in the study (year 1). In addition, the Research Assistant will be responsible for performing library and computer searches (years 1–5), accompanying the field coordinator during the one-on-one interviews (years 2 and 4), creating, maintaining, and updating of the computerized database files for the proposed project while generating reports and letters pertaining to the data input, and assisting the principal investigator with the preparation of dissemination materials (year 5).

Fringe Benefit Rate and Indirect Cost Rate

The fringe benefit rate consists of the following legally required benefits, which includes worker's compensation, unemployment insurance, and severance allowance; insurance and retirement benefits, which include major medical, group life insurance, and retirement annuity; and noncash benefits consisting of vacation, sick time, and other time off with pay. The fringe benefit rate for the project staff is 29% of salaries and wages in project years 1–5. The indirect cost is calculated at 68% of the modified total direct cost for years 1–5. Cost of living inflation adjustments are calculated at 3%.

Consultants

Xavier Miller Ph.D., who will serve as a consulting investigator on the proposed research project, is Director of the Pesticide and Fertilizer Program with the Kansas Department of Agriculture. Dr. Miller's research interests include developing preventive interventions for agricultural studies, pesticide risk assessment methodologies, and developing intervention approaches that can be implemented in resource-poor settings. Dr. Miller is the principal investigator for a five-year longitudinal study funded by the U.S. Department of Agriculture that seeks to develop an intervention aimed at increasing crop productivity and efficiency in rural farm areas by developing ways to improve protection against pests and diseases.

In the proposed research, Dr. Miller will assist in pilot testing the instrument to ensure that it adheres to contemporary principles of the agricultural industry. Dr. Miller will also provide scientific advisory and guidance on the field trial research project and will assist in ensuring that the interview assessment is appropriate for the study. Dr. Miller may also serve as a collaborator in manuscript preparation, publications, and presentations. He will be compensated for three consulting days/year in all years of the proposed study at a rate of $500/day ($1,500 per project year).

Equipment

SuperXYZ Machine ($8,000 – year 1 only)

Funds are being requested to purchase **one** new SuperXYZ Machine (model no. X87-Z478) from Equipment, Inc. The SuperXYZ machine is designed chemically formulate and reproduce mass batches of treatment X for distribution to the farmers. A copy of the product manual is included in the Appendix.

The proposed expense will cover the cost to purchase the SuperXYZ machine and all of its peripherals, including annual calibration of the machine, diagnostic fees, independent power source, and regular maintenance of the machine. The quote from Equipment, Inc. also includes 50 traps and toxicology kits, which will be used by Dr. Blocks to trap the Japanese beetles at randomly selected farm sites. The captured pests will be collected, tested, and evaluated by Dr. Blocks before and after treatment X administration. These projected expenses are based upon actual quotes received from the vendor.

Supplies

SuperXYZ Machine Supplies ($278 – year 1 only)

Funds are being requested to purchase all of the supplies (listed in the accompanying table) for the SuperXYZ machine in year 1 instead of spreading the cost in subsequent years of funding. We are proposing this measure to increase cost savings by eliminating annual inflation costs. The materials being purchased are nondegradable and will not lose value or quality by purchasing them in the initial year of funding.

Supplies from Vials U.S.A., Inc.			
Item	Quantity	Cost per Unit	Total Cost
28 × 117 mm 50-mL polypropylene transport tubes	100*	$0.26	$26.00
Custom labels for vials	60	$0.50	$30.00
Preprinted package insert/vial	60	$0.75	$45.00
One-gallon polyurethane jugs with hose attachment	20	$3.75	$75.00
Lubricant for SuperXYZ	3	$10.00	$30.00
Customized disinfectant for SuperXYZ	6	$12.00	$72.00
TOTAL			$278.00

*We estimate that a total of 60 vials will be distributed to the farmers in the course of the proposed 5-year project. However, Vials U.S.A., Inc. sells the vials in bulk and not individually.

Treatment X Concentrate ($300/year in project years 2 and 4 and $600 in year 5)

Funds are being requested to formulate 150 mL of concentrated treatment X solution/year to distribute to the **10** farmers in the experimental group in project years 2 and 4. Each farmer in the experimental group will be given a 10 mL vial of concentrated treatment X during the one-on-one interviews conducted at the farm sites. We will retain 50 mL of the concentrated treatment X solution in the lab in the event that the vials shipped are lost or destroyed during shipment. The cost to reproduce the solution in concentrated form is $2.00/mL. Therefore, we are requesting $300 in years 2 and 4 to reproduce the batches for distribution. The cost is computed as follows: $2.00/mL 150 mL = $300. As per the research protocol, at the conclusion of the study, all **20** farmers will receive a free batch of treatment X in year 5 (i.e., $2.00/mL × 15 mL^g × 20 vials = $600). The 15 ml batches are less concentrated and would be the standard practice in delivery of this treatment at mass distribution levels.

Food Coloring ($35 in year 2 only)

Funds are being requested to purchase one gallon of highly concentrated canary yellow food coloring, which will be prepared for distribution to the **10** farmers in the control group in project years 2 and 4 of the proposed research. Each farmer in the control group will be given a 15 mL vial of the food coloring during the one-on-one interviews conducted at the farm sites. The purchase of the food coloring is necessary to mock the color of treatment X so that the farmers cannot determine whether they are in the treatment group or in the control group of the study.

Evaluation Surveys ($80/year in years 2 and 4 and $40/year in years 3 and 5)

Funds are being requested to print questionnaires and evaluation materials for the farmer surveys. The optical survey costs $2.00 each to print. All of the farmers will be surveyed twice/year in project years 2 and 4 during their participation in the in-depth one-on-one interviews (i.e., 20 surveys × 2 data collection points × $2.00/survey = $80.00). The focus groups will occur once per year in project years 3 and 5 (i.e., 20 surveys × 1 data collection point × $2.00/survey = $40.00).

	Project Year				
	Year 2	Year 3	Year 4	Year 5	
Control Group	10 farmers; 1:1 interview	10 farmers; focus group	10 farmers; 1:1 interview	10 farmers; focus group	**Before Treatment X (first 6 months)**
Experimental Group	10 farmers; 1:1 interview	10 farmers; focus group	10 farmers; 1:1 interview	10 farmers; focus group	
Control Group	10 farmers; 1:1 interview		10 farmers; 1:1 interview		**After Treatment X**
Experimental Group	10 farmers; 1:1 interview		10 farmers; 1:1 interview		
No. of surveys	40	20	40	20	
Cost/unit	$2.00	$2.00	$2.00	$2.00	
TOTAL	**$80.00**	**$40.00**	**$80.00**	**$40.00**	

The accompanying table provides the detail for the survey costs, which are based upon comparable studies conducted by the Weill Medical College of Cornell University.

Soil pH Test Meter ($250 – year 1 only)

Funds are being requested to purchase 10 Electronic Soil pH Meters at $24.95/unit to evaluate the acidity and alkalinity of the soil before and after administering treatment X to the farmers crops. The soil quality tests will be conducted by the field coordinator and research assistant during their one-on-one interviews at the farm sites. As per the research protocol, determining these factors will aid the biometrician in determining if other external environmental factors may have an impact on the Japanese beetle prevalence in the crops not treated with treatment X.

Research Supplies ($280 year 1)

Funds are being requested to purchase project specific supplies in years 1–5 of the proposed research project. We estimate that the research supplies for year 1 will cost $280, allotting each project staff person a $40 supply budget/year (i.e., $40 supply budget × 7 project staff). A 3% inflation cost is factored into the budget to purchase research supplies in the out years of the budget.

Travel

Travel to Farm Sites ($2,000/year in years 2 and 4 only)

Funds are being requested for the field coordinator and research assistant to travel to the farm sites in years 2 and 4 to conduct the one-on-one interviews. All of the farm locations are accessible via ground transportation. The field coordinator and research assistant will conduct two one-on-one interviews per day (20 consults/year) for the pre- and post-treatment X (control and experimental) groups. In addition, they will conduct the pH soil tests and train the farmers to administer treatment X to their crops. The daily reimbursement rate for ground transportation and meals per consult day is $50 ($25 for round-trip ground transportation and $25 for meals). The costs breakdown as follows: ($50/interview day) × (20 interview days) × (2 staff members) = $2,000/year.

Travel to Focus Groups ($500/year in years 3 and 5 only)

Funds are being requested for the field coordinator to travel to the annual Farmers Convention in Kansas that takes place twice each year. The farmers are required to attend one of the two conventions annually in order to maintain their licensing with their local agricultural state departments. The farmers can opt to attend one of two focus groups, which will take place concurrent to the convention dates. Each one-day trip includes a round-trip domestic flight to Kansas

($125) plus the cost of meals and other incidentals ($125). The cost breakdown is as follows: (2 focus groups) × ($250/trip) = $500/year.

Other Expenses

Overnight Shipment of Vials ($300 – year 5 only)

Funds are being requested to overnight 20 vials to the farmers who complete the study in year 5. Per the research protocol, each farmer will be entitled to receive a free 15-mL batch of concentrated treatment X at the conclusion of the study. The estimated cost to ship the vials is $15/vial. The cost breakdown is as follows: (20 vials) × ($15/vial) = $300.

We Do Focus Groups, Inc. ($10,000/year – years 3 and 5 only)

Funds are being requested to compensate We Do Focus Groups, Inc. to conduct two focus groups per year in project years 3 and 5 only. These two focus groups will take place during the annual Farmers Convention in Kansas. A breakdown of the firms costs are provided in the accompanying table:

Breakdown of Focus Group Expenses	
Activity	Cost
Rental of room to conduct focus group at convention site (equipped with audiovisual supplies)	$2,000
Audio and video recording for 1.5 hours	$1,000
Refreshments	$100
Data tabulation and data processing	$900
Moderator fee	$1,000
TOTAL (per focus group)	**$5,000**

Keypunching/Scanning ($70/year, project years 2 and 4; $35/year, project years 3 and 5)

After data are collected and cleaned, the questionnaires will be keypunched and optically scanned. We estimate in project years 2 and 4 that 40 surveys (i.e. 20 pretest surveys and 20 posttest surveys) will be keypunched and optically scanned at $1.75/survey at a cost of $70/year. We estimate in project years 3 and 5 that 20 focus group surveys/year will be keypunched and optically scanned at $1.75/survey at a cost of $35/year. These projected expenses are based upon comparable studies conducted by the Weill Medical College of Cornell University.

Incentives

One-on-One Interview Incentives

Funds are being requested to offer a $75 cash incentive to the farmers who participate in the in-depth one-on-one interviews in years 2 and 4 (i.e., $50 will be offered at the completion of the pretest survey and $25 will be offered at the completion of the posttest survey).

One-on-One Farmer Interview Incentives				
			Incentive Amount	
	Activity	N=	Year 2	Year 4
One-on-One Interview Incentives	Pretest survey and training (control group)*	10	$500	$500
	Pretest survey and training (experimental group)*	10	$500	$500
	Posttest treatment X survey (control group)**	10	$250	$250
	Posttest treatment X survey (experimental group)**	10	$250	$250
TOTAL			**$1,500**	**$1,500**

*$50/farmer for completion of pretest survey
**$25/farmer for completion of posttest survey

Focus Group Incentives

In addition, $50 will be offered to the farmers who participate in one of the two focus groups being conducted in project years 3 and 5.

Focus Group Farmer Incentives				
			Incentive Amount	
	Activity	N=	Year 3	Year 5
Focus Group Farmer Incentives	Focus group #1*	10	$500	$500
	Focus group #2*	10	$500	$500
	TOTAL		**$1,000**	**$1,000**

*$50/farmer for focus group participation

Computer ($2,000 year 1 only)

Funds are being requested to purchase one computer for the principal investigator to expand the capacity of data analysis on the research project. Specifically, the new system will enhance Dr. Anderson's ability to clean data, manage and archive large data files, evaluate biometric and intervention analysis of the data, and test the developmental hypothesis.

Consortium

Funds are being requested to establish a consortium with Biometrics Consulting, LLC. Please refer to the accompanying consortium budget pages for a complete description of their activities to the project. The $25,000 overhead charge for executing the subcontract and other administrative matters for the consortium is included in the modified total direct cost base for WCMC in year 1 only.

Principal Investigator/Program Director (Last, First, Middle): Anderson, Jacob P., Ph.D.

WCMC Checklist Page

CHECKLIST

TYPE OF APPLICATION *(Check all that apply.)*

☒ NEW application. *(This application is being submitted to the PHS for the first time.)*

☐ REVISION/RESUBMISSION of application number: _____

    (This application replaces a prior unfunded version of a new, competing continuation/renewal, or supplemental/revision application.)

INVENTIONS AND PATENTS
(Competing continuation/renewal appl. only)

☐ COMPETING CONTINUATION/RENEWAL of grant number: _____

    (This application is to extend a funded grant beyond its current project period.)

☐ No   ☐ Previously reported

☐ SUPPLEMENT/REVISION to grant number: _____

☐ Yes. If "Yes,"   ☐ Not previously reported

    (This application is for additional funds to supplement a currently funded grant.)

☐ CHANGE of principal investigator/program director.

    Name of former principal investigator/program director: _____

☐ CHANGE of Grantee Institution.   Name of former institution: _____

☐ FOREIGN application   ☐ Domestic Grant with foreign involvement   List Country(ies) Involved: _____

1. PROGRAM INCOME *(See instructions.)*

All applications must indicate whether program income is anticipated during the period(s) for which grant support is request. If program income is anticipated, use the format below to reflect the amount and source(s).

Budget Period	Anticipated Amount	Source(s)
N/A	N/A	N/A

2. ASSURANCES/CERTIFICATIONS *(See instructions.)*

In signing the application Face Page, the authorized organizational representative agrees to comply with the following policies, assurances and/or certifications when applicable. Descriptions of individual assurances/certifications are provided in Part III. If unable to certify compliance, where applicable, provide an explanation and place it after this page.
•Human Subjects Research •Research Using Human Embryonic Stem Cells •Research on Transplantation of Human Fetal Tissue •Women and Minority Inclusion Policy •Inclusion of Children Policy •Vertebrate Animals•

•Debarment and Suspension •Drug- Free Workplace *(applicable to new [Type 1] or revised/resubmission [Type 1] applications only)* •Lobbying •Non-Delinquency on Federal Debt •Research Misconduct •Civil Rights (Form HHS 441 or HHS 690) •Handicapped Individuals (Form HHS 641 or HHS 690) •Sex Discrimination (Form HHS 639-A or HHS 690) •Age Discrimination (Form HHS 680 or HHS 690) •Recombinant DNA Research, Including Human Gene Transfer Research •Financial Conflict of Interest •Smoke Free Workplace •Prohibited Research •Select Agent Research •PI Assurance

3. FACILITIES AND ADMINSTRATIVE COSTS (F&A)/ INDIRECT COSTS. See specific instructions.

☒ DHHS Agreement dated: 06/07/06   ☐ No Facilities And Administrative Costs Requested.

☐ DHHS Agreement being negotiated with _____ Regional Office.

☐ No DHHS Agreement, but rate established with _____ Date _____

CALCULATION* *(The entire grant application, including the Checklist, will be reproduced and provided to peer reviewers as confidential information.)*

a. Initial budget period:	Amount of base $ 318,161	x Rate applied	68.00 % = F&A costs	$	216,349
b. 02 year	Amount of base $ 399,495	x Rate applied	68.00 % = F&A costs	$	271,657
c. 03 year	Amount of base $ 382,829	x Rate applied	68.00 % = F&A costs	$	260,324
d. 04 year	Amount of base $ 417,688	x Rate applied	68.00 % = F&A costs	$	284,028
e. 05 year	Amount of base $ 418,296	x Rate applied	68.00 % = F&A costs	$	284,441

TOTAL F&A Costs $ **1,316,799**

*Check appropriate box(es):

☐ Salary and wages base   ☒ Modified total direct cost base   ☐ Other base *(Explain)*

☐ Off-site, other special rate, or more than one rate involved *(Explain)*

Explanation *(Attach separate sheet, if necessary.)*:

Principal Investigator/Program Director (Last, First, Middle): Anderson, Jacob P., Ph.D.

Biometrics Consulting, LLC - Subcontract

DETAILED BUDGET FOR INITIAL BUDGET PERIOD DIRECT COSTS ONLY						FROM 4/1/08		THROUGH 3/31/09	

PERSONNEL (Applicant organization only)		Months Devoted to Project				DOLLAR AMOUNT REQUESTED (omit cents)			
NAME	ROLE ON PROJECT	Cal. Mnths	Acad. Mnths	Sum. Mnths	INST.BASE SALARY	SALARY REQUESTED	FRINGE BENEFITS	TOTAL	
JJ Hewitt, Ph.D.	Principal Investigator	3.60			$155,000	$46,500	$13,020	$59,520	
Shellie Mack, M.S.	Research Assistant	1.80			$45,000	$6,750	$1,890	$8,640	
SUBTOTALS						$53,250	$14,910	$68,160	

CONSULTANT COSTS

EQUIPMENT (Itemize)

SUPPLIES (Itemize by category)

TRAVEL
PI travel to New York City to attend annual investigators meeting at WCMC (twice/yr $1,500/trip) $3,000

PATIENT CARE COSTS	INPATIENT	
	OUTPATIENT	

ALTERATIONS AND RENOVATIONS (Itemize by category)

OTHER EXPENSES (Itemize by category)

CONSORTIUM/CONTRACTUAL COSTS		DIRECT COSTS	
SUBTOTAL DIRECT COSTS FOR INITIAL BUDGET PERIOD (Item 7a, Face Page)			$ 71,160
CONSORTIUM/CONTRACTUAL COSTS		FACILITIES AND ADMINISTRATIVE COSTS	$17,790
TOTAL DIRECT COSTS FOR INITIAL BUDGET PERIOD			$ 88,950

Principal Investigator/Program Director (Last, First, Middle): Anderson, Jacob P., Ph.D.

Biometrics Consulting, LLC - Subcontract

BUDGET FOR ENTIRE PROPOSED PROJECT PERIOD
DIRECT COSTS ONLY

BUDGET CATEGORY TOTALS		INITIAL BUDGET PERIOD (from Form Page 4)	ADDITIONAL YEARS OF SUPPORT REQUESTED			
			2nd	3rd	4th	5th
PERSONNEL: *Salary and fringe benefits. Applicant organization only.*		$68,160	$70,205	$72,311	$74,481	$76,714
CONSULTANT COSTS						
EQUIPMENT						
SUPPLIES						
TRAVEL		$3,000	$3,000	$3,000	$3,000	$3,000
PATIENT CARE COSTS	INPATIENT					
	OUTPATIENT					
ALTERATIONS AND RENOVATIONS						
OTHER EXPENSES						
CONSORTIUM/ CONTRACTUAL COSTS	DIRECT					
SUBTOTAL DIRECT COSTS *(Sum = Item 8a, Face Page)*		$71,160	$73,205	$75,311	$77,481	$79,714
CONSORTIUM/ CONTRACTUAL COSTS	F&A	$17,790	$18,301	$18,828	$19,370	$19,929
TOTAL DIRECT COSTS		$88,950	$91,507	$94,139	$96,851	$99,643

TOTAL DIRECT COSTS FOR ENTIRE PROPOSED PROJECT PERIOD	$ 471,089

JUSTIFICATION. Follow the budget justification instructions exactly. Use continuation pages as needed.

See attached continuation page for budget justification.

BIOMETRICS CONSULTING, LLC SAMPLE BUDGET JUSTIFICATION

*Disclaimer

This sample budget justification is for instructional purposes only. If any names or entities referenced bears resemblance to the name and/or function of an actual person or entity, it is purely by coincidence.

Personnel

All personnel are listed in alphabetical order, with Principal Investigator listed first.

Principal Investigator

J.J. Hewitt, Ph.D., will serve as the Biometrician, and his responsibilities will include analyzing the data collected by the project staff at WCMC for trends and underlying relationships. Dr. Hewitt received his B.A. in Statistics from the University of Pennsylvania, his M.Sc. in Biometry at the University of Reading, and his Ph.D. in Applied Statistics from the University of Pittsburgh. Dr. Hewitt's research has focused on investigating links between environmental exposures and disease and devising clinical trials on new crop varieties. Dr. Hewitt currently holds an adjunct professorship with the Medical University of South Carolina and has served in an advisory capacity to numerous universities and federal government agencies on his important research endeavors. Dr. Hewitt is a national expert on the design and analysis of randomized clinical trials.

Dr. Hewitt will devote **3.60 person-months** to the proposed research project in all years of requested support. Dr. Hewitt will be responsible for providing quality control measures and will employ statistical methods using SPSS and SAS software to understand trends in crop development with and without the use of treatment X. In addition, his responsibilities will include evaluating the trends of survival of the Japanese beetles before and after administering treatment X to the crops, and interpreting qualitative data collected from the farm sites during the one-on-one interviews and the focus groups.

Research Assistant

Shellie Mack, M.S., will serve as the Research Assistant and Junior Research Biostatistician, and her responsibilities will include performing statistical design and data analysis and assisting in database design and data management. Ms. Mack received a Bachelor of Applied Science degree in Mathematical and Computer Modeling from Pennsylvania State University and her Master of Science in Statistics and Operations Research at the Pennsylvania State University.

Ms. Mack joined Biometrics Consulting, Inc. firm in the fall of 2003 and currently has ongoing collaborations with the Medical University of South Carolina Department of Biometry. Ms. Mack will devote **1.80 person-months** to the proposed research project in all years of requested support, and her responsibilities will include streamlining the data management procedures, examining evaluation methods, and assisting with statistical analyses.

Fringe Benefit Rate and Indirect Cost Rate

The fringe benefit rate consists of the following legally required benefits, which includes worker's compensation, unemployment insurance, and severance allowance; insurance and retirement benefits, which include major medical, group life insurance, and retirement annuity; and noncash benefits consisting of vacation, sick time, and other time off with pay. The fringe benefit rate for the project staff is 28% of salaries and wages in project years 1–5. The indirect cost is calculated at 25% of the modified total direct cost for years 1–5. Cost of living inflation adjustments are calculated at 3%.

Travel

Funds are being requested for Dr. Hewitt to travel to attend two investigator meetings at WCMC. Each two-day trip will cost $1,500 to cover the costs of round-trip airfare ($500), car rental ($175/day), lodging ($250/night), meals ($50 per diem/day), and other incidental expenses ($50).

Biometrics Consulting, LLC Checklist page

CHECKLIST

TYPE OF APPLICATION *(Check all that apply.)*

☒ NEW application. *(This application is being submitted to the PHS for the first time.)*

☐ REVISION/RESUBMISSION of application number:
(This application replaces a prior unfunded version of a new, competing continuation/renewal, or supplemental/revision application.)

INVENTIONS AND PATENTS
(Competing continuation/renewal appl. only)

☐ COMPETING CONTINUATION/RENEWAL of grant number:
(This application is to extend a funded grant beyond its current project period.)

☐ No   ☐ Previously reported

☐ SUPPLEMENT/REVISION to grant number: ☐ Yes. If "Yes,"   ☐ Not previously reported
(This application is for additional funds to supplement a currently funded grant.)

☐ CHANGE of principal investigator/program director.

Name of former principal investigator/program director: _____

☐ CHANGE of Grantee Institution.   Name of former institution: _____

☐ FOREIGN application ☐ Domestic Grant with foreign involvement   List Country(ies) Involved: _____

1. PROGRAM INCOME *(See instructions.)*
All applications must indicate whether program income is anticipated during the period(s) for which grant support is request. If program income is anticipated, use the format below to reflect the amount and source(s).

Budget Period	Anticipated Amount	Source(s)
N/A	N/A	N/A

2. ASSURANCES/CERTIFICATIONS *(See instructions.)*
In signing the application Face Page, the authorized organizational representative agrees to comply with the following policies, assurances and/or certifications when applicable. Descriptions of individual assurances/certifications are provided in Part III. If unable to certify compliance, where applicable, provide an explanation and place it after this page.
•Human Subjects Research •Research Using Human Embryonic Stem Cells •Research on Transplantation of Human Fetal Tissue •Women and Minority Inclusion Policy •Inclusion of Children Policy •Vertebrate Animals•

•Debarment and Suspension •Drug- Free Workplace *(applicable to new [Type 1] or revised/resubmission [Type 1] applications only)* •Lobbying •Non-Delinquency on Federal Debt •Research Misconduct •Civil Rights (Form HHS 441 or HHS 690) •Handicapped Individuals (Form HHS 641 or HHS 690) •Sex Discrimination (Form HHS 639-A or HHS 690) •Age Discrimination (Form HHS 680 or HHS 690) •Recombinant DNA Research, Including Human Gene Transfer Research •Financial Conflict of Interest •Smoke Free Workplace •Prohibited Research •Select Agent Research •PI Assurance

3. FACILITIES AND ADMINSTRATIVE COSTS (F&A)/ INDIRECT COSTS. See specific instructions.

☒ DHHS Agreement dated: 06/06/06   ☐ No Facilities And Administrative Costs Requested.

☐ DHHS Agreement being negotiated with _____ Regional Office.

☐ No DHHS Agreement, but rate established with _____ Date _____

CALCULATION* *(The entire grant application, including the Checklist, will be reproduced and provided to peer reviewers as confidential information.)*

a. Initial budget period:	Amount of base $ $71,160	x Rate applied 25.00	% = F&A costs	$ 17,790
b. 02 year	Amount of base $ $73,205	x Rate applied 25.00	% = F&A costs	$ 18,301
c. 03 year	Amount of base $ $75,311	x Rate applied 25.00	% = F&A costs	$ 18,828
d. 04 year	Amount of base $ $77,481	x Rate applied 25.00	% = F&A costs	$ 19,370
e. 05 year	Amount of base $ $79,714	x Rate applied 25.00	% = F&A costs	$ 19,929
			TOTAL F&A Costs	$ 94,218

*Check appropriate box(es):

☐ Salary and wages base   ☒ Modified total direct cost base   ☐ Other base *(Explain)*

☐ Off-site, other special rate, or more than one rate involved *(Explain)*
Explanation *(Attach separate sheet, if necessary.):*

16

Documenting Human Subjects Protections and Procedures

Danny R. Hoyt

The public will support science only if it can trust the scientists and institutions that conduct research.

—Institute of Medicine and National Research Council, *Integrity in Scientific Research: Creating an Environment That Promotes Responsible Conduct*

Grant proposals for research involving human subjects must include a narrative to address the protection of the research participants. An investigator is expected to provide the description of protocols that will be implemented to ensure adequate federal protections. A fundamental error in preparation of a research grant is to treat the human subjects section as a minor detail that may be written at the last minute. It is imperative that the human subject protocols are consistent with the study design. Indeed, human subject considerations generally influence elements of the research design (e.g., consenting, laboratory procedures, specimen handling). The human subject research section of the grant proposal is placed immediately following the research design and method section. A standard PHS 398 NIH application designates this section E.

It is readily apparent to a grant reviewer when there are inconsistencies between the research design and the protections afforded to human subjects. A well-designed human subjects narrative represents an opportunity to address potential reviewer concerns and provide details on the implementation of the research design. In addition to addressing required elements, careful attention to this section reinforces the presentation of a well-designed, integrated research proposal.

Two broad requirements must be addressed in the human subject research section. The first is a requirement to demonstrate compliance with the federal Department of Health and Human Services (DHHS) standards for the conduct of ethical research. The second element is the documentation of responses to the NIH requirements regarding the inclusion of women, minorities, and children. For research involving clinical trials, there will be additional requirements associated with the NIH policies on data and safety monitoring plans (DSMPs). The key is to provide the reviewers with sufficient information that they can determine if the proposed research adequately meets these requirements. Failure to completely respond to the required elements in this section of your proposal can result in a human subjects hold or concern being placed on your grant. This portends more paperwork, having another round of review within the institute or center, and certainly additional headaches.

ETHICAL GUIDELINES AND REGULATIONS

It is apparent when conducting reviews of human subject research sections in grant applications that some investigators have partial or incorrect understanding of the ethical guidelines and regulations. The ethical standards are the foundation for the human subject protection regulations, and these regulations provide an important framework for writing a human subjects plan that is responsive to the required elements. The importance of the ethical guidelines and regulations for the design and conduct of human subjects research has been reinforced through the mandatory training guidelines established by the NIH. Effective October 1, 2000, the NIH requires that the principal investigator (PI) and all other "key personnel" on a grant be certified by their organizational research compliance office as having completed formal training in the protection of human subjects. The documentation of this training must be submitted prior to the release of any grant funds as part of the just-in-time procedures.

An investigator should not assume that the mandated training provides all of the information needed to design a responsive human subject research protocol. One concern is that the training content is determined independently at each respective host institution, thereby providing considerable variability pertaining to the coverage of topics. In addition, the training is usually structured to minimize time requirements by the PI and is often delivered using Internet Web sites. The format and delivery generally mean that more specialized topics that are relevant to many grant protocols are not directly addressed. Also, since the training documentation is not required at the time of grant submission, investigators may hold off completion of the training until such time as they prepare the human subjects protocols for review by their respective institutional review board (IRB). Both the content variability and timing considerations suggest that, despite being mandatory, human subjects training will provide insufficient background for a complete and thorough rendition of this grant proposal section.

In light of this, the optimal strategy suggests that an investigator approach the human subject research section with the same level of proactive planning and preparation applied to the rest of a grant proposal. The Office for Human Research Protections (OHRP) is an excellent source of information and guidance for research involving human subjects. The OHRP Web site (www.hhs .gov/ohrp/) provides a number of useful resources and links regarding general ethical concerns as well as primary source documents and guidance on the federal regulations for human subject protection.

On an important note, the OHRP Web site includes links to documents that track the development of ethical standards in human subject research. The Nuremberg Code and the Declaration of Helsinki provide historical context, particularly with respect to medical research on human subjects. The 1979 Belmont Report, *Ethical Principles and Guidelines for the Protection of Human Subjects of Research*, also provides a more contemporary extension of these earlier ethics statements (www.hhs.gov/ohrp/humansubjects/guidance/belmont.htm). This report, released by a federally sanctioned governing body, the National Commission for the Protection of Human Subjects of Biomedical and Behavioral Research, defines the ethics principles of respect for persons, beneficence, and justice that collectively serve as the foundation for current regulations on the protection of human subjects in research. The report also provides guidance on the application of these principles. Specifically, the applications elaborate on the extension of the ethical principles to the processes of informed consent, assessment of risk and benefits, and the selection of subjects. Investigators wishing to have successful careers and minimize obstacles from their IRB should make these reports and documentation essential reading.

The regulatory standards associated with the ethical guidelines are published in the *Code of Federal Regulations*, Title 45, Part 46, Protection of Human Subjects, revised June 23, 2005 (www.hhs.gov/ohrp/humansubjects/guidance/45cfr 46.htm). This document provides the definitions and guidance used as the foundation for the research compliance systems. The code, also known as the Common Rule, includes criteria for institutional assurance of compliance, outlines the structure and function of the IRB, and provides details on informed consent processes. It also provides guidance regarding additional protections required for vulnerable populations (e.g., pregnant women, prisoners, and children).

One of the main challenges associated with the interpretation of Common Rule is that, by design, it provides a modicum of flexibility. This openness represents an important issue and provides an IRB with the latitude to take into consideration various elements of research protocols in the assessments of risks, benefits, and the level of protections required. However, this flexibility also can lead to investigators interpreting the regulations more liberally than their IRB, and potentially instigating discordant views during grant reviews. Thus, while a familiarity with the Common Rule will help an investigator determine the proper responses to the required elements of the human subjects research section of their grant, the best strategy is to take the time to verify their interpretations with other individuals knowledgeable about the federal regulations on human subject protection. Your own institutional IRB is one obvious source for getting this type of input.

HUMAN SUBJECTS

The NIH provides a general set of instructions to help with the human subject narrative: Supplemental Instructions for Preparing the Human Subjects Section of the Research Plan, which can found at grants.nih.gov/grants/funding/phs398/instructions2/phs398instructions.htm. These instructions point to five questions that need to be answered in order to determine the necessary components to be included in the narrative. The first question addresses whether any of the research involves human subjects. While this may appear to be obvious, there are some distinctions that are not readily apparent to the prospective investigator.

The definition for what constitutes human subjects is provided in the Common Rule (45 CFR Part 46):

> *Human subject* means a living individual about whom an investigator (whether professional or student) conducting research obtains (1) data through intervention or interaction with the individual, or (2) identifiable private information.

For most behavioral science research, it is obvious that the study involves human subjects. However, there are areas where this distinction is less than clear. For example, observational research that takes place in public settings, where there is no reasonable expectation of privacy regarding the behavior being observed, and where the investigator takes no actions to influence or manipulate that behavior would not typically be considered human subjects research. On the other hand, there are also times when the investigator has no direct contact with research subjects, but it would still constitute human subjects research. The OHRP policy on coded specimens and data (www.hhs.gov/ohrp/humansubjects/guidance/cdebiol.pdf) indicates that bodily materials, residual diagnostic specimens, and private information in data files (e.g., medical records) from living individuals who are individually identifiable to the investigators should be considered human subjects data. It does not matter who collected the data or specimens (i.e., they can be obtained through secondary data analysis). If the investigator, or any of the key personnel on the grant, has the ability to determine the identities of living individuals, then these participants are human subjects. This interpretation also applies to secondary data analysis where through deductive disclosure the investigator could logically determine the individual identity of at least some living individuals who participated in the original research. OHRP provides a decision chart that can be helpful with making these distinctions at www.hhs.gov/ohrp/ humansubjects/guidance/decisioncharts.htm.

If the investigator determines that the research proposal does not involve human subjects, then the "No" box should be checked in section 4 for human subjects on the NIH grant face page. The NIH supplemental instructions recommend that the investigator should still create a section E heading for human subjects research and add the following statement: "No human subjects research is proposed in this application." If data or specimens that were previously collected from individuals are being used, and it has been determined that they do not meet the standard for human subjects, then the investigator should add an explanation for this interpretation.

EXEMPT RESEARCH

Most behavioral science research submitted to the NIH involves human subjects. Once qualification of this issue is made, a second question in the NIH supplemental instructions concerns whether the research meets one of the criteria that would make it exempt from the regulations. The Common Rule defines six exemptions from the DHHS regulations (45 CFR Part 46.101(b)). The first exemption addresses research in educational contexts that is limited to educational practices:

> (1) Research conducted in established or commonly accepted educational settings, involving normal educational practices, such as (i) research on regular and special education instructional strategies, or (ii) research on the effectiveness of or the comparison among instructional techniques, curricula, or classroom management methods.

A common error on the part of investigators claiming this exemption is using very liberal definitions of normal educational practices. Not all activities carried out in schools, with the oversight of school officials, would necessarily fit the criteria. For example, studying bullying behaviors during school recess would not typically be considered exempt. This same study could be posed as a naturalistic observational study with the number of bullying behaviors observed by researchers indicated on tally sheets with no personal identifiers used, and this "might" qualify the study for an exemption.

The second category is likely to be the most frequently claimed exemption. It is inclusive of a broad range of social and behavioral data collection methods:

(2) Research involving the use of educational tests (cognitive, diagnostic, aptitude, achievement), survey procedures, interview procedures or observation of public behavior, unless: (i) information obtained is recorded in such a manner that human subjects can be identified, directly or through identifiers linked to the subjects; and (ii) any disclosure of the human subjects' responses outside the research could reasonably place the subjects at risk of criminal or civil liability or be damaging to the subjects' financial standing, employability, or reputation.

Research does not qualify for this exemption if the subject has the potential to be identified *and* the nature of the data collected could produce harm if individual responses were disclosed. Thus, research that collects sensitive data where the subjects are known, but kept confidential, would not qualify for this exemption. It is also important to note that this exemption does not apply to children as research subjects. In effect, survey-based studies of children in classrooms, even using anonymous data collection practices with no personal identifiers, do not qualify for exemption under this portion of the Common Rule.

The other frequently claimed exemption is for public domain or otherwise "de-identified" data obtained from human subjects:

(4) Research involving the collection or study of existing data, documents, records, pathological specimens, or diagnostic specimens, if these sources are publicly available or if the information is recorded by the investigator in such a manner that subjects cannot be identified, directly or through identifiers linked to the subjects.

One important caution worth noting is that this type of data requires the investigator to ensure that the subjects cannot be identified indirectly through the merging of other data files with the data being used in the grant (this is often possible with U.S. Census files containing block identifiers and geo-coded segment-level data; see, e.g., www.census.gov). If such a potential exists, even if only through deductive disclosure, and there are noted risks for a subset of subjects, then this exemption would not apply.

The remaining exemptions cover research on public officials and candidates for public office (exemption 3), evaluation research, and demonstration projects associated with public benefit or service programs (exemption 5), and food quality, taste, and consumer acceptance studies (exemption 6). These are less common exemptions, particularly for research that is likely to be reviewed at the NIH.

If the research meets one of the exempt categories, the "Yes" box in section 4a on the NIH grant face page should be checked. The investigator should also enter the number of the exemption that is being claimed for the study. The human subject research section of the grant application (section E for the NIH) should be used to provide a justification for why the selected exemption is appropriate for the proposed research project. Be sure that the narrative clearly shows the how the research fits within the scope of a particular exemption. A local or institutional IRB may be a good place to seek an initial critical reading of this narrative to help the investigator identify necessary details. It is important to give peer reviewers sufficient information to evaluate the justification of the exemption. Depending on the exemption claimed, the investigator also may need to include narrative on the inclusion of women and minorities and the inclusion of children in the human subject research section.

CLINICAL RESEARCH AND CLINICAL TRIALS

The remaining set of questions in the NIH supplemental instructions concern whether or not the proposed research is clinical research and, if so, whether it also involves clinical trials. Clinical research includes (1) patient-oriented research, (2) epidemiological and behavioral studies, and (3) outcomes research and health services research. If the study is clinical research, then the "Yes" box in section 4c on the NIH grant face page should be checked. All clinical research requires the addition of a DSMP in the human subjects research section.

Clinical trials are defined by the NIH as prospective biomedical or behavioral research studies designed to determine if biomedical or behavioral interventions are safe, efficacious, and effective. There are four phases in the progression of clinical trials. An initial phase is designed for smaller studies predominantly geared to evaluate safety. A second phase involves a larger study where the focus rests with determining efficacy. A third phase studies efficacy with large samples of human subjects including experimental comparison to other interventions. A fourth phase measures the effectiveness of interventions in the general population (i.e., translational studies). If the proposed research meets criteria for the NIH-defined phase 3 clinical trial, then in addition to the DSMP, the investigator will need to address whether there are likely to be clinically important differences in the intervention effect across gender and/or race. If the study is an NIH-defined phase 3 clinical trial, the "Yes" box in section 4d on the NIH grant face page should be checked.

PROTECTION OF HUMAN SUBJECTS

With the exception of research that does not include human subjects, and studies where the research is exempt, the human subject research section should include a subheading on the protection of human subjects. Box 16.1 shows an outline for the recommended content of this section.

Box **16.1**

E. Human Subjects Research
1. Protection of Human Subjects
  a. Risks to the subjects
    1. Human subjects involvement and characteristics
    2. Sources of materials
    3. Potential risks
  b. Adequacy of protection against risks
    1. Recruitment and informed consent
    2. Protection against risk
  c. Potential benefits of the proposed research to the subjects and others
  d. Importance of the knowledge to be gained
  e. DSMP plan

Risks to Subjects

This first subheading under the protection of human subjects has three re-commended components. The first component is a description of the human subjects to be involved in the proposed research. The narrative needs to be consistent with what has been described in the research design and methods section (section D, also called Experimental Design). An investigator should include information on study inclusion and exclusion criteria, protocols for selection of study participants, and the expected characteristics of the resulting sample. The description of the characteristics should minimally include information on the expected number of research subjects, age range, gender, and racial composition. If there are any protected classes of subjects planned for inclusion in the proposed research, the investigator should provide justification. This would include children, pregnant women, fetuses, prisoners, individuals with diminished capacity, and other vulnerable groups.

An investigator also should provide a description of the site, or sites, where the human subject research will be conducted. The role of any collaborating sites in performing the research should be described. Letters of support, documenting any issues that may be related to access to the research populations, should be provided as appendix materials for each collaborating site.

The next component in this section, sources of materials, is used to describe the research materials (e.g., survey data, records, specimens) that will be obtained from the human subjects as part of the research. The narrative should address both the types of data that will be gathered and the possible linkages to subjects by personal identifiers in the data. Be sure to describe who will have access to information containing the identity of research subjects and how access is handled as part of the standard or normal operating procedures in the laboratory. Specifics should be included if datasets are mounted on networks or university computing systems that may be accessible by parties outside of the research group. In particular, describe limitations covering access by nonresearch personnel, graduate students, or other investigators, with specific descriptions of firewall protection, and any additional security protections (password or file encryption) that would prohibit linkages of personal identifiers with actual sensitive data.

The final component in this section is the specification of risks. The investigator should provide a description of any potential risks that could reasonably be anticipated for the proposed research. For each type of risk considered, it is important to provide an assessment of both the seriousness and the likelihood. Where the risks of the proposed procedures are appreciable, it may be beneficial to provide a description of alternative procedures and the related risks to the research subjects.

Adequacy of Protection Against Risk

In the first component of this section an investigator should describe how subjects are going to be recruited. It is important that this narrative be consistent with the inclusion criteria and the description of subject characteristics. The recruitment processes must be designed in such a way that they do not require the inappropriate disclosure of private information about potential subjects. This is often a concern in studies where the subject population is difficult to locate. For example, it is inappropriate for an investigator to get the names of potential subjects from a third party that involves disclosing private information on these subjects. An alternative would be to have the third party distribute information regarding the study. In this manner, subjects who have an interest in participation in the research could be notified, but their eligibility based on private information would be known only to the investigator through direct disclosure by the prospective subject. Investigators contemplating conducting follow-up studies where subject tracking is essential should consult various authorities on this matter who are cognizant of these rules and regulations. Many commercial enterprises that use credit card information or other personal electronic tracking information are not abiding carefully by these HIPPA privacy regulations.

This section also should describe the process for obtaining consent. The investigator should describe how prospective subjects should document consent and how the study is explained to potential subjects. This should include specification of who will administer the consent process, the information that will be provided to the potential subject, and how consent will be documented. Typically the documentation of consent involves signed consent forms with copies retained by both the subject and the investigator. Consent forms must be written in plain language with reading indices appropriate for a person with a sixth-grade education. No confusing or obfuscating language is permissible. Many investigators get their consent forms returned by their respective IRB because the form is not intelligible to the average person on the street. Keep in mind that certain key phrases have no meaning outside of the ivory tower research community and that alternative expressions (common language) must be found and used.

If the study includes children, or other subjects with diminished capacity to give consent, then consent has to be provided by a parent or legal guardian (i.e., informed consent). In this context, the investigator needs to describe the process for getting consent from the parent or guardian, and the subsequent process for obtaining child assent. The definition for children that is relevant to the human subjects consent process is specific to age of majority in the research location. Again, the child assent form has to be written in a language that is comprehensible to children. Have children read the consent form prior to submission to your IRB so that you are assured that the children understand the language. Submit the forms to a sixth-grade teacher to ensure that the language is developmentally appropriate.

Some investigators provide copies of the proposed consent and, when appropriate, assent forms in an appendix for the grant application. It is not a requirement that consent forms be submitted as part of the documentation of this narrative on recruitment and consent. Academic institutions and research think tanks have IRBs to provide oversight on these forms, and the federal government registers all IRBs (both those housed at academic centers and those in commercial IRBs) and requires an assurance of compliance with the federal regulations. Thus, the federal government does not expect an investigator to submit consent and assent forms, but rather to describe the procedures for consenting in detail. If consent or assent forms are submitted along with the application, the investigator should take painstaking care to ensure that the required elements of consent, as detailed in the Common Rule (45 CFR Part 46), are covered in the consent form. Similarly, there is no requirement that the consent process or forms be reviewed and approved by the host institution IRB prior to the submission of the proposal. There is a window upon which the IRB materials and approval must be forwarded to the NIH institute prior to release of any funds or a notice of grant award.

The next element to be addressed in this section of the narrative is to describe the protections against risk in the study protocols. An investigator should provide a description of procedures that will be used to minimize potential risks to the subject. The protocols should specify what will be done to prevent risk that could be reasonably anticipated in the conduct of this research. This section should include a treatment of risks associated with breaches of confidentiality and how those would be minimized. It is a good strategy also to include an assessment of the probable effectiveness of the protections outlined in this section. If the investigator has prior experience with similar risk management that supports the effectiveness of the proposed approach, it is a good strategy to reference this in the narrative.

It is very important that investigators not inherently assume there are no risks associated with their research, merely because they infer the survey or testing format is innocuous. This is overly simplistic and has caused great consternation among many investigators conducting behavioral science research. Even in the situation where a survey using fixed-choice responses is being used with high school students, there may be content in the questions that evokes emotional material in the students. A student may become flustered or begin crying, wish to see a counselor, and so on. All of this may have been provoked by a simple question asking whether youths spend any quality time with their parents (a parent may be abusive, which provokes the excited state). Stating there are no anticipated risks is not the same thing as preparing for the event there are risks associated with introduction of the survey questions into the lives of youth.

If there is some reasonable expectation of health or mental health risks associated with participation, then this section should include a description of plans for appropriate level of medical assistance or professional intervention. Again, going back to the earlier point about unanticipated risks, students may become overly obsessive or ruminate about certain thoughts and require a brief period of counseling. Stating that counseling services are available at the school and including a section that shows the researchers will advise students of the availability of the counseling services may satisfy the IRB on all counts. If the study is a clinical trial involving a biomedical or behavioral intervention, then a DSMP will be required to enhance protection of the research subjects. The required elements and structure of this plan are provided in a subsequent sub-heading in the protection of human subjects section.

Potential Benefits of the Proposed Research to the Subjects and Others

This section is important in helping the grant reviewer understand the risk-to-benefits ratio involved in the research. The risk elements and protections were delineated in the prior section, and this narrative is an opportunity to balance those concerns with a discussion of the anticipated benefits. The higher the risks, the more important it becomes to effectively identify important benefits that could reasonably be expected to come from the research. These benefits do not have to be identified solely for the subjects in the study. Indeed, the strongest benefits may be associated with long-term implications of the research for similar populations. It is incumbent on the investigator to describe the benefits to society as a whole, venturing forth to consider how we all benefit from knowing more about the subject at hand, the success of an intervention, the comparison of two modalities, introduction of a therapeutic regimen, and so on.

Be sure to provide a direct discussion of how, in the context of the benefits, the risks are reasonable and appropriate. Do not leave it to the grant reviewer to infer that comparison from the risk and benefits discussion. It is important to put the risks in context and to provide the reviewer with an argument to evaluate.

Importance of the Knowledge to Be Gained

In this section, the investigator needs to provide an overview of the importance of the knowledge to be gained. This should be relatively easy because it effectively addresses the same topic as the significance narrative in the body of the proposal. Here again, the investigator has the opportunity to reinforce important points made earlier in the grant and show that the human subjects considerations are consistent with the project description and plan.

This section of the human subject research narrative is also important in providing a context for evaluation of the potential risks. A fundamental point that the investigator should make here is that any anticipated subject risks are reasonable in the context of the increment in knowledge that is expected as a result of the research.

Data and Safety Monitoring Plan

This section should be added to the protection of human subjects outline if the research includes a clinical trial. The NIH policy requires that each institute and center have in place a system for the oversight and monitoring of clinical trials to ensure the safety of subjects (grants.nih.gov/grants/guide/notice-files/not98-084.html). If it is a multisite clinical trial involving an intervention with potential risk to the subjects, the establishment of a data safety monitoring board is also required.

The DSMP should include a description of the reporting mechanisms for any adverse events to the IRB, the institute or center, and the NIH. The specific reporting requirements vary by institute and center, and depend on the level of clinical trial. Monitoring should be relative to degree of risk, and the size and complexity of the intervention. In phase 1 and phase 2 clinical trials where the risk is low, close monitoring by the PI with clear and quick reporting to the IRB and the NIH may be adequate and appropriate. Moving to higher risk protocols, and to larger and more complex interventions, requires more rigorous monitoring in the form of data and safety monitoring boards.

INCLUSION OF WOMEN AND MINORITIES

Every application that proposes to involve human subjects must contain a section outlining inclusion of women and minorities (unless using existing specimens or data that meet the criteria for exemption 4). There are four basic elements that must be addressed in this section. The first of these is completion of the targeted/planned enrollment table. Second, you must provide a description of the procedures used to select the subjects. It is important in this section of the narrative that you make it clear how the selection procedures meet the stated scientific objectives and are consistent with the proposed study design. Third, if there is any exclusion on the basis of gender or racial/ethnic group, the investigator needs to provide a justification. It is also important here to provide a description of projected subject pools that might have little or no representation of some racial/ethnic groups due to the population base from which the subjects are drawn. For instance, Native Americans may be hard to recruit in certain geographical regions of the country, and likewise, there may be a study on male infertility that does not require participation by females. The investigator only needs to include a brief but reasonable justification tied to the study design or population at hand. The investigator should document procedures for attempting to ensure adequate representation by gender and racial/ethnic groups among the subjects. Here, it is important that it be clear that every reasonable effort is made to be inclusive in the composition of the human subjects in the proposed research.

If the research qualifies as a phase 3 clinical trial, the investigator is required to provide a narrative regarding the potential for clinically significant gender and/or race/ethnicity differences in the intervention outcomes. This discussion should include specific analysis plans designed to detect potential significant differences in the effects of the intervention across gender and race/ethnicity. If prior studies suggest gender or race/ethnicity effects, the analytic plan should include appropriate statistical controls for these demographic factors. Moreover, the investigator needs to make clear in the analysis section there will be efforts to tease apart whether there are mean differences on select variables of interest or proportional differences for key variables of interest. Another alternative would be to conduct a series of analyses using gender and race subgroups (e.g., multiple group analyses to show different factor structures between males and females on some neuropsychological measure would satisfy this requirement). Regardless of the specific analysis choice, there has to be some recognition that testing for demographic differences is built into the study design.

INCLUSION OF CHILDREN

Every research application involving human subjects must address the inclusion of children (unless using existing specimens or data that meet the criteria for exemption 4). For the purpose of the NIH guidelines, a child is person who is younger than 21 years of age. Guidance on this particular section may be found at grants.nih.gov/grants/funding/children/children.htm. OHRP guidance on children may be found at www.hhs.gov/ohrp/children/. An investigator must provide a description of the plans to include children. This narrative should specify the age range of the children to be included in the proposed study. A justification for the inclusion of children within the specific age range should be provided.

If any of the children are under the age of majority at the sites where the research is to be conducted, then there should be appropriate considerations for child assent and parent consent in the protection against risk narrative. Note that it is possible to have a research design including subjects who may be considered children when documenting inclusion under this definition, but not include any minors.

If children are not to be included in the proposed research, the investigator needs to provide justification for this exclusion. The NIH supplemental instructions for the preparation of the human subjects section of the proposal provide some examples of possible exclusion justifications (grants.nih.gov/ grants/funding/phs398/instructions2/phs398instructions.htm). Naturally, if the study would be inappropriate if conducted with children, this would satisfy exclusion.

KEY MISTAKES

The most common mistake made in the preparation of the human subject research section of the grant proposal is when investigators approach it as simply a technical matter of responding to required elements. The narrative should provide responses that go beyond the minimal required documentation. This is an opportunity to demonstrate to the reviewers that the grant team understands the human subject considerations in the proposed research and has designed an appropriate approach. Moreover, it is important to provide justifications for decisions regarding human subject protocols. Inadequate, incomplete, or otherwise poor documentation of procedures and justifications can result in a "human subjects concern" raised by one or more reviewers. This is effectively a determination that some component of the human subjects protocol is unacceptable and will result in a hold (a "bar," in NIH lingo) being placed on any funding until the inadequacy is resolved. It is useful for a prospective investigator to read the human subject reviewer guidelines (grants1.nih.gov/grants/peer/ hs_review_inst.pdf) prior to preparing this section. These guidelines make it clear that reviewers will be looking for detailed plans and justifications in this portion of the grant narrative.

While the primary purpose of this section of the grant proposal is to document the human subjects concerns, protections, and procedures, it is also an opportunity to provide additional detail that is supportive of the body of the grant proposal. For example, a detailed description of initial contact, subject recruitment, and consent processes meets the requirements of adequately describing human subject protection protocol as well as reinforces the grant narrative on sampling or related concerns in the research design and methods narrative. An investigator who approaches the human subject narrative section with an orientation toward providing minimal responses misses the opportunity to enhance and strengthen the overall proposal.

| Box **16.2** | Some Common Mistakes in Protocols |

Statement

We are just gathering survey questionnaire data, so it will be exempt research.

Response and Guidance

The definition of exempt research is guided by risk consideration, not research methods (www.hhs.gov/ohrp/policy/index.html#exempt).

Statement

We will get a waiver of parental consent for the children in the study.

Response and Guidance

While waivers may be granted by the IRB, they are not routinely given and the investigator must document four specific criteria related to level of risk, impact on rights, lack of a practical alternative, and information to be provided to subjects (www.hhs.gov/ohrp/humansubjects/guidance/45cfr46.htm). If all four criteria are met to the satisfaction of the IRB, a waiver might be granted. Any human subject research protocol that suggests a waiver will be sought should provide the reviewer with documentation on the four criteria.

Statement

We will obtain a list of potential subjects from the clinic patient records.

Response and Guidance

The DHHS has issued the Privacy Rule to implement elements of the Health Insurance Portability and Accountability Act (HIPAA). The Privacy Rule sets standards by which "protected health information" may be released. This would include information regarding who is seeking health care. The ability of the investigator to get this information would depend on the releases obtained at the proposed study site. Guidance on privacy issues in general may be found at privacyruleandre search.nih.gov/. This Web site is also replete with information on international re-search considerations. More specific information regarding the HIPAA Privacy Rule is available online at www.hhs.gov/ocr/privacysummary.pdf.

It should be apparent from the preceding comments that when documenting the protection of research subjects, it is not adequate to simply indicate that the investigator will seek IRB approval before starting the research. This is a common error on the part of many new investigators. While this section may not contain the level of detail of an IRB application, the human subject narrative needs to address specific concerns and with sufficient detail. Absence of these critical details may lead the grant reviewers to wonder whether the prospective investigator has the administrative expertise necessary to carry out the proposed research.

Finally, it is important that investigators do the necessary research into special circumstances that may apply to their research. An investigator needs to understand the regulations associated with various aspects of research with human subjects. A key mistake evident in many human subjects research protocols is recommending procedures that are not consistent with the NIH and OHRP requirements. There is ample guidance available on the OHRP and the NIH Web sites for many of the more common questions that arise in human subjects. Three examples of some common mistakes in protocols and where one could seek appropriate guidance are provided in box 16.2.

Each of the examples in box 16.2 shows simple statements that are typical of the type seen in abbreviated treatments of human subject research narratives. Without additional documentation, these statements represent basic mistakes by the prospective investigators. They fail to provide the grant reviewer with the information needed to determine if the plan is appropriate and realistic. These are just a few examples of the types of mistakes seen in human subject narratives. At best, they are correct but not adequately documented. At worst, they are indicators of a lack of awareness of the complexity of the issue and the associated risk and protection concerns. The OHRP and the NIH sites on human subjects provide links to the source documents and specific guidance on most of the issues that an investigator is likely to encounter in considering human subjects protections. However, it is important to recognize that there is a degree of flexibility, or perhaps ambiguity, built into many of the regulations and guidance documents. It is always a wise decision to seek advice of others with experience in matters of human subject protocols when trying to interpret the guidelines and develop an effective plan.

17

Navigating the Maze

Electronic Submission

Mark R. Green

Obviously, computers have made differences. They have fostered the development of spaceships—as well as a great increase in junk mail.

—Tracy Kidder, *The Soul of a New Machine*

Electronic submission is part of an ongoing process to create a fully paperless grant process from receipt to review to grant administration. The paper-based application process is wasteful of time and resources. Applications for the typical PHS 398 paper submission start with an investigator preparing an application electronically, using word-processing, spreadsheet, and other software. These files are converted to paper and shipped to the NIH, where key information from the paper application is keyboarded into an NIH administrative database and entire applications are scanned back into electronic media. The process cycles an electronic format to paper then back to electronic format—its time to eliminate the middleman. Also, think about a process that produces five copies for each of more than 75,000 paper applications submitted to the NIH per year. If you think of your application as hand delivered by courier to a staff person at the NIH who signs for it, you need to think more in terms of loading docks and a warehouse.

Beyond savings millions of pages of paper, there are a number of other benefits that are expected to accrue, including efficiencies that may allow the NIH to shorten the review cycle, use of electronic validations to improve data quality, reductions of scanning, printing, and data-entry costs, creation of a comprehensive repository of data that can be mined by knowledge management and other tools, and a reduced administrative burden on the federal grants community.

Beyond simply making good sense, converting to an electronic process is the law, Public Law 106-107, the Federal Financial Assistance Management Improvement Act of 1999. The law aims to improve the effectiveness and performance of federal financial assistance programs, simplify federal financial assistance application and reporting requirements, and improve the delivery of services to the public. Also, the Office of Management and Budget set the following FY 2006 goal for agencies: post 75% of funding opportunities in Grants.gov.

Grants.gov is a Web-based grant submission site already used by more than two dozen government agencies that handles hundreds of grant programs. Since this is a shared site, it is not tailored specifically to the NIH. It utilizes processes and forms that must serve a wide community and cannot have the specificity to the NIH that the prior paper submission process provided. The NIH is fully committed to a process that successfully joins the Grants.gov portal with its own electronic research administration (eRA) system for managing grants.

To meet the challenge of combining two systems, the NIH is closely watching the progress of the integration with Grants.gov and working to improve system performance. There are continuous outreach activities for the applicant community through Web sites and hands-on training sessions. Even long-standing "traditions" have been changed, such as revising traditional receipt dates, to spread out workloads to manage system demand efficiently.

E-submission began in 2005, and converting grant mechanisms from paper submission to this new process has been implemented in stages. The NIH hopes to have all grant mechanisms converted to e-submission by October 2007. It is critical to keep in mind that this is a process undergoing changes. Modifications are necessary to incorporate accumulating experience into system improvements, to deal with the increasing numbers of applications using electronic methods, and to integrate changes in NIH policies that are evolving at the same time. For this reason, this chapter does not delve deeply into the details of the process because they may become quickly outdated. It does, however, refer to Web sites that are continually updated to have the most current information, and it provides an overview and tries to shed some light on those parts of the process where the transition to the e-submission process requires special attention from applicants.

Anyone planning to submit an application electronically must check for the most current information available. Information or electronic forms that are months old could easily be outdated. The NIH maintains a Web site at era.nih.

gov/ElectronicReceipt/index.htm that provides up-to-date information about electronic submission:

- The full electronic submission process
- The most common errors
- Frequently asked questions
- Links to places to find help
- Links to listservs that provide news of changes in electronic submission

THE SUBMISSION PROCESS

The main features of the e-submission process are outlined below, providing details on how to

1. Find out how your institution has implemented e-submission
2. Be sure that registrations for Grants.gov and the NIH Commons are in place
3. Be sure that you have the required software operational on your computer
4. Find a funding opportunity announcement (FOA) for your application
5. Prepare your application
6. Send the application to your authorized organizational representative (AOR) to submit to Grants.gov
   - After the application is successfully processed by Grants.gov, it is transferred to the NIH Commons.
   - In the NIH Commons, the application is electronically validated according to the NIH business rules.
   - An image of the application is generated if the application passes the NIH Commons validations. A list of errors or warnings may also be generated.
7. Log onto the NIH Commons and inspect the application image
   - Only the signing official (SO) has two days to reject an application before it moves forward.
   - After two days in the Commons, if there are no errors, applications are forwarded to the Center for Scientific Review.

A more complete description of the process can be found at era.nih.gov/ElectronicReceipt/process.htm.

Step 1: Find Out How Your Institution Has Implemented E-Submission

During the initial year of e-submission most institutions are relying on forms-based submission. Organizations using forms-based submission will rely on the PureEdge Viewer, provided free of charge by Grants.gov. A limited number of organizations use system-to-system transfer of data, although this number is expected to grow as the process matures. Organizations desiring a systems-to-systems approach can work with Grants.gov to develop their own data exchange system (XML datastream). Investigators need to know which form of submission is being used at their institution.

E-submission presents not only a change in the interaction between applicants and the NIH, but also a change in interactions within an applicant institution. A major issue is that electronic applications are not submitted by individual investigators; they must be submitted by an authorized organization representative (AOR), which is the Grants.gov term for the official designated by an organization to electronically submit NIH grant applications. The NIH term for this function is signing official (SO), although it is possible for the AOR and the SO to be different people.

Efficient communications between investigators and their AORs are critical to ensure a smooth application submission process. Investigators need to remember that the receipt date is no longer their deadline for submission—it is the deadline for the AOR to submit. Investigators can no longer make revisions until the last express courier pickup the day before the receipt date. Institutions have to develop internal deadlines so the AOR has materials in time to submit the application. However, there are new receipt dates for all grant mechanisms that you need to be aware of. In most but not all cases, dates have been pushed back. For example, new R01 applications formerly had three standing receipt dates of February 1, June 1, and October 1. The new receipt dates are February 5, June 5, and October 5. The new dates vary by type of grant and are listed fully in the *NIH Guide for Grants and Contracts* at grants.nih.gov/grants/guide/notice-files/NOT-OD-07-001.html.

Investigators also need to be aware that notification of successful transmission of an application to Grants.gov only goes to the AOR, so it is important for an institution to have a process to track applications submitted to Grants.gov. Only after an application makes it to the NIH Commons will the investigator receive any notification.

There is also an increased importance for version control. With a potential need to edit or revise applications after initial submission to the AOR, investigators will have to establish adequate version control to make sure that the correct version of the application is submitted by the AOR.

Step 2: Be Sure That Registrations for Grants.gov and the NIH Commons Are in Place

E-submission requires two registrations: Grants.gov and the NIH Commons. Your institution must be registered on Grants.gov so that the AOR can submit applications. Both the institution and the investigator need to be registered on the NIH Commons to view an application after submission. These are separate registration processes that can be done simultaneously. All registrations must be completed prior to application submission. Failure to complete the required registrations prior to application submission may result in delay of review assignment and funding consideration. It is critical for institutions to begin these registrations at least two to four weeks before applications are due.

Grants.gov registration for applicant organizations is a one-time-only registration and it is good for electronic submission to all federal agencies. Grants.gov registration requires institutions to obtain a DUNS (Data Universal Numbering System) number and register in Central Contractor Registry (CCR). Detailed instructions are provided at grants.gov/GetStarted.

Applicant organizations must be registered in the eRA Commons before an account can be established for an individual investigator. An institution's NIH Commons SO can create user accounts, register the institution, and update institutional profiles. The SO should create a separate account for the investigator. Registration with Commons can take two to four weeks. If not already registered, be sure to have plenty of time to complete the process prior to the application submission deadline.

If an investigator is affiliated with multiple institutions or has moved to a new institution, the business office of the sponsoring organization must affiliate the investigator's Commons account with the organization. Each organization will see only its own applications/grants, whereas an investigator will see all of his or her own applications and grants regardless of which organization was the sponsor. Please remember that investigators are responsible for maintaining their own profiles through eRA Commons.

Investigators who have been registered to participate in the peer review process and Internet-assisted review will need a separate registration to fully use the NIH Commons for application submission and other grant related activities.

The following resources for the NIH Commons should be of assistance in the process:

- Home page for registration and updates: commons.era.nih.gov/commons/
- Frequently asked questions: commons.era.nih.gov/commons/faq.jsp
- Commons helpdesk: (866) 504-9552 or commons@od.nih.gov

Step 3: Be Sure That You Have the Required Software Operational on Your Computer

Applicants need to have PureEdge software to view the online forms; it can be downloaded for free from the Grants.gov site. Unfortunately, the PureEdge software is not currently Mac compatible, although a Mac-compatible version has been promised sometime in the near future along with a limited special edition Mac Viewer for PPC and Intel. Mac users can download from the Grants.gov site a free Citrix server to remotely launch a Windows session and submit an application. Grants.gov does have plans to move to platform-independent software that should facilitate the process for Mac users. There is more detailed information for Mac users at www.grants.gov/MacSupport.

Applicants also need PDF conversion software because the NIH requires that all application attachments be submitted in this format. These files may initially be created using any word-processing program; however, they must be converted to PDF format prior to attaching to your application. Attachments generated from the PureEdge forms (e.g., R&R Subaward Budget attachment form) should *not* be converted to PDF. The electronic submission Web site has tips on creating PDF files that will be accepted, and there is a list of PDF generators that produce documents that can be processed by the NIH. Scanning printed text to an image should not be used because it will impede automated processing of your application. However, scanning to an image is acceptable for things that are not part of the application body, such as letters of support.

Step 4: Find a Funding Opportunity Announcement for Your Application

Once you have the software downloaded, you can begin to search for an FOA; this term is replacing the NIH terms such as program announcement and request for applications. You do not need to be registered with Grants.gov to search for FOAs or to download and fill out application forms. Only submission of an application by the AOR requires registration on Grants.gov.

The NIH will simultaneously post FOAs online in the *NIH Guide for Grants and Contracts* and in Grants.gov Find. The NIH guide is located at grants.nih .gov/grants/guide/index.html.

While FOAs may be found either through the Grants.gov site or through the *NIH Guide*, current experience indicates that use of the *NIH Guide* is the easiest way to search for FOAs. When you find an FOA of interest, scroll down a little to find the "Apply for Grants Electronically" button (see figure 17.1). Clicking this button will automatically take you to the Grants.gov site and directly to the application package that is specific for the FOA selected. From this page, you should download both the application instructions and the application package. Be sure to save them to your computer's hard drive so that you can work on them.

All e-applications *must* be submitted in response to an FOA; there are FOAs that deal with specific topics of interest, and there are also FOAs that do not include programmatic content. This latter group of FOAs are program-neutral and are referred to as "parent announcements." They enable applicants to submit an electronic investigator-initiated application for a single grant mechanism, for example, the Exploratory/Developmental Research Grant Program (parent R21) FOA. If you are interested in looking only for parent FOAs, there is a search criterion on the

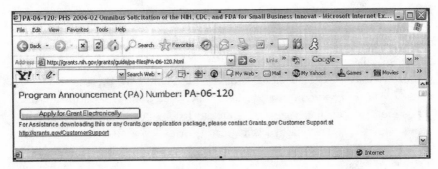

Figure 17.1. Program Announcement

Advanced Search page of the *NIH Guide* that will retrieve all of the parent FOAs. Investigators need to be aware that not all NIH institutes participate in all FOAs.

Within any FOA, pay special attention to the Key Dates section. Once "posted," an application package can be downloaded and started, but it cannot be submitted to Grants.gov until after the "opening date." This is especially important for newly transitioned grant programs where the FOAs are posted at least eight weeks in advance of the receipt date, but the open date is four weeks in advance of the receipt date.

As application packages are updated, the old packages are expired and are no longer accepted by Grants.gov. It is important to use the latest application package (forms and application guide) prior to filling out an application, especially when applying to opportunities with multiple receipt dates.

To ensure you are using the application guide appropriate for the opportunity, download the application guide *and* the application package at the same time.

You have the option to sign up for notification of changes to the application package. It is highly recommended that you sign up for these notifications so you are always aware of changes to the package. These changes could result in critical changes in submission requirements.

Step 5: Prepare Your Application

There are essentially two places to find instructions for e-submission. First is the application guide, which is posted and downloadable with every FOA in Grants. gov. Second is the FOA itself. Program-specific application requirements will continue to be part of the actual announcement and supersede instructions in the application guide.

It is recommended that applications be prepared using a word-processing program, followed by cutting and pasting sections into the proper forms. This is a preparation method investigators are used to and will keep track of the page limits. When material is converted to PDF and pasted into the various forms, there may be a "white space" created that does not count toward the page limits.

Use the page count in the word-processing program to make sure that page limits are not exceeded.

Within the application forms, all Grants.gov mandatory fields will be highlighted in yellow and will have an asterisk. There are additional fields that are mandatory for the NIH but not mandatory for Grants.gov. These fields are not marked yellow or with an asterisk. Remember that Grants.gov forms are used across multiple federal agencies with different requirements, so the NIH requirements cannot always be reflected as mandatory fields on the form. The application guide will provide instruction for which fields are required by the NIH for the FOA.

Be sure to save a copy of your completed application locally to your computer. If applications are being completed by investigators, they will need to save the package and then work with their office of sponsored research and the AOR to submit the application on their behalf. Saving the application is critical in case there are submission problems and you have to revise and resubmit the material.

The two errors that have most commonly shown up during the early phases of e-submission are failure to put the NIH Commons user ID of the principal investigator (PI) in the credential field on the R&R Senior/Key Person Profile and failure to use the PDF format for all non-PureEdge attachments that make up the body of the application.

The NIH electronic submission Web site has a page on avoiding common errors (era.nih.gov/ElectronicReceipt/avoiding_errors.htm) and frequently asked questions specifically regarding PDF format (era.nih.gov/ElectronicReceipt/faq_prepare_app.htm#2e), as well as many other resources.

Step 6: Send the Application to Your Authorized Organizational Representative to Submit to Grants.Gov

This process is controlled by the applicant institution. The set of filled out forms can be emailed as attachments or your institution may have a centralized service to handle processing of applications to create submission packages.

After the Application Is Successfully Processed by Grants.gov, It Is Transferred to the NIH Commons

Once submitted to Grants.gov, the AOR will receive an immediate confirmation online with a Grants.gov tracking number and a date/time stamp of receipt. This information should be kept for reference. If you need to contact the help desk staff, they will need this information.

Grants.gov performs basic form validations and a virus check on submitted application. Over the 24–48 hours after submission, the AOR will receive multiple e-mails. (Grants.gov does not contact the PI since he/she is not registered with Grants.gov.) The first email will confirm receipt of the application by the Grants.gov system, and the second will indicate that the application has either been successfully validated by the system prior to transmission to NIH or has been rejected due to error. If your application is successfully submitted to Grants .gov and subsequently retrieved by NIH, an email is sent by Grants.gov indicating the agency has retrieved it.

After successful submission to Grants.gov, the application moves to the NIH Commons for NIH validation. The Commons sends status emails to both the AOR and the investigator. The Commons generally has a one-business-day response time after receipt of the application from Grants.gov.

In the NIH Commons, the Application Is Electronically Validated According to NIH Business Rules

The eRA software performs NIH business rule validations on the submitted application and the NIH notifies the PI and SO by email to check the eRA Commons for results of NIH validations.

An Image of the Application Is Generated If the Application Passes NIH Commons Validations (a List of Errors or Warnings May Also Be Generated)

The PI and SO find out if the grant application passed or failed the NIH validation check by logging on the Commons. There may be either errors or warnings listed. Warnings can be fixed at the applicant's discretion but do not require action for the application to move on to the next step. For example, an application with a budget year exceeding $500,000 in direct costs would get a warning indicating that prior approval is needed. If you have prior approval for the budget request, no action is necessary. On the other hand, errors must be addressed and the entire application resubmitted before the application image can be created. One source of errors is the absence of data in required fields. Once all errors are corrected and the application resubmitted, a grant image is generated and made available for viewing by the PI and AOR/SO.

Step 7: Log Onto the NIH Commons and Inspect the Application Image

Both the investigator and the AOR/SO can view the application image to check it for accuracy, to check that each PDF attachment is formatted correctly, and to check that each attachment has been included. Viewing the application image on the NIH Commons is a critical step because it provides the only opportunity to see the grant application just as a reviewer will see it. There is a two-day window to view the application. After this time, any changes to the application must be made through and with the permission of the assigned scientific review administrator, which can potentially delay the processing of the application.

There may be protocols at your institution indicating who has responsibility for inspecting the application, but it is recommended that the investigator view the image. If it is the investigator who must correct any warnings or errors, he/ she must work with the AOR because the *entire* application must be resubmitted again through Grants.gov, and only the AOR can submit the corrected version.

Only the Signing Official Has Two Days to Reject It Before It Moves Forward

After the image of the application is available in Commons, there is a two-weekday viewing window for the AOR/SO to reject an application that has system formatting errors. Investigators must work through their AOR/SO to reject an application in order to make corrections. While weekends are not counted as part of the two-day window for rejections, any holidays that occur on a weekday do count. So if July 4 falls on a weekday, it would count as part of the two-day window.

If the two-day window falls *prior* to the receipt date, the AOR/SO can "reject" the assembled application and submit a changed/corrected application within the two-day viewing window. This option should be used if it is determined that warnings should be addressed. Keep in mind that warnings do not stop further application processing. If an application submission results in warnings (but no errors), it will automatically move forward if no action is taken. Please remember that some warnings may not be applicable or may need to be addressed after application submission.

If the two-day window falls *after* the receipt date, the AOR/SO will have the option to "reject" the application if, due to an eRA Commons or Grants.gov system issue, the application does not correctly reflect the submitted application package (e.g., some part of the application was lost or did not transfer correctly during the submission process). The AOR/SO should first contact the eRA Commons help desk (ithelpdesk.nih.gov/eRA/) to confirm the system error, document the issue, and determine the best course of action. The NIH will not penalize the applicant for an eRA Commons or Grants.gov system issue.

If the AOR/SO chooses to "reject" the image after the receipt date for a reason other than an eRA Commons or Grants.gov system failure, a changed/corrected application still can be submitted, but it will be subject to the standard NIH late policy guidelines and may not be accepted. The reason for this delay should be explained in the cover letter attachment.

After Two Days in the Commons, If There Are No Errors, Applications Are Forwarded to the Center for Scientific Review

If the application has no errors and is not rejected by the AOR during the two-weekday viewing window, it will automatically proceed to receipt and referral in the Center for Scientific Review. There it will be processed by the NIH staff and assigned to an institute for potential funding and to a review committee for evaluation. There will still be administrative reviews by NIH staff during and after referral where problems with an application may require action by an applicant. Investigators should continue to follow the status of their application via the NIH Commons.

HELPFUL RESOURCES

- General information on electronic submission and the SF424 (R&R): era.nih.gov/ElectronicReceipt
- Questions about Grants.gov registration, submission, and the PureEdge Viewer: grants.gov/CustomerSupport
- eRA Commons registration and postsubmission questions on Commons functionality: go to either the Support Page (era.nih.gov/commons/index.cfm) or the eRA Commons help desk (Web support: ithelpdesk.nih.gov/eRA/; email: commons@od.nih.gov; phone: 866-504-9552 or 301-402-7469)
- Forms transition and questions on the NIH overall plan for electronic receipt: go to NIH Grants Information (email: grantsinfo@nih.gov; phone: 301-435-0714)

There are also NIH electronic mailing lists providing updates on the e-submission process:

- To subscribe to the listserv targeting investigators, leave the subject line blank and send a plain text email message to Listserv@list.nih.gov including only the words "Subscribe NIH_eSUB_PI-L" in the body of the message.
- To subscribe to the listserv targeting institutional officials, leave the subject line blank and send a plain text email message to Listserv@list .nih.gov including only the words "Subscribe NIH_eSUB_AOR_SO-L" in the body of the message.

18 Revisions and Resubmissions

Thomas N. Ferraro & Lawrence M. Scheier

Permanence, perseverance and persistence in spite of all obstacles,
discouragement, and impossibilities: It is this, that in all things distinguishes
the strong soul from the weak.

—Thomas Carlyle

It is only fitting that a chapter covering the art of writing revisions and resubmissions comes at the end of the book. By now the reader has a more complete and refined picture of how to construct a well-written grant. Furthermore, earlier chapters of this book have discussed at great length the essential guidelines for the grant submission process. Coupled with this factual information, several contributors to this volume have highlighted the importance given to establishing contact and communication with NIH program staff. Also stressed has been the importance of following application guidelines, making sure the paperwork supporting a grant application is in order, and submitted in a timely manner. Different grant mechanisms have been outlined, and different tactics and strategies for developing top-notch applications have been proffered.

Another essential component in the grant submission process revolves around acquiring a deeper respect for the full range of grant resubmission tactics. It should be well understood by now that not every grant will be funded on the first submission (or even the second). Chapter 1 examining the status quo and peer review process at NIH (and duly noted in other chapters, as well) emphasizes the low success rate for grants. When we consider the overall NIH funding rates of the present and recent past, it is possible to predict that the vast majority of all grants in any given cycle (80–90%) will not be funded. Particularly with grants that are submitted and "unscored" (theoretically, 50% of all submitted applications), applicants are well advised to "get over the hurt" and prepare a resubmission. In light of this scenario and the impetus to get funded, it is essential to develop a comprehensive strategy for crafting revisions.

A story comes immediately to mind when thinking about grant submission and revisions. One of the authors of this chapter was awarded an NIDA FIRST (R29) award as his first grant, but not on the first try. The priority score for the first submission was above 200, and given the funding lines at that time, the grant required revision and resubmission. The first activity after receiving this disappointing priority score was to send a copy of the critique to a consultant with the simple query, "Why did this grant not fare better at the review?" The consultant, who had extensive grant-writing experience, provided the following response: "The grant needs a simpler statement of the problem, a more coherent set of hypotheses, greater attention to power, and a more refined (detailed) statistical analysis plan. In essence, the grant needs better organization." This advice basically meant that a major overhaul of the grant was required. However, once revised according to these important suggestions, the grant priority score improved substantially at the subsequent review, and the grant was eventually funded. Interestingly, this very R29 grant served as a springboard for a promising area of study, led to other successful grants (including an R01), and also infused a modicum of hope in the principal investigator (PI)—belief in the peer review process and the importance of paying close attention to the critiques.

BASIC RULES OF RESUBMISSIONS

With the exception of grants submitted in response to an official institute request for applications, essentially any grant that is reviewed and not funded may be revised and resubmitted. In a practical sense, there are several issues pertinent to revisions that should be considered. Research grant applications submitted to NIH are limited to two revised or amended resubmissions (termed A1 for the first and A2 for the second resubmission). Both on the critique (written or electronic) and during review, the application is sequentially numbered to reflect the submission sequence (see figure 1.10). This allows the reviewers to monitor the submission timing of applications and address whether the applicant has repackaged the application within a year's time frame or the resubmission is the third and final submission of a particular application. There is no statute of limitations with respect to the timing of resubmissions (i.e., amended applications), and thus it is possible to delay resubmission as long as necessary in order to strengthen the application (e.g., collection of additional preliminary data). NIH provides guidelines regulating timing windows for resubmissions, which can be found at grants.nih.gov/grants/guide/notice-files/not97-011.html, and is also graphically portrayed in figure 1.9. Investigators should consider, however, that when the time period between submissions is lengthy, there is a need for the application to be current with any advances or recent publications in the field.

Assuming an application is eligible for resubmission, the decision to prepare a revised application should still be made cautiously and in consultation with co-investigators and consultants and, importantly, after discussion with the appropriate institute program official. Once an applicant makes the decision to resubmit, there are a number of steps to follow. This chapter outlines these steps and provides a template outlining how to construct revised grants. Not all grants will or should follow this template. However, it is worth considering the information presented as it applies to the reader's situation.

ESSENTIAL STEPS FOR HANDLING REVISIONS AND RESUBMISSIONS

All revised applications should be based first and foremost on the comments provided by the internal review group (IRG), also known as a "study section," in the summary statement. Written evaluations provided by members of the IRG are collated by the scientific review administrator (SRA) who presided over the meeting. These comments and the discussion from around the table by reviewers are synthesized by the SRA into an overall evaluation, which is provided to the applicant in the summary statement along with individual reviewers' comments. It should be noted that while peer review study sections are composed of several dozen members (both standing and ad hoc members), any single application is assigned specifically to two or three reviewers. The "primary," "secondary," and "tertiary" (if there is one) reviewers provide written critiques of the application. Sometimes, an additional reviewer or "discussant" is assigned to an application. Discussants are utilized to provide an alternate viewpoint or additional expertise that may be required for a complex application; however, it should be noted that discussants are not required to compose an official set of comments; rather, they may simply present their opinions during the discussion. Therefore, comments and concerns voiced by discussants or other committee members (which can have a strong influence on scoring) are reflected only through the SRA's summary of the proceedings.

Until recently, summary statements were mailed to investigators six to eight weeks following the study section meeting. Beginning in the calendar year 2006, however, summary statements must be retrieved by the applicant after registering at the NIH Commons Web site (commons.era.nih.gov/commons). This change has allowed a slight decrease in the time it takes to gain access to grant reviews, and thus five- or six-week turnaround times are feasible. It can be somewhat unnerving to log onto Commons in anticipation of receiving grant scores and critiques, but it is prudent to acquire this material as soon as it becomes available in order to expedite the resubmission process. Additional information on how to access NIH Commons is presented in appendix 1 at the end of this book.

In considering the comments provided by an IRG in the summary statement, the applicant should confer with collaborators, consultants, mentors, and also, as mentioned, with the designated program official. The importance of contacting the program officer was highlighted in chapter 2, which outlines specifically the reasons to maintain an open line of communication with NIH staff and institute program officials. It is essential to maintain visibility at the institute level. This is particularly true if you are a junior faculty member and just submitted your first grant. Most established investigators will have already solidified their standing within an institute (and perhaps across several institutes where research lines cross) and likewise developed a relationship with program staff. The distinction of high visibility will help put a voice (face) to your application and enable you to reason with the program official about the focus, content, and style of your grant. You may find out, for example, that a particular division chief or even the institute director does not favor grants of this scope. Likewise, changing currents at NIH may necessitate that you incorporate a new area in your design and specifically address a pressing issue confronting both the scientific community and the institute (with regard to their stated funding agenda). Historically, drug abuse research has been reactive when a new, virulent or deadly form of a drug appears on the market (e.g., rohypnol, GHB, MDMA, and ecstasy). Likewise, funding for mental health studies has shifted along with the tides of public health interest (e.g., schizophrenia and the use of antipsychotic medication). Remember, program staff at every institute is in constant contact with leaders and pioneers in the field who themselves are only a phone call away to both the applicant and program officials.

INTERPRETING THE SUMMARY STATEMENT

Summary statements contain written commentary on many different aspects of an application based usually on the framework and specific guidelines developed by NIH (see chapter 3). Comments may range from comprehensive evaluation of experimental details to general criticism of central hypotheses and strategies. In a worst-case scenario, the summary statement may indicate little enthusiasm for the science contained in an application. This perspective may be shared by multiple reviewers who highlight substantive weaknesses in the scientific plan as the main reason for the poor priority score. Such sentiment is generally presented very clearly in the summary statement. Likewise, if the aims are not articulated clearly or supported by the proposed methodology as detailed in the approach, the summary statements should reflect this problem as well. In addition to weak or insufficient details in approach, several chapters in this book emphasize the need (especially for fellowship and/or K-series mentorship applications) to have oversight provided by mentors and the importance of obtaining input from colleagues prior to submission. As often happens, summary statements indicate openly if an application appears not to have been prepared carefully and to lack the final brush stroke of a mentor or more experienced colleague. In such cases, it may be best to identify a different mentor or, alternatively, to have the current mentor apply him- or herself more diligently to the application (mentorship affects F awards, K awards, and T awards, to name a few examples).

The summary statement may raise not only scientific concerns regarding significance and approach, but also issues related to budget, personnel (including choice of consultants or mentors), as well as productivity of the investigator, environment, and institutional support, among others. Some of these factors are not amendable to change, whereas others can be remedied with little fuss. For example, short of ensuring that reviewers have duly noted all the contributions that the PI and the research team have made to the literature and the scientific community at large, there is little that can be done to address the issue of lackluster past productivity. Papers that are pending submission or in press works that have been recently accepted for publication should be listed and this information highlighted to address shortages of publications. If reviewers point to lackluster support from the institution as a main area of concern, it is possible to garner stronger levels of institutional or departmental support. It also may be the case that grammatical and editorial problems (and we attend to this below in greater detail), including disjointed text, herald poor science. Summary statements that pick up on the disjointed nature of an application will indicate so partly by nitpicking on an assortment of problems, but also by showing lack of enthusiasm for the proposed research plan. In fact, this may occur during review because the application is confusing and the absence of clarity surfaces as a flaw (although it is worth noting that grammar problems do not indicate a fatal flaw).

CONTACTING YOUR PROGRAM OFFICIAL

Program staff within an institute or center represents a key point of contact for several reasons. Whereas colleagues can advise on the scientific criticisms leveled at an application, program officials can advise on less tangible elements. For example, although the summary of the SRA is intended to capture the full sentiment of the committee, it sometimes falls short due to differences in interpretation of the discussion, especially if the discussion is highly technical or revolves around a subtle point of contention. If a program official, or institute emissary, was in attendance, additional insight can sometimes be gained by requesting to the program official review the notes from the meeting. An applicant may find that the program official does not have complete grasp of the proposed scientific approach and does not see clearly the shades of gray that are often highlighted by reviewers. It is thus rarely worthwhile to debate the merits of the scientific review with the program official as they relate to experimental details (i.e., approach). It is usually more productive to seek advice related to general strategy and focus, particularly with respect to the "infrastructure" of the application. With the exception of career scientist awards and several special funding mechanisms (where budgets are fixed), the budget is a prime infrastructural element of all applications (and this fact is duly noted in chapter 15 addressing financing science). Program officials can yield good advice in the event that concerns were raised over budgetary issues. It goes without saying that economic aspects of an application can affect levels of enthusiasm. Getting the "biggest bang for the buck" may be a cliché, but it is no less real when it comes to the way in which funding agencies operate.

Program officials also can be of assistance by virtue of the broad perspective they have on their own institutional portfolio. Thus, whereas an application may have been welcomed by a given institute during a particular funding cycle, it is possible that in the time between initial submission and review a similar application was in fact funded. The decision to resubmit in such a case may be dependent upon a shift of focus in order to avoid duplicative studies. Although it is true that replication is the hallmark of good science, practical (financial) considerations often constrain or hinder any institute's desire to support purely confirmatory studies. Alternatively, it is possible that, along with the shifting tides of scientific endeavor, the funding priorities of a particular institute change and, as a result of this ebb and flow, applications that were previously encouraged are now less attractive. Such a turn of events could very well influence the decision to resubmit an application, and program staff can certainly be of value in identifying such "climactic changes."

Thus, when considering the submission of a revised application, a critical step is to call your program official and discuss the critique in detail, including issues that potentially exist "between the lines" of the summary statement. The phone call between the applicant and the program official will necessitate some careful listening. Applicants need to determine whether the institute maintains interest in the science embodied in the grant. While it is of course important to determine whether the institute is interested in the science *before* initial submission, it is not too late to shape the application so that it may dovetail with current institute needs and themes. Also included in the discussion about scoring is what happened during review. Asking this question up front has tremendous probative value and can lead to immeasurable insight for the applicant. In other words, what went on in the room during the discussion of your grant? Did both reviewers agree on the score? Did one reviewer present a slightly different take on the grant and feel more or less favorable than the other? Were the scores divergent at the beginning of the discussion and come together ultimately to approximate each other? Conversely, were scores initially concordant only to then drift apart as the critique developed? While much of this information will be clear by reading the summary statement, it is also important to gain insight based on the general tenor of the conversation that transpired during the review. All of this relevant background noise plus more should unfold naturally during conversation with the program official.

FORMULATING THE INTRODUCTION IN A REVISED APPLICATION

After discussing the summary statement with your program official, you must decide how to frame the three-page (maximum) section that introduces a revised A1 or, if necessary, A2 application. It is worth considering that you can use all 25 pages of a revised application to address the reviewers' comments; however, you have three additional "Introduction to Revised Application" pages in which to outline specifically how the revised submission has changed. These three pages are critical elements of a resubmission for several reasons. The introduction provides a means to highlight the changes in the application and state explicitly how the changes address the comments made by reviewers. You can do this by writing in a point-by-point manner or using a more general phrase "in response to the reviewers' concern ..." Box 18.1 presents a template showing an acceptable

---

Box **18.1**   Sample Opening Paragraph

Introduction to Revised Submission

This is a second revised submission of an R21 application titled, "Validity of Ethnic Identity and Adolescent Drug Use." The application details a program of empirical research emphasizing the role of social and cultural factors in the etiology of drug use among ethnic minority youth. The original proposal was reviewed by ZRG1 NIH SNEM-1 (01) and received a priority score of 200. A revised application received a priority score of 170 with major improvements noted by the reviewers [ZRG1 SNEM-1 (05)]. Summating across both reviews, there was an element of enthusiasm for the proposal, noting strengths in the principal investigators track record, the innovative use of associative memory techniques in the construction of cultural identification scales, the development of an integrated program of research examining drug etiology, and a high level of responsiveness to the Program Announcement's goals (PA-02-043: Social and Cultural Dimensions of Health). Notwithstanding, there were several noted weaknesses, which are addressed in this second revision. The three-page introduction provides a brief overview of the proposed changes, all of which are further detailed in the body of the proposal. To facilitate review of this revised application, **[bold]** text reflects changes that specifically address the most recent reviewers' concerns.

---

manner in which to create an opening paragraph acknowledging the review score and detailing how changes are duly noted in the revised application.

EXPECT HEADACHES ASSOCIATED WITH NEW REVIEWERS

Often a revised and resubmitted application may be assigned to one or more new reviewers. If possible, SRAs may try to maintain some consistency across review cycles by assigning revised applications to at least one individual who reviewed it previously. This gesture makes it possible for review continuity, so that reviewers can determine if the changes in structure and/or format merit new enthusiasm. It is also possible that two or three new individuals may be assigned to review the revised application and contribute reviews "de novo." For instance, individuals who attended the previous review cycle may not be available to attend a subsequent review session or for any of myriad reasons may not get assigned the application. Should this occur, a second set of reviewers will be assigned the A1 or A2 application and thus encounter the application for the first time. Whether an application receives a fresh set of eyes or the same reviewers from a previous cycle, it is imperative that the applicant outline all changes clearly in the introduction.

Consider also that a new set of reviewers may raise a completely different set of issues; in essence, they are not "bound" by the comments and concerns that were raised during a previous review. Applicants should be aware that reviewers assigned an A1 or A2 revised application also receive a copy of the previous summary statement. This helps them to determine the degree to which an applicant has revamped the proposal and responded to the comments from past reviewers, and whether the application contains formidable as opposed to cursory changes. Even with an acceptable slate of changes, new reviewers, seeing the application for the first time, are free to raise additional concerns and introduce new comments and criticisms. While this can cause some consternation among applicants, it is an essential piece of the peer review process.

Reviewers need to feel unhindered in making their own assessment and cannot be tied to comments generated by a previous set of reviewers. New reviewers may acknowledge the importance of previous comments outlined in a summary statement but move in a different direction when dissecting an application. Regardless of whether a revised application is assigned to new or former reviewers, adhering to the basic guidelines of grant writing outlined in this book will help to avoid common pitfalls. Essentially, we encourage readers to implement the tactics offered in this book for constructing grants and to make sure the application addresses the comments and concerns outlined in the critique.

This latter point may be crucial and is worth considering in greater detail. In many respects, applicants should determine whether they have chosen the optimal methodological and analytic strategies that support the specific aims, whether the research hypotheses capture the focal scientific relationships, and whether the analytic strategies will be fruitful and elucidate the statistical relations of concern. Applicants also need to consider whether alternative approaches and modifications to the design detract from the science or strengthen the science in ways not previously considered. These few points are considered the backbone of basic grant writing and resonate as key items throughout this book. Applicants need to consider whether they are wedded to their own experimental design and whether their design optimally reflects the state-of-the art science. Under certain conditions, it may be better to repackage the science in a resubmission and showcase these wholesale changes as part of the revision process.

SMALL CORRECTABLE PROBLEMS REVOLVING AROUND STYLE

A number of tips and suggestions are useful for formatting revised applications. First, reviewers need to be able to distinguish all major (and even some minor) changes in substance from previous grant material. One common means to handle this is to add vertical lines in the margin adjacent to new or revised text. Alternatively, new text can be indicated through the use of [brackets] or it can be highlighted with the use of **boldface** type, or through the use of *italics*. Regardless of stylistic choice, the applicant should rely on a consistent form to indicate changes in the text, and this, along with any other stylistic nuances, should be made clear in the Introduction section.

An effective strategy for formatting the Introduction with respect to addressing previous reviewers' comments involves the use of direct quotes taken from the summary statement coupled with specific responses. If space permits, it is useful to state the exact location in the body of the revised grant (page and line numbers) where a given modification occurs (e.g., Section 3.3 "Sampling" found on pages 25–26 describes the revised sampling plan in greater depth). More minor changes can be tackled in the body of the grant. Lengthier discussion that requires more space and clarification should be addressed in the body of the grant and duly noted in the introduction. When adopting a direct "criticism/response" format, it is useful to distinguish criticisms from responses with bold or italics. The sample revisions offered in box 18.2 showcase this latter approach.

IS IT ART OR SCIENCE?

From the very outset, applicants should know there is an art to constructing revised resubmissions. This fact is well known to both authors of this chapter, who have participated as reviewers on various NIH review panels. Therefore, some good and useful advice follows. Don't be overly ingratiating, but find ways to be humble. Don't be pedantic, but find ways to be polished and erudite. Don't

Box **18.2** Sample "Criticism/Response" Format

Introduction to Revised Application

We thank the reviewers very much for their comments. The following section addresses the changes made in the application in response to the reviewers' specific comments. All new text in the body appears in Times Roman font. Original text is in Arial.

Reviewer 1:

Comment

"The investigator has carefully addressed all of the major criticisms of the previous critique. He has modified or amended experiments in response to reviewer recommendations."

Response

I thank the reviewer for this positive comment. The major criticisms previously focused upon the fact that the overall project was premature since there were as yet no mapping data and also because there was no progress in the development of drug assays. The previous (A1) application thus included QTL mapping data for the Balb/cJ (129X1/SvJ cross as well as documentation of development of a reliable assay to measure valproic acid levels in brain and blood.

Comment

"The investigator mentions recent nomenclature changes for the 129 strain, but this nomenclature remains quite confusing as presented in this application since the different nomenclatures are used simultaneously. A single nomenclature should be used throughout to avoid confusion."

Response

It is true that nomenclature for 129 substrains can be confusing, particularly in light of recent changes. Nonetheless, after the changes were described in the previous "Introduction to Revised Application" (i.e., the old 129/SvJ is now 129X1/SvJ and the old 129/IMSvJ is now the 129S1/IMSvJ), the currently approved (new) substrain designations were then used throughout the text of the application. The exception to this usage was in the figures (and their accompanying legends), which retained the old strain designations. I have now changed the figures and legends to be as consistent as possible. Some of this confusion will also now be avoided since proposed experiments to study crosses between 129 substrains have been removed from the Research Plan as suggested by the reviewer (see below).

grovel, but delineate the changes clearly and concisely. Keep in mind that you can revise the 25-page application to any extent you wish, from minor tweaking to a major overhaul. You can modify your study design (approach), institute new statistical methods, add or drop measures, revise existing experiments—even drop/add whole aims, introduce new co-investigators and/or consultants, eliminate personnel (both key and otherwise), change your budget (this should be carefully defended and most likely discussed with the project officer before-hand), change your institution (people do relocate now and then), and even alter your focus if it is in keeping with the goals of the particular institute where the application was submitted for review. Whatever you do, however, the first three pages must hail these changes in an organized and meaningful fashion. The first paragraph should restate the scoring received, mention the name of the assigned committee that reviewed the first (or second) submission, specify which review cycle produced this score, and also note if the application was submitted for a special Program Announcement.

Reviewers should always be able to say something positive about an application: the application's strengths should be clearly signaled. Highlighting the strengths of an application in the introduction is not regarded generally as brag-gadocio, but rather as an important tool that helps refresh reviewers with regard to the core science of an application. These positive comments are often combined with less favorable comments (weaknesses) that can detract from the overall score of an application. It is important that both the positive and negative points raised in the body of the critique be highlighted in the introduction so that reviewers are assured that the applicant (investigator) read through the reviews thoroughly and has developed a clear sense of why the application received the assigned priority score (or, for that matter, was unscored). Since it is an art to provide a thorough, comprehensive, and informative review, it is also an art to glean from these comments what are the most important components of the grant that require polishing and further modification. Box 18.3 shows a combined approach from a very seasoned grant writer who also serves as a grant reviewer. This particular investigator is well aware of the importance of intro-ductions to the review process. As noted, the prose in box 18.3 heralds a unique opportunity for the applicant, who openly straddles a fence between applicant and reviewer. In fact, the investigator first acknowledges the overall importance of the introduction to revised submissions and then follows this statement by reinforcing the point-by-point manner of the introduction. This approach will in effect make sure that any new reviewer feels comfortable reading the revised submission.

Once the content of the summary statement has been absorbed and circu-lated among collaborators and consultants, the applicant should delve into each and every point raised by the reviewers. All major concerns should be addressed in the introduction to the revised application, even if it is to simply acknowledge

---

Box 18.3 Addressing Both Positive and Less Favorable Comments

---

Introduction to Revised Application

From past grant reviewing experience, I realize that this Introduction sets the tone for the rest of the proposal. Reviewers often desire an understanding of how the applicant improved the grant. Our team thanks the IRG members for their suggestions. Revisions are noted in this application in **bold text**. Peccadilloes found during the revision process were changed for better readability but not noted in bold.

Summary

We wanted new (and former) reviewers to be apprised of the comments on the summary statement, so this section individually reviews comments of reviewers. Numerous strengths were noted relevant to the methods, which we appreciated, given the methodological nature of our work. Weaknesses reduced reviewers' enthusiasm, which resulted in this resubmission. It is our hope that reviewers will agree that this submission is stronger and could contribute more significantly to the field. Areas of strength retained:

- The discrepancy interview protocol and debriefing interview—innovative aspects of our design that allow us to understand why answers may differ on separate occasions to improve reliability of assessments and ultimately match users to treatment
- Qualitative methods appreciated—now better defined
- Test/retest/validity components, with more focused populations
- Nosological analyses—focused on issues salient to the DSM V and ICD XI Substance Related Disorders Workgroup
- A great team and environment (!)

---

that the grant has been modified in response to a single identified deficiency. Based on the three-page limitation, it may be necessary to restrict discussion in the introduction to the most critical perceived flaws. When all is said and done, the three-page introduction should contain detail on every change proposed in the revised application. This effort will allow the reviewer a chance to summarize the changes mentally and then determine whether these changes address adequately the comments embodied in the initial review. If a synopsis of the summary statement indicates that a total of 10 weaknesses in the study design or methodology were noted by reviewers, the investigator should then duly note that 10 changes were instituted in the application, as part of his or her effort to show reviewers the statements were contemplated in a serious matter. Appendix 18.1 at the end of this chapter contains the full text of an introduction to a revised application that eventually resulted in a funded R21 grant.

Applicants should also consider that not every comment by reviewers necessitates a revision to the research plan. Grant reviewers are regularly cautioned by NIH program staff to not "tutor" applicants or rewrite their grants in the review; however, it is inevitable that reviewers' suggestions for improvement find their way into summary statements. When an applicant chooses not to heed the recommendation of a reviewer that is made in the spirit of offering ways to strengthen the grant, the reviewer comments should not simply be ignored in the introduction. Rather, the applicant should craft a polite but erudite response that provides a solid rationale defending this position. The careful and well-written defense of a research plan embodied in the introduction to the revised application serves as a keystone that links together the narrative that follows. The importance associated with the introduction materials and the proper defense of a research plan cannot be overstated.

If the applicant has provided an attractive, comprehensive, and systematically organized introduction, reviewers will be sensitive to these changes, note their relevance to the full text, and attempt to integrate them with their overall reading of the application. In other words, the introduction goes a long way toward providing the reviewer with a sense of how important are past reviewers' comments in getting the attention of the applicant and how deeply these comments are folded into the revised application. Again, the process of gleaning this information from the summary statement and incorporating it into a revised application is as much art as it is science. How much value a particular reviewer places on the degree to which an application is changed as opposed to the quality of the science is also difficult to generalize. Reviewers are instructed to consider each grant on its own merit, based strictly on what is presented in the application itself, and not to measure its worth using yardsticks defined by previous scores or levels of enthusiasm for previous versions. Thus, it is important to realize that every word that goes into the application is meaningful and that each thought should be expressed with due care and consideration.

Another important point to consider is that, regardless of whether the applicant agrees or disagrees with the tone and tenor of the review, great tact is needed when the revised introduction is written. A carefully composed introduction should allay major criticisms raised by reviewers. In essence, there should be a statement that articulates how the revisions lead to an improved and more organized application, highlighting how the overall science of the application has benefited from the reviewer's concerns, and noting how the study is stronger as a result of incorporating the recommended changes. The grant mechanism (R21) used to exemplify some of these issues also included an important paragraph attending to a design change. Box 18.4 provides an example of how a reviewer expressed concern regarding sampling issues that could, if not corrected, represent a major and potentially fatal flaw. The argument posed by the reviewer is certainly worth considering, and the investigator responded in a positive

---

Box 18.4 Reviewer's Concern Regarding Sampling Issues

It seems as if the study will consist of a large majority of two racial groups, i.e., Blacks and Hispanics. If this is true, the study will provide only limited support of the contention because the study results will not demonstrate whether, or to what extent, ethnic identity reduces racial/ethnic variations in behavioral, emotional, and developmental outcomes of early drug use/abuse. Inclusion of a comparable size of a white sample would be instrumental. This omission can introduce **a flaw** because the associations of ethnic identity and major constructs of the study can be spurious.

---

manner, taking the time to outline modifications to the sampling design. Box 18.5 shows how the investigator carefully responded to the reviewer's concerns, altering the study design and acknowledging how the study is vastly improved as a result of this modification. One important point at the end of this rebuttal section showcases how the investigator believed it worthy enough to mention that the budget was not adversely affected by the expanded sampling plan. Consistent with chapter 15, this shows the investigator had the foresight to remind the reviewers that science and budgetary considerations go hand in hand.

The introduction section is also a good place to note any modifications that address design or methodological issues raised by reviewers. In essence, this is the place to set the record straight regarding comments made about the science of a grant (e.g., technical merit, approach, design concerns, statistics, measurement, power). Sometimes reviewers misinterpret what was proposed or develop alternative interpretations of preliminary data. Applicants can use the introduction section carefully to explain their thinking; it is, in this regard, the place to highlight why the revised application is significant and innovative.

Regardless of whether an application has undergone minor or substantial changes, the introduction serves as a place to acknowledge the importance of the peer review process. In effect, you are telling the anonymous reviewers that you appreciate their comments and that your application has benefited from their review. Keep in mind that reviewers never make any decisions about funding; in fact, at numerous occasions during reviews, reviewers are sternly reminded by NIH program staff not to mention the "F" word (funding). Nonetheless, reviewers do want to feel they have some input on whether good science is reviewed fairly and promoted with integrity. This is perhaps the most rewarding part of the review process; it is the place where your peers recognize that their labors, careful reading, and thoughtful comments become ingrained as part of scientific endeavor, a solution rather than a problem, a credible scientifically based response to the human condition.

To summarize, the three-page introduction section of a revised application has to clearly set forth a synopsis of changes, summarize the strengths of the

| Box **18.5** | Response to Reviewer's Concern Regarding Sampling Issues |

It is worth noting that **Critique #2** endorsed the sampling strategies and data collection procedures (claiming that efforts to maximize the response rate were "sound"). Notwithstanding, the same reviewer expressed concern that, absent a sample of white or non-minority youth, structural processes reflecting the influence of psychosocial functioning (or behavior, for that matter) attributed to minority youth might be spurious. We concur and have now revised the proposal to include a comparable sample of white youth (N=200 for implicit memory task and N=500 for the longitudinal study), matched on various socio-demographic indicators (the school district has made available an electronic file with various school characteristics [e.g., rates of truancy, race breakdowns, and free-lunch status]) and student proficiency scores. This fundamental design change will make it possible to draw inferences regarding minority-specific developmental risks and their association with identity development and drug use. We have been able to offset the expenses associated with the inclusion of white (non-minority) youth (e.g., extra assessment forms, data collectors in the schools, and follow-up assessments for hard-to-reach and truant youth) spread over the three-year study and thus maintain the integrity of our proposed budget.

application, and very carefully and tactfully acknowledge that the comments raised by previous reviewers have helped to reshape the application, making it more formidable and helping the investigator advance toward better science.

MOLDING WEAKNESSES INTO STRENGTHS

Up to this point in the chapter, we have described the relative importance of the introduction in a revised application and suggested that applicants consider the introduction as a major marketing tool. The next step should be to consider making wholesale revisions to the body of the application and specifically addressing (at much greater length) any concerns expressed by reviewers. A story comes to mind that recounts an incident that occurred to one of the authors while attending a junior tennis tournament in Las Vegas with his teenage daughter. Mike Agassi, a legend among tennis gurus and father of tennis great Andre Agassi, was promoting his new book *The Agassi Story*. During a book signing that coincided with a junior tournament registration, Mr. Agassi asked this 14-year-old tennis neophyte, "What is the weakest part of your game?" She responded in a shy manner, "I guess my serve," to which Mike Agassi responded, "Then you should make this the strongest part of your game." Ever so curious a father, I then asked, "What was the weakest part of Andre's game when he was an aspiring junior tennis player?" Mr. Agassi responded, "His return of serve." I thought hard about his response because I knew that a strong component of Andre Agassi's tennis success over his illustrious tennis career was his quick and powerful return of serve. In fact, Andre's trademark return of service had effectively reduced many a serve and volley player to a mere quiver. Mike Agassi then went on to state, "And we made that his strength."

The kernel of truth in this story highlights the importance of working diligently to convert any noted weaknesses in your grant (both those raised by colleagues prior to submission and those contained in summary statement) into strengths. If weaknesses are detected, it is most effective to reach out to other capable investigators and colleagues for advice and assistance. Some of the best discussions many of us have ever had with respect to our research career ended up scribbled on napkins or as hand-drawn figures faxed back and forth until they emerged as well-developed and complete grants. Importantly, do not hesitate to let other scientists review your writing style to make sure the ideas embodied in your grant come across in a scientifically credible and coherent manner. The long and arduous road to writing successful grants traverses the painful realization that salesmanship is a crucial underlying factor to why some grants are scored better than others. Salesmanship considers factors such as linking up with highly acclaimed researchers with powerful investigative careers who serve as consultants. Related to this point, it is useful for applicants to increase their visibility in the field through networking with colleagues. Junior faculty should attend national conferences and make themselves visible through poster or plenary sessions.

Grant applications that show clear evidence of input from mentors or senior investigators come out of the gates flying faster than grants constructed laboriously by investigators writing in isolation and without needed support by senior colleagues. Moreover, many applications from new or junior investigators build on the arduous work of more senior colleagues. This relationship is strengthened when the more senior investigator provides a glowing endorsement of the application rather than a weak or ineffective letter of support.

THE TENOR AND LANGUAGE OF A REVISED SUBMISSION

Invariably, applicants will note that certain comments in the summary statement will seem to be unjustified, inappropriate, or simply lacking scientific credibility. It is rarely useful or even prudent to become animated, and "raise one's heckles." The introduction is the last place you want to take umbrage with a reviewer; there are other more verdant fields (and publications) where you can harvest or promote your ideas. However, it is worth noting that reviewers are people and along with this territory come certain quirks and downsides. It is best not to generate hostility, express anger, or become argumentative using the grant as a platform for diatribe. Generally speaking, the most prudent approach to "holding one's ground" when composing a revised application necessitates using clear, concise scientific writing, writing that is devoid of any hint of anger, frustration, or indignant tone. Applicants should take painstaking care to explain all their ideas carefully and not mince words. Principles and key theoretical ideas should be hammered home in an erudite manner. If it is obvious that reviewer have made a scientific error or used poor judgment in the critique, it is wise not to be blunt or rub their nose in it. Rather, elucidate clearly your stated position and support it with original data or citations from the literature. Nothing ever changes the fact that solid, well-written, and scientifically meritorious grants always stand out from the rest of the pack. The art of writing revisions and resubmitting grants is to learn to recognize why an application failed to accomplish this in its previous submission.

LACK OF INVESTIGATIVE STRENGTH

One of the more difficult and perhaps intangible review comments to deal with arises when a reviewer criticizes the investigative strength of an application. Such commentary can be directed at the PI, the investigative team, the consultants supporting execution of the grant, or all of the above. When the application in question takes the form of a mentoring grant (K-award or fellowship), criticism of investigative power is often lodged at the mentor and less so at the investigator, although both individuals can be the focal target. It is not uncommon for junior investigators to receive low priority scores because their application reflects too much hubris and not enough grant administration experience. A junior investigator planning a large-scale field trial must show connections to more senior investigators who will support budgetary and administrative decisions, lend credence to theoretical and practical issues under scrutiny based on their own work, and provide overall logistic support. Randomized field trials and clinical laboratory research are messy, and junior investigators have limited experience handling the day-to-day finagling that occurs in the field. A piece of advice, in this instance, is to query more senior investigators prior to submission on the following points

1. What components (sections) of the grant application should be highlighted
2. Which strengths of the investigative team providing logistic support should be noted
3. How best to showcase a brief and integrated picture of past research and publications
4. How to accentuate differences between this application and other applications that have emanated from the same laboratory (this is partic-

ularly true of shops that rely on specific assay techniques in their experimental paradigm or distinct theoretical or treatment approaches to
behavioral science)

5. How to delineate the unique features of the proposed science and address the influence of the proposed study on the scientific event
horizon

Query 1 detailing the importance of highlighting different sections of an
application may come into play because junior investigators base their submission on work conducted by a particular scientific group from an identified laboratory. This can occur when the applicant is making a transition from a postdoctoral position outside the laboratory to a junior faculty position. In this
instance, investigators may wish to highlight their training and educational
background as stepping stones that create a natural progression toward their
specific research goals. This tactic emphasizes their transition and showcases the
strengths of the laboratory in the preliminary studies section. It also serves to
provide a historically accurate synopsis of the institutional history that preceded
their joining the laboratory without diminishing their own research achievements. Specific aims of the application may also borrow from aims used in
previous R01 applications or dovetail with aims put forth in a P30, P50, or P60
Center. Centers, as discussed in chapters 9 and 10, serve as a career springboard
for junior investigators, who can incrementally grow, mature, and blossom under
the tutelage of more senior investigators. Otherwise, when an investigator extends ongoing studies at a center, new aims must be emphasized and details
provided on how they depart from previous program projects. This is sometimes
necessary to avoid the criticism of "piecemealing."

Query 2 highlighting team strengths calls for a detailed statement about
mentoring, the proven track record in training postdoctoral fellows or junior
faculty, and the ability to place high-quality scientists in successful research
positions. Mentors should keep detailed records on job placement for their
protégés and consider providing a table to detail this information. Query 3 involves showcasing past accomplishments and may be accomplished by using
some boilerplate material heralding the laboratory's perspective on its technique
or theory and integrating this material into the new approach defined in the
revised application.

For query 4, to distinguish an application from a slew cropping up from the
same laboratory, delineate the research steps needed in the refinement of a
technique, theory, or a particular model of human behavior. Each step is defended as the necessary or requisite components of scientific inquiry. In this case,
investigators highlight the laboratory paradigm and then defend their choice to
either incrementally improve on a particular method or move entirely in a different direction. While this can be risky, the advent of new assay techniques or

cross-fertilization with technical advances from other laboratories often helps promote use of new approaches. Query 5 regarding uniqueness can be addressed by distinguishing between old and new and weaving together a story about prior concerns affecting the field and new areas of exploration. When all is said and done, the crux of any application is the scientific premise that attempts to solve an existing problem or underscore the potential for new ones.

CONCERNS WITH THE RESEARCH ENVIRONMENT

Tied to concerns regarding investigative strength is the question of whether the research or university environment supports the applicant's scientific goals. This question usually arises when an individual scientist or research group does not curry favor because of a lack of high-quality research training, evidence of poor mentorship, failure to provide adequate laboratory or training resources, or a general malaise by reviewers that accompanies reviews of an organization that may be guilty of being overambitious or trying to overextend itself. It may seem improbable that applicants seeking NIH funding would have problems securing the necessary resources (logistic, mentoring, or laboratory) to support their research endeavor, particularly given that their professional goals require actively pursuing funding. However, as many of us know first hand, smaller universities and colleges place a greater emphasis on teaching and university service and less emphasis on independent research (though successfully funded applicants can secure protected research time in any environment). Notwithstanding, reviewers often give worse priority scores to grants that do not show promise with regard to the environment. Potentially useful advice to new or more junior applicants who cannot muster strong environmental support is to link efforts with recognized giants in the field, arguing that training on-site in the larger university and more research-friendly environment will promote better science. Other avenues to pursue include coursework at summer institutes (usually part of larger training environments), associating with existing funded centers, shopping out labor-intensive field work to larger organizations with more extensive experience, and similar tactics that help share or reduce any research burden. Therefore, it pays to review the basic constituent elements of the research environment and possibly gain further insight into why certain grants run into trouble on this very important review criterion (chapter 3 provides a more in-depth analysis of factors that fuel scoring applications with regard to environment).

SUMMARY OF MAIN POINTS

The responsibility of all applicants contemplating submission of a revised grant is to make sure they have a clear picture of why their original application did not fare well during review. Revising an application cannot be conducted a week prior to the submission deadline, nor can it be done months before and then shelved without further concern. The revisions take time and entail communicating with program officials (this is best done when ideas are fresh), and application materials need to be disseminated to colleagues and consultants. Most important, the revised application needs to address all of the points raised by reviewers even if there is some debate about the scientific merit of certain criticisms. In the long run, using a point-by-point rebuttal system best highlights the responses contained in the revision, although there is no single best way or accepted format to detail such changes. The applicant must ensure that the revised grant addresses all concerns expressed by reviewers both in the introduction and in the body of the application. This necessitates a careful reading and helps develop a logic flow to the application. Specific aims need to be clearly articulated, defended at some later point in a coherent and cogent research plan, addressed in the statistical analysis section, and described formatively as an essential piece of science in the background and significance section. Such an approach will prevent the application from appearing disjointed and will help to avoid serious editorial flaws.

The strongest component of any application, new or revised, should be the formulation and presentation of ideas in an erudite manner. Applications should read informatively and authoritatively, and the lead investigator should have a keen sense that seasoned veteran reviewers (who are themselves scientists) will read a revised application with the intent of determining the degree to which the application has improved and is meritorious. Although cautioned by program staff to evaluate each application on its own merit without reference to previous iterations, reviewers will still ask how the has application responded to the previous criticisms provided in the summary statements. This evaluative stance taken by reviewers should also be of great concern to the applicant and can be employed as a metric in reconstructing an application. The critique represents a formal outline of noted strengths and weaknesses; however, it is up to the applicant to use these comments to synthesize a coherent response and revised application. Ultimately, the ability of a PI to digest the comments in the summary statement, make the necessary changes in experimental strategy, and present them in an organized and systematic fashion will determine the success of the vast majority of all grants. We hope that this chapter has provided information on ways to facilitate this arduous yet necessary and important process.

Appendix **18.1**   SAMPLE INTRODUCTION TO REVISED GRANT APPLICATION

INTRODUCTION TO REVISED SUBMISSION

This is a second revised submission of an R21 application titled "Validity of Ethnic Identity and Adolescent Drug Use." The application details a program of empirical research emphasizing the role of social and cultural factors in the etiology of drug use among ethnic minority youth. The original proposal was reviewed by ZRG1 NIH SNEM-1 (01) and received a *priority score of* 200. A second revised application received a *priority score of* 170 with major improvements noted by the reviewers [ZRG1 SNEM-1 (05)]. Summating across both reviews, there was an element of strong enthusiasm for the proposal noting strengths in the principal investigators track record, the *innovative* use of associative memory techniques in the construction of cultural identification scales, the development of an integrated program of research examining drug etiology, and a high level of responsiveness to the Program Announcement's goals (PA-02-043: *Social and Cultural Dimensions of Health*). Notwithstanding, in the revised application there were several noted weaknesses, which are addressed more thoroughly in this second revision. The three-page introduction provides a brief overview of the proposed changes, all of which is further detailed in the body of the proposal. To facilitate review of this revised application, [**bold**] text reflects changes that specifically address the most recent reviewers' concerns.

First, the Clark County School District's research and human subject approval procedures have undergone major revision since our last submission. Staffing has been increased at CCSD to permit greater emphasis on research in the nation's sixth largest school district, which also contains the fastest growing middle school population. Twelve new schools are under construction each year and more than 255,000 students currently attend CCSD. Paralleling this burgeoning growth is an explicit need to improve drug and violence prevention efforts, which dovetails with our stated research interests. In the time since our last submission, we have met with various school and district personnel to iron out a sampling mechanism that will enable us to obtain a high rate of student participation in the experimental portion of the study (involving recruitment through a variety of school and home-based approaches). School personnel will now provide class lists for phone sampling along with student identifier numbers and personal data (e.g., name, phone, and home address). In addition, recruitment for the implicit cognition tasks involves flyers sent home with students, school and PTA announcements, in-school presentations during homeroom and recess, and information packets sent home to students in select minority-rich schools (to over sample ethnic minorities). Moreover, we have the support of regional superintendents (the district now contains four geographic regions) to conduct this project, and we fully expect a high level of success in the recruitment stage. These same procedures netted a 78% retention rate in the PI's one-year longitudinal study of ethnic identity processes in New York City.

It is worth noting that **Critique** #2 endorsed the sampling strategies and data collection procedures (claiming that efforts to maximize the response rate were "sound"). Notwithstanding, the same reviewer expressed concern that, absent a sample of white or non-minority youth, structural processes reflecting the influence of psychosocial functioning (or behavior for that matter) attributed to minority youth might be spurious. We concur and have now revised the proposal to include a comparable sample of white youth (N=200 for implicit memory task and N=500 for the longitudinal study), matched on various socio-demographic indicators (the school district has made available an electronic file with various school characteristics [e.g., rates of truancy, race breakdowns, and free-lunch status]) and student proficiency scores. This fundamental design change will make it possible to draw inferences regarding minority-specific developmental risks and their association with identity development and drug use. We have been able to offset the expenses associated with the inclusion of white (non-minority) youth (e.g., extra assessment forms, data collectors in the schools, and follow-up assessments for hard-to-reach and truant youth) spread over the three-year study and thus maintain the integrity of our proposed budget.

Related to the issue of sampling, the experimental procedure (i.e., implicit cognition tasks) also collects data on self-reported drug use and psychosocial functioning. The experimental procedure is now fully computerized, and we are currently pilot testing a small group of middle and high school students from a minority rich school in Las Vegas. Students providing data for the experimental procedure *are not tested* as part of the short longitudinal follow-up study (these "panel" students are unbiased by the experimental procedure). Data for the short-longitudinal study are collected by an independent research team trained by the PI and data collection takes place over a two-day period. We rely on the same protocols and data collection methods used at the Multiethnic Drug Abuse Prevention Research Center (Cornell University), which have been continually refined over a 10-year period (including detailed video training tapes outlining data collection procedures). A research assistant/project coordinator is appropriately budgeted and graduate students plus per diem workers assist in data collection, collation, and keypunching. The two-day assessment procedure is not regarded as burdensome to students and has been a staple part of our school-based etiology and prevention studies underway in New York and now in Las Vegas. Teachers are compensated for their classroom participation through incentives for high rates of survey returns and students also receive financial incentives commensurate with their participation.

Second, reviewers also expressed some concern with certain "ambiguities" they encountered describing the experimental procedures using self-generated outcomes. It is worth nothing the experimental portion of the study using implicit cognition tasks assessing ethnic identity offers a remedy to traditional psychometric approaches attempting to either create "de novo" or cull existing reliable and valid self-report items. Again, rather than having subjects endorse researcher-generated items using fixed response formats and then applying traditional data reduction techniques (i.e., factor analysis), we ask students to "generate" their own "accessible" responses to minimally cued probes. Since the last submission, we have developed a fully computerized protocol, which allows us to obtain additional data on response latency. An initial set of questions are used (unbeknownst to the student) to obtain a baseline for response latency. Application of a few nonspecific or generic questions enables us to measure response latency, which is controlled statistically in subsequent analyses (a portion of variability in latency may reflect unfamiliarity with computers or typing speed). Self-generated outcomes are categorized based on frequency distributions after scanning for key words (i.e., "self"). In the case of ties or self-generated outcomes that do not fall into clear categories, we use expert raters (experts in racial or ethnic identity) and compute kappa concordance statistics based on obtained ratings. The final categories and self-generated outcomes are then used to develop a multi-axial assessment. An important element of the present study is the ability to validate the new "self-generated" items against existing ethnic identity scales using confirmatory factor analysis procedures.

Third, it is worth noting the use of an implicit cognitive task paradigm offers an alternative line of inquiry that may help to settle questions regarding method variance and construct validity. If self-report paper-and-pencil information regarding ethnic identity and self-esteem converge with information obtained from implicit cognition tasks, we may be able to conclude that a common cognitive-evaluative process underlies these seemingly disparate constructs. More important, if we find that psychometric information derived from implicit cognition tasks regarding ethnic identity differentiates itself clearly from the measurement of self-esteem, we offer the unique possibility that ethnic identity taps self-evaluative processes (self appraisals) that are different from "global self-worth" suggesting in turn a more refined view of ethnic-specific identity. The factors in the now revised $2 \times 4 \times 3$ between subject design includes "gender," "order of presentation" (racial vs. ethnic vs. cultural vs. self-esteem), and "racial group" (white students, black students, and Hispanic students).

Fourth, reviewers asked "why ethnic identity would be related to adolescent substance use in the first place," commenting further that "there is a conceptual gap." In part, we believe this concern dovetails with additional issues regarding "how ethnic identity is different from self-esteem." Reviewers also felt the "analytic plan does not really seem to get at this issue." Importantly, there exist a number of conceptual models of self-esteem, but a general consensus suggests that self-esteem regards "global self-worth," or a "self-attitude" tapping an evaluation of the self (how the person feels about himself or a personal judgment of worthiness). More recently, researchers have articulated a model of self-esteem based on self-evaluation of one's effectiveness in different societal roles, reinforcing that self-esteem is part of a "reflected appraisal." Our model of identity processes suggests that, for minority youth, several "ethnic-specific factors" may contribute to "reflected self-appraisal" including cognitive processes that tie together familial, cultural, peer, school, and personal reward mechanisms. Accordingly, the foundation underlying individual differences in ethnic identity may rest on race or identity-specific cognitions. A number of additional concerns were raised attending to conceptual and measurement problems linking self-esteem, identity, and drug use. We propose three platforms or vantage points from which to explore these relations. *First*, evidence is accumulating that self-esteem contributes uniquely to early-stage drug use. The precise mechanisms of this predictive relation remain unclear, but enough evidence has accumulated to implicate self-reflective processes in drug etiology. Because self-esteem may capture reflective appraisal processes, youth who do not feel socially accepted by their immediate peer group, or who cannot establish strong ties to conventional institutions may feel despair and loneliness generated by their felt rejection. In turn, lacking peer or family-based social support mechanisms, these youth may embark on a trajectory of drug use as a form of palliative or emotion-focused coping. *Second*, peer influences play a large role in the early-stages of drug use and these linkages have been elaborated well by theories of peer socialization and peer selection mechanisms. Developmental studies provide clear evidence that social processes (including peers) contribute to the construction of self-esteem over time and that self-esteem may vary with regard to level of peer socialization. It is possible that peer selection mechanisms contribute to self-esteem and simultaneously generate feelings of group affinity (i.e., ethnic identity) that is generated in the context of early-stage drug use.

Third, and somewhat related to this latter point, both ethnic identity and self-esteem relate empirically to drug use, and one common thread shared by these psychological constructs may involve mediation through peer social relations. Social identity theory may provide a useful framework for understanding these relations. A major component of social identity theory revolves around the prominent role of reflected appraisals of the social world. Two integrated components fuel this appraisal: (1) social comparison involving "social cognitions" regarding group membership and comparisons of self vs. other and (2) group categorization, involving evaluation of group affinity and bonding (attachment). Social comparison can foster peer selection mechanisms that either serve to protect youth through enhanced group attraction and bonding or increase vulnerability as youth develop a growing sense of disaffection and self-denigration when they perceive themselves as outcasts (i.e., race-based group comparison). Self-esteem may attenuate when group affinity is low and peer support mechanisms wane. Thus, the social component of ethnic identification (based on group selection and affinity mechanisms) fosters changes in self-esteem. Reductions in self-esteem based on problems with ethnic identification (group categorization and comparison) may place some youth at developmental risk for drug use.

There are additional factors that may link self-esteem and ethnic identity and in turn create a common developmental pathway to drug use. Family influences, for instance, also play a large role in the selection of friends and thus indirectly influence peer social relations and self-esteem. Supportive, nurturing parents who monitor their child's behaviors may indirectly assist in peer selection mechanisms thus contributing to social self-esteem and ethnic identification. Another overlooked component regards the role of school factors. We previously reported differences in the magnitude of clustering estimates based on peer influences for cigarette and alcohol use. The analyses clearly indicated that clustering varied depending on school with racially heterogeneous samples (66% Black in one case, 85% Hispanic in another, and 91% White in a third sample). Very few, if any studies, have indicated that school-level factors contribute to self-esteem or ethnic identification, although school and neighborhood level factors have been shown to uniquely predict drug use. Thus, the literature has not advanced with respect to developing a more detailed understanding of macro-level influences that may influence psychosocial functioning and contribute to early-stage drug use.

In order for the field to progress with regard to a better understanding of ethnic-specific risk mechanisms, we first must elucidate what ethnic identity is (measurement) and then second, elaborate how it relates to drug use (structural). Our research program suggests one of two possible mechanisms: (1) ethnic identity is a component of social self-esteem involving group social comparison and group categorization (via the tenets of social identity theory) or (2) ethnic identity is distinct from self-esteem and third-variable alternatives including peer selection mechanisms connect these two processes. If this is the case, once third-variable alternatives are controlled, the magnitude of relations between self-esteem and ethnic identity should diminish. Either way, the research program outlined in our proposal moves us closer in the direction of ascertaining a correct measurement model for ethnic identity (based on explicit and implicit cognition) and the short-longitudinal design should move us closer to a more refined understanding regarding the predictive role of identity formation in minority drug etiology.

Finally, the revised proposal now includes a more well-defined model testing strategy. We hope that the rich theoretical context of the present proposal coupled with an innovative use of experimental procedures and rigorous analyses will lend itself to a more detailed examination of ethnic-specific identity processes.

19 Concluding Remarks

The Bottom Line

Lawrence M. Scheier & William L. Dewey

> *It is proper to the role of the scientist that he not merely find new truth and communicate it to his fellows, but that he teach, that he try to bring the most honest and intelligible account of new knowledge to all who try to learn.*
>
> —J. Robert Oppenheimer, "*Prospects in the Arts and Sciences*"

IN HIS BOOK *Phenomenology of Mind*, philosopher Georg Wilhelm Friedrich Hegel introduced the concept that what drives mankind forward in our living, thinking, and daily activities is a struggle for recognition. This emphasis on recognition stands in stark contrast to economic models that purport we are driven by consumption and utility (i.e., satisfaction) or motivational models popular in psychology that neatly disassemble us into cognitions, emotions, and atavistic instincts. According to Hegel, the struggle for recognition exists because we are social creatures; we are, in essence, "other directed," looking to each other for praise and paying considerable attention to what our peers think of us. As strange a philosophy as it may seem, the struggle for recognition is what prompts soldiers to give up their lives while storming a hill during a fierce battle or to sacrifice themselves by placing their body over a hand grenade thrown into a tent that would have surely killed their fellow comrades. The struggle for recognition is what pushes history forward and keeps us tethered to the concepts, ideologies, and political machinations that turn the world. If you think carefully about this point of view, it is the very core reason we write grants for a living. Self-recognition is the impetus for revising an application and mulling over the summary statements in a quiet moment of reflection. It is, at the very least, the core reason that man strives for excellence.

Striving for excellence is not foreign to most of us. It has been the very kindling that has kept our own fires of desire and professional growth lit and moving in the directions we seem to "choose." The journey of our "scientific" lives has been guided by signposts along a road of success. These signposts have taken shape as grants, indicating to us where to turn, when to pull over, when to rest, when to add fuel to the vehicle. This has been the road most of us have traveled, and it is the recognition that this road is part of a larger map that gives us some idea or an overall picture of the territory we travel. For many of us, grants have provided a sense of direction, and using them carefully as a guide, we have learned that they truly point toward the ultimate goal of science, the goal of seeking knowledge and a piece of the truth about that which makes us uniquely human.

As many of us look back on our own careers and cobble together the bits and pieces of memory that make up our professional lives, a few salient themes seem to surface that are worth exploring on the road to success. First and foremost, most of us wanted to write, in addition to the many clinical, administrative, supervisory, and laboratory responsibilities we accrued. Writing for many of us seems so strange given that we wanted to be hard core scientists. However, the contributors to this volume hail from a fairly diverse set of backgrounds, including chemistry, biology, physics, pharmacology, sociology, medicine, education, and many different branches of psychology, including clinical, developmental, social, quantitative, and cognitive. Despite our different training and educational backgrounds, we still ended up doing the same thing, or nearly close to the same thing, for a living. We ended up writing and learning how to convert scientific endeavors and practices into articles, books, chapters, commercial products, manuals, and reports. That is part of the natural beauty of things, how we traveled different educational paths and yet ended up focused on the same topic, or applying a similar set of skills.

The physicist J. Robert Oppenheimer, whose words appear at the beginning of this chapter, leaves us with a slightly different message about our backgrounds and ultimate professional goals. He encourages us to invest in "teaching." In effect, science can do no good unless we spend some of our resources on sharing knowledge and bridging science and practice. This is the second glaring fact about our careers and career paths. We all ended up, in some manner or another, teaching and focusing on practice. There is a shared or consensual belief by all of the contributors that the process of sharing our knowledge and assuring ourselves that there will be a future rests with the investment we place in the full retinue of our graduate students, pre- and postdoctoral fellows, and junior investigators. Through their efforts, we can assure ourselves that our scientific endeavors and research enterprise will be continued. We invest in the future so that the inductive and deductive methods that guide our daily scientific practices can help uncover the truth we all seek. We hope that the interventions we develop and the programs we refine will actually work and make a difference in someone's life. We hope that the brain–behavior mechanisms we fastidiously work to unravel will ultimately inform us about human behavior. Just by happenstance, we hope that maybe, just maybe, one of our own protégés will discover where time goes.

Teaching is the essence of why we wrote this book; it is the fabric that connects all of us together as colleagues, weaves together a story from chapter to chapter, and prompted us to collect the materials and knowledge that comprise each chapter, each grant, and each article we ever constructed. We came to this point in place and time because we recognize our own heavy investment in the process of teaching. We are grateful to our own mentors who shared their knowledge and helped sharpen our own minds and hone our skills and gave us the chance to succeed. We now understand to a greater degree what Oppenheimer advises us to do, and we have a better sense, a better grasp of the map, and a clearer picture of where the road of our professional life leads.

There is another common side to our professional backgrounds that is worth noting: our attraction to the scientific methods that help organize our search for truth and knowledge. Even though we may be involved in breaking apart the smallest atomic particles into smaller and more defined units, there is still a very human quality to our research. A good deal of what lies at the heart of our success is shaped by these human qualities and the personality we bring to the mix. It should also be noted that we are, in fact, attracted to dealing with some of the most intractable problems that plague the human condition, including drug abuse, alcoholism, crime, child abuse, violence, senility, mental health problems, and, more generally, problems in living. We are, in essence, whether we admit it or not, politically charged individuals, actively lobbying for a better life, if not for ourselves, then for the constituents out there who make up the masses and who can benefit from arduous scientific discovery.

In addition to the general philosophical tenor that connects each chapter, there also were specific hallmarks or features that surface in each chapter, mostly reinforcing the importance of attending to detail. In fact, one of the most important messages cropping up in the various chapters of this book is that a good deal of attention needs to be paid to the preparation of grant applications. It is not uncommon to find that very successful investigators with ample funding have set aside no less than three months for the preparation of grant applications. This is particularly true of the more competitive grant mechanisms, including K05, T32, R01, P50, P20, and P30 applications. At one point in time, the first author of this chapter spent three months outlining a P30 Core Center grant and then another six months actually writing up the contents of a single core. This project required the services of several collaborators, each with a different expertise in biometrics, quantitative methodology, and psychometrics, all of which came together under the aegis of a single Methodology Core. The single most impressive part of our collaboration was the friendships that surfaced along with the deep respect for each other's work. It also is worth mentioning that we are collectively aware that by happenstance we designed a very successful business model for a beltway bandit consulting company.

So, in tying together the loose ends of this book, one of the first things we realized is that it has been a joy to write it. We also realize that we have been given a gift in terms of our careers and the opportunities that mark the roadside of our professional journeys. It also has been a gift to share our passion and our thirst for knowledge. The best thing, perhaps, is that the sharing of this passion has taken shape through teaching and cultivating younger minds. Most important, the greatest gift has been our friendships, the companionship along the journey. It is really a deep level of respect for each other that binds us to the peer review system and keeps our hopes alive. Last but not least, we are grateful for the pleasures that science bears, for us now, and for the future.

CHAPTER 2

1. National Academy of Sciences (2004). *Bridging to independence: Fostering the independence of new investigators in biomedical research.* Washington, DC: National Academies Press.
2. University of Washington (2005a). *Mentoring: How to mentor graduate students—a faculty guide.* Seattle: University of Washington Graduate School.
3. University of Washington (2005b). *Mentoring: How to obtain the mentoring you need—a graduate student guide.* Seattle: University of Washington Graduate School.

CHAPTER 3

1. Bandura, A. (1977). Self-efficacy: Toward a unifying theory of behavioral change. *Psychological Review, 84,* 191–215.
2. Bandura, A. (1986). *Social foundations of thought and action: A social cognitive theory.* Englewood Cliffs, NJ: Prentice-Hall.
3. Bandura, A. (1997). *Self-efficacy: The exercise of control.* New York: W. H. Freeman.
4. Jessor, R., & Jessor, S. L. (1977). *Problem behavior and psychosocial development: A longitudinal study of youth.* New York: Academic Press.
5. Heyduk, R. G., & Fenigstein, A. (1984). Influential works and authors in psychology: A survey of eminent psychologists. *American Psychologist, 39,* 556–559.
6. Twain, M. (1924). *Mark Twain's autobiography.* A. B. Paine (Ed.). New York: Harper and Bros.
7. Substance Abuse and Mental Health Services Administration. (2006). Results from the 2005 National Survey on Drug Use and Health: National Findings (Office of Applied Studies, NSDUH Series H-30, DHHS Publication No. SMA 06-4194). Rockville, MD: Author. Available at www.samhsa.gov and www.oas.samhsa.gov.

B1. Cross, W. E. (1991). *Shades of black: Diversity in African American identity.* Philadelphia, PA: Temple University Press.

8. Donner, A. (1984). Approaches to sample size estimation in the design of clinical trials: A review. *Statistics in Medicine*, 3, 199–214.

9. Murray, D. M. (1998). *Design and analysis of group-randomized trials.* New York: Oxford University Press.

10. Murray, D. M., & Short, B. (1996). Intraclass correlation among measures related to alcohol use by school aged adolescents: Estimates, correlates and applications in intervention studies. *Journal of Drug Education*, 26, 207–230.

11. Scheier, L. M., Griffin, K. W., Doyle, M. M., & Botvin, G. J. (2002). Estimates of intragroup dependence for drug use and skill measures encountered in school-based drug abuse prevention trials: An empirical study of three independent samples. *Health Education and Behavior*, 29, 83–101.

12. Baron, R. M., & Kenny, D. A. (1986). The moderator-mediator variable distinction in social psychological research: Conceptual, strategic, and statistical considerations. *Journal of Personality and Social Psychology*, 51, 1173–1182.

13. Scheier, L. M., Miller, N. L., Ifill-Williams, M., & Botvin, G. J. (2001). Perceived neighborhood risk as a predictor of drug use among ethnic minority adolescents: Moderating influences of psychosocial functioning. *Journal of Child and Adolescent Substance Abuse*, 11, 67–105.

14. Scheier, L. M., Botvin, G. J., & Griffin, K. W. (2001). Preventive intervention effects on developmental progression in drug use: Structural equation modeling analyses using longitudinal data. *Prevention Science*, 2, 89–110.

15. Kuhn, T. S. (1970). *The structure of scientific revolutions.* Chicago: University of Chicago Press.

16. Rosenstock, I. M. (1974). Historical origins of the Health Belief Model. *Health Education Monographs*, 2, 328–335.

17. Becker, M. H. (1974). *The Health Belief Model and personal health behavior.* San Francisco, CA: Society for Public Health Education.

18. Becker, M. H., Drachman, R. H., & Kirscht, J. P. (1974). A new approach to explaining sick-role behavior in low income populations. *American Journal of Public Health*, 64, 205–216.

19. Palmgreen, P., Donohew, L., Lorch, E., Pugzles, H., Rick, H., & Stephenson, M. T. (2001). Television campaign and adolescent marijuana use: Tests of sensation seeking targeting. *American Journal of Public Health*, 91, 292–296.

20. Sternberg, R. J. (1992). Psychological Bulletin's top 10 "Hit Parade." *Psychological Bulletin*, 112, 387–388.

21. Campbell, D. T., & Fiske, D. W. (1959). Convergent and discriminant validation by the multitrait-multimethod matrix. *Psychological Bulletin*, 56, 81–105.

22. Newcomb, M. D., Scheier, L. M., & Bentler, P. M. (1993). Effects of adolescent drug use on adult psychopathology: A prospective study of a community sample. *Experimental and Clinical Psychopharmacology*, 1, 1–28.

23. Bentler, P. M., & Bonett, D. G. (1980). Significance tests and goodness of fit in the analysis of covariance structures. *Psychological Bulletin*, 88, 588–606.

24. Bentler, P. M. (1992). On the fit of models to covariances and methodology to the Bulletin. *Psychological Bulletin*, 112, 400–404.

25. Wiers, R. W., & Stacy, A. W. (Eds.) (2006). *Handbook of implicit cognition and addiction.* Thousand Oaks, CA: Sage Publications.

26. Legal advice was provided by R. Scott Weide, J.D., of Weide & Miller, Ltd., an intellectual property law firm located at 7251 W. Lake Mead Blvd., Suite 530, Las Vegas, NV 89128; telephone (702) 382-4804; fax (702) 382-4805; email sweide@weidemiller.com.

27. American Psychological Association (2001). *Publication manual of the American Psychological Association*, 5th ed. Washington, DC: Author.

28. Huxley, T. H. (2005). *On the method of Zadig*. Whitefish, MT: Kessinger Publishing.

CHAPTER 4

1. Feng, Z., & Thompson, B. (2002). Some design issues in a community intervention trial. *Controlled Clinical Trials*, 23, 431–449.

2. Pocock, S. J., Geller, N. L., & Tsiatis, A. A. (1987) The analysis of multiple endpoints in clinical trials. *Biometrics*, 43, 487–498.

3. Cohen, J. (1988). *Statistical power analysis for the behavioral sciences*, 2nd ed. New York: Academic Press.

4. Fleiss, J. L., Levin, B., & Paik, M. C. (2003). *Statistical methods for rates and proportions*, 3rd ed. Hoboken, NJ: John Wiley & Sons.

5. Murray, D. M. (1998). *Design and analysis of group-randomized trials*. New York: Oxford University Press.

6. Kelsey, J. L., Whittemore, A. S., Evans, A. S., & Thompson, W. D. (1996). *Methods in observational epidemiology*, 2nd ed. New York: Oxford University Press.

7. Meinert, C. L. (1986). *Clinical trials*. New York: Oxford University Press.

8. Schlesselman, J. J. (1982). *Case-control studies: Design, conduct, analysis*. New York: Oxford University Press.

9. Hannan, P. J., & Murray, D. M. (1996). Gauss or Bernoulli? A Monte Carlo comparison of the performance of the linear mixed model and the logistic mixed model analyses in simulated community trials with a dichotomous outcome variable at the individual level. *Evaluation Review*, 20, 338–352.

10. Diggle, P. J., Heagerty, P., Liang, K. Y., & Zeger, S. L. (2002). *Analysis of longitudinal data*, 2nd ed. New York: Oxford University Press.

CHAPTER 6

1. National Institutes of Health. (2005). About NIH. Available at www.nih.gov/about.

2. National Institutes of Health. (2000, June 1). National Research Service Awards for individual postdoctoral fellows (F32). Available at grants.nih/gov/grants/guide/pa-files/PA-00-104.html.

3. Whitman, N.A. (1987). Reducing stress among students. Available at www.the-memoryhole.org/edu/eric/ed284526.html.

4. Austin, J. (2002). Stress rising for college students. Available at www.dfw.com/mld/dfw/news/ local/4394018.html.

5. National Opinion Research Center. (1998). *Doctorate recipients from United States universities: Summary report*, 1998. Chicago: National Opinion Research Center.

6. National Institutes of Health. (2004). NIH competing applications, fiscal years 1998–2003. Institute/center and research category. Available at grants1.nih.gov/grants/awards/success/icact9803.xls.

CHAPTER 9

1. Fuqua, J., Stokols, D., Gress, J., Phillips, K., & Harvey, R. (2004). Transdisciplinary collaboration as a basis for enhancing the science and prevention of substance use and abuse. *Substance Use and Misuse*, 39, 1457–1514.

CHAPTER 13

1. Legal advice was provided by R. Scott Weide, J.D., of Weide & Miller, Ltd., an intellectual property law firm located at 7251 W. Lake Mead Blvd., Suite 530, Las Vegas, NV 89128; Telephone (702) 382-4804; fax (702) 382-4805; email sweide@weidemiller.com.
2. Flesch, R. (1948). A new readability yardstick. *Journal of Applied Psychology*, 32, 221–233.
3. Kincaid, J. P., Fishburne, R. P., Rogers, R. L., & Chissom, B. S. (1975). *Derivation of new readability formulas (Automated Readability Index, Fog Count and Flesch Reading Ease Formula) for Navy enlisted personnel*, Research Branch Report 8-75. Millington, TN: Naval Technical Training, U.S. Naval Air Station, Memphis, TN.

CHAPTER 14

1. Arthur, M. W., & Blitz, C. (2000). Bridging the gap between science and practice in drug abuse prevention through needs assessment and strategic community planning. *Journal of Community Psychology*, 28, 241–255.
2. Backer, T. E. (2000). The failure of success: Challenges of disseminating effective substance abuse prevention programs. *Journal of Community Psychology*, 28, 363–373.
3. Biglan, A., Mrazek, P. J., Carnine, D., & Flay, B. R. (2003). The integration of research and practice in the prevention of youth problem behaviors. *American Psychologist*, 58, 443–440.
4. Biglan, A., & Taylor, T. K. (2000). Increasing the use of science to improve child-rearing. *Journal of Primary Prevention*, 21, 207–226.
5. Kumpfer, K. L., & Kaftarian, S. J. (2000). Bridging the gap between family-focused research and substance abuse prevention practice: Preface. *Journal of Primary Prevention*, 21, 169–183.
6. U.S. Department of Health and Human Services. (1999). *Mental health: A report of the surgeon general*. Rockville, MD: DHHS/SAMHSA/CMHS and NIH/NIMH.
7. Institute of Medicine—Committee on Quality of Health Care in America. (2001). *Crossing the quality chasm: A new health system for the 21st century*. Washington, DC: National Academy Press.
8. Mrazek, P. J., & Haggerty, R. J. (1994). *Reducing risks for mental disorders: Frontiers for preventive intervention research*. Washington, DC: National Academy Press for the Institute of Medicine, Committee on Prevention of Mental Disorders.
9. Kumpfer, K. L., Alvarado, R., & Whiteside, H. O. (2003). Family-based interventions for the substance abuse prevention. *Substance Use and Misuse*, 38, 1759–1789.
10. National Institutes of Health. (2005). *Strategic plan*. Office of Behavioral and Social Sciences, Office of the Director.e Available at obssr.od.nih.gov/about/plan.html.

11. Mihalic, S., & Irwin, K. (2003). Blueprints for violence prevention: From research to real-world settings—factors influencing the successful replication of model programs. *Youth Violence and Juvenile Justice*, 1, 307–329.

12. Rohrbach, L. A., Grana, R., Sussman, S., & Valente, T. W. (2006). Type II translation: Transporting prevention interventions from research to real-world settings. *Evaluation and Health Professions*, 29, 302–333.

13. Rogers, E. M. (2003). *Diffusion of innovations*, 5th ed. New York: Free Press.

14. Bandura, A. (1989). Human agency in social cognitive theory. *American Psychologist*, 44, 1175–1184.

15. Dusenbury, L., Brannigan, R., Falco, M., & Hansen, W. B. (2003). A review on fidelity of implementation: Implications for drug prevention in school settings. *Health Education Research*, 18, 237–256.

16. Jansen, M. A., Glynn, T., & Howard, J. (1996). Prevention of alchohol, tobacco, and other drug abuse. *American Behavioral Scientist*, 39, 790–801.

17. Greenwald, P., & Cullen, J. W. (1985). The new emphasis in cancer control. *Journal of the National Cancer Institute*, 74, 543–551.

18. Park, M., & Kumpfer, K. L. (2005). Qualities of an effective family group leader. Master's Thesis. Salt Lake City: Department of Health Promotion and Education, University of Utah.

19. Ringwald, C. R., Ennett, S., Vincus, A., Thorne, J., Rohrbach, L., A., & Simons-Rudolph, A. (2002). The effectiveness of substance use prevention curricula in U.S. middle schools. *Prevention Science*, 3, 257–265.

20. Cook, T. D., & Campbell, D. T. (1979). *Quasi-experimentation: Design and analysis issues in field settings*. Chicago: Rand-McNally.

CHAPTER 15

1. Office of Management and Budget. (2006). *Budget of the United States government (fiscal year 2007). The budget system and concepts*, chap. 26. Retrieved July 21, 2006, from www.whitehouse.gov/omb/budget/fy2007/pdf/concepts.pdf.

2. Office of Management and Budget. (2004, May 10). Circular No. A-21: Cost principles for educational institutions. Available at www.whitehouse.gov/omb/circulars/a021/a21_2004.pdf (retrieved July 21, 2006).

3. National Institutes of Health. (2003, December 1). NIH Grants Policy Statement. Available at grants1.nih.gov/grants/policy/nihgps_2003/nihgps_2003.pdf (retrieved July 21, 2006).

4. U.S. Department of Health and Human Services Public Health Service. (2006). Grant application (PHS398) part I instructions (interim revision April 2006). Available at grants1.nih.gov/grants/funding/phs398/phs398.pdf (retrieved August 16, 2006).

5. National Institutes of Health, Office of Extramural Research. (2006, May 12). Frequently asked questions regarding the usage of person months. Available at grants1.nih.gov/grants/policy/person_months_faqs.htm (retrieved July 21, 2006).

6. Weill Medical College Cornell University. (2003, April 25). *Service provider payments (independent contractor/consultant) policy and guidelines*. (Available from the Weill Medical College of Cornell University, Finance Department, 100 Broadway, 8th Floor, New York, NY 10005).

7. U.S. Department of Health and Human Services Public Health Services. (2006, July 5). Grants.gov application guide SF424 (R&R) version 2. Available at grants1.nih.gov/grants/funding/424/SF424_RR_Guide_General_Ver2.pdf (retrieved July 21, 2006).

8. Cornell University, Office of Sponsored Programs. (2006). *Guide to budgeting and costing of sponsored projects.* Available at www.osp.cornell.edu/ProposalPrep/Costing-guide.html (retrieved August 9, 2006).

9. RAND Corporation. (2000, August 25). *Paying for research facilities and administration. Background: How universities recover F & A Costs from the federal government,* chap. 2. Available at www.rand.org/pubs/monograph_reports/MR1135-1/MR1135.1.chap2.pdf (retrieved August 15, 2006).

1   Appendix: The NIH Web Sites

Jennifer N. Lapin

This appendix provides more detailed information for all of the Web sites cited throughout this edited volume. We felt this would be helpful to readers after poring through the individual chapters that are so full of information. From this appendix, readers can summarize the Web site information, jot down notes in the page margins, and copy these sites into a Web browser. Web sites were last accessed June 15th, 2007 and may periodically change content, URL, or become inactive. For updates, check with the LARS Web site (www.larsri.org) for any errata and updates to *The Complete Writing Guide to NIH Behavioral Science Grants*. Where appropriate, we included a paragraph containing a brief description of a Web site. For some Web sites, the title clearly explains the Web site content, so no further information is included. Some descriptions include links to other areas of the parent Web site that may be of interest to readers.

The NIH Homepage

www.nih.gov

The NIH Mission

www.nih.gov/about/

The NIH Budget

grants1.nih.gov/grants/award/research/rgmechact9905.pdf

This Web page reports on the NIH budgets for competing and noncompeting grants—for the period from 1999 to 2005.

NIH eRA Commons

commons.era.nih.gov/commons/

The Electronic Research Administration (eRA) Commons is a virtual meeting place where NIH extramural grantee organizations, grantees, and the public can receive and transmit information about the administration of biomedical and behavioral research. The eRA Commons has both unrestricted and restricted sections that provide for exchange of public and confidential information, respectively. Information given at this Web site is directed toward handling electronic submissions of applications and allows investigators to make corrections to an application once it has been submitted. Summary statements regarding scoring of applications will now be available to investigators using eRA Commons, and peer reviews are also handled using this Web site. Readers should be aware that in order to access certain information, an eRA Commons user name and password are required.

The primary features associated with the eRA Commons (1) allow principal investigators to review the current status of all their grant applications and information associated with their grants, (2) allow an institution to review noncompeting grant data and submit a progress report online, (3) allow reviewers to submit critiques and preliminary scores for applications they are reviewing, (4) allow for submission of financial information related to grant, and (5) allow an institution to create and manage user accounts associated with the institution. A number of links are also associated with this Web site, in particular, era.nih .gov/Electronic Receipt/tips_tools.htm, which is a Web site dedicated to help candidates learn about the most frequent application errors.

eRA: Avoiding Common Errors

era.nih.gov/ElectronicReceipt/avoiding_errors.htm

This Web page lists the most common errors made by applicants, offers resolution to these frequently encountered problems, and describes the process for resubmitting a corrected application.

eRA Help Desk

ithelpdesk.nih.gov/eRA/

eRA Commons Frequently Asked Questions (FAQ)

commons.era.nih.gov/commons/faq.jsp

eRA Commons Electronic Application Process

era.nih.gov/ElectronicReceipt/process.htm

This Web site provides links to all the necessary steps in submitting an electronic application. Consider this a must-use Web site for your first time using electronic submission.

Center for Scientific Review

cms.csr.nih.gov/

The Center for Scientific Review (CSR) Web site contains a wealth of information outlining the operational and organizational structure of CSR, describes the process of review for a grant, and also contains links to various resources for applicants. The CSR is a portal for NIH grant applications and their review for scientific merit. Up to 70% of all research grant applications are evaluated by the CSR's peer review groups that it organizes. The CSR receives nearly 80,000 applications each year and recruits more than 15,000 external experts to review its portion of those grants. The primary goals of the CSR are stated as being to shorten the review process, recruit and retain the best reviewers, foster a culture more favorable to innovative applications, address the concern that clinical research is not properly evaluated, and increase the transparency, accountability, and uniformity of the NIH peer review.

The CSR Web site provides an in-depth description for potential applicants as to what happens to an application following submission. Essentially, an application is assigned to a scientific review group consisting of experts in the field detailed in the application. The experts in this group (both standing members and ad hoc members) convene either by phone or in person and collectively decide on a score. Their written comments (and those raised during review) are sent to the investigator in the form of a summary statement. The expert panel (internal review group) also provides the parent institute with a priority score (ranging from 1.0 to 5.0).

Center for Scientific Review: Resources for Applicants

cms.csr.nih.gov/ResourcesforApplicants/

Center for Scientific Review—published peer review notes

www.csr.nih.gov/prnotes/prnotes.asp

The Center for Scientific Review publishes peer review notes to inform reviewers, the NIH program and administrative staff, and the general public of news related to the grant application review policies, procedures, and plans.

NIH Standard Postmark/Submission Dates for Competing Applications

grants.nih.gov/grants/funding/submissionschedule.htm

This NIH Web page, sponsored by the Office of Extramural Research, outlines the submission dates for numerous competing grant applications. These dates are broken down for each cycle in which applications are due for a total of three dates for each application. Submission dates for applications are broken up into non-AIDS applications and AIDS and AIDS-related applications. Researchers need to take note that their requested start date for a project in their application may not always be honored by the awarding institute. Therefore, applicants should make no commitments or obligations until they have official confirmation from NIH or their respective funding agency grants management of the start date.

The Web page also provides an overview of paper submission polices which include mailing, dates, special receipt dates, and procedures for handling late applications. Important points for applicants to remember are that applications may not be delivered by the individuals, an application is considered on time if it is postmarked/courier-dated by the date listed on the Web site, late applications are accepted only on extenuating circumstances, and permission for a late submission will not be granted in advance.

NIH Bioengineering Consortium (BECON) 2003 Symposium on Catalyzing Team Science

www.becon.nih.gov/symposium2003.htm

This Web site describes the 2003 BECON Symposium on Catalyzing Team Science. Included are links to the final report, contents all the plenary sessions, and other information related to the symposium.

NIH Roadmap for Medical Research

nihroadmap.nih.gov/

The purpose of the NIH Roadmap is to identify major opportunities and gaps in biomedical research that all of the NIH must address, to have the largest and most beneficial impact on the progress of medical research. Developed on the basis of input from meetings with more than 300 nationally recognized leaders in academia, industry, government, and the public, the NIH Roadmap provides a framework for the priorities of NIH and gives some indication what NIH must address in order to optimize its entire research portfolio. The Roadmap lays out a vision for a more efficient and productive system of medical research, and identifies the most compelling opportunities in three main areas: new pathways to discovery, research teams of the future, and reengineering the clinical research enterprise.

New Investigators Program

grants.nih.gov/grants/new%5Finvestigators/

The NIH Web site for new investigators sponsored by the Office of Extramural Research provides information and support to facilitate investigators receiving an R01 award earlier in their research career. Support includes the Pathway to Independence Award, NRSA Individual and Institutional Training Awards, Career Development Awards, Research Project Grant Program, and NIH Institute and Center Practices and Resources for New Investigators.

K Kiosk—Information About NIH Career Development Awards

grants.nih.gov/training/careerdevelopmentawards.htm

The Career Development Award Program Web site at NIH provides a listing of different grant award types by doctorate type. Individuals with a research doctorate are directed to an area of the Web site outlining at least eight different award types, including the Career Transition Award (K22) for researchers early in their career, the Mentored Research Scientist Development Award (K01), and the Scientist Award (K0-2). Individuals with a health-professions doctorate are directed to a different area of the Web site that outlines nine different award types, including the Mentored Clinical Scientist Developmental Program Award (K12), the Mentored Clinical Scientist Award (K08), and the Mentored Patient-Oriented Research Career Development Award (K23).

MENTORED RESEARCH SCIENTIST AWARD

grants.nih.gov/grants/guide/pa-files/PA-95-049.html

This award is for research scientists who need an additional period of sponsored research experience as a way to gain expertise in a research area new to the candidate or in an area that would clearly enhance the candidate's scientific career. Following this award, it is expected that the recipient would have the ability to pursue an independent and productive research career.

Mentored Patient-Oriented Research Career Development Award

grants.nih.gov/grants/guide/pa-files/PA-05-143.html

This award provides support for three to five years of supervised study and is designed to support researchers who are committed to focus their research on patient-oriented research. Applicants must justify their need for mentored research experience and make the case that the support will enhance their career as an independent investigator in patient-oriented research. The Web site provides links to all the information necessary to apply for the K23 award.

Mentored Grants for Quantitative Skills

grants.nih.gov/grants/guide/pa-files/PA-06-087.html

This Web site provides links for all the information necessary to apply for the K25 award, which is designed to attract quantitative researchers, whose careers have been focused in other areas, to NIH-relevant research. The program provides mentored research experiences that provide expertise in a new research area or an area that will enhance an investigator's research capabilities. Ultimately, the program experience will lead to and independent and productive research career.

Independent Scientist Award

www.nih.gov/grants/guide/pa-files/PA-95-050.html

This award is intended to foster the development of outstanding scientists and enable them to expand their potential to make significant contributions to their field of research. This award replaces two career development awards, the Research Scientists Development Award (K02) and the Research Career Development Award (K04).

Midcareer Investigator Award in Patient-Oriented Research

www.nih.gov/grants/guide/pa-files/PA-98-053.html

This award provides support for clinicians, allowing them protected time to devote to patient-oriented research and to act as mentors for beginning clinical investigators. Candidates for this award are within 15 years of their specialty training, demonstrate a need for a period of intensive research focus as a means of enhancing their clinical research careers, and are committed to mentoring new clinical investigators focusing on patient-oriented research.

Senior Scientist Award

www.nih.gov/grants/guide/pa-files/PA-95-051.html

The Senior Scientist Award (K05) provides support to outstanding scientists who have demonstrated a sustained, high level of productivity and whose expertise, research accomplishments, and contributions to the field have been and will continue to be critical to the mission of the particular NIH center or institute. The award provides salary support for award periods of five years.

Individual Predoctoral National Research Service Awards for M.D./Ph.D. Fellowships

www.nih.gov/grants/guide/pa-files/PA-99-089.html

This Web page contains program announcements for individual predoctoral Research Service Awards for graduate students currently enrolled in accredited M.D./Ph.D. programs to help ensure that highly trained physician/scientists will be available in research areas and fields to meet the nation's mental health, drug abuse and addiction, alcohol abuse and alcoholism, and environmental health sciences research needs.

National Research Service Award for Individual Predoctoral Fellowships

www.nih.gov/grants/guide/pa-files/PA-99-017.html

This program is for individuals currently enrolled in accredited research doctorate (Ph.D. or D.Sc.) programs only and have sponsorship from their institution. The program is designed to help ensure that highly trained scientists will be available in research areas and fields to meet the nation's mental health, drug abuse and addiction, and alcohol abuse and alcoholism research needs.

National Research Service Award for Individual Postdoctoral Fellowships

www.nih.gov/grants/guide/pa-files/PA-99-025.html

Requirements for this award include receipt of doctorate (M.D., Ph.D., D.O., etc.) from an accredited institution and a sponsoring institution as well as a sponsoring individual. The program is designed to help ensure that highly trained scientists will be available in the biomedical research to meet the nation's biomedical research needs.

Budget and Just-in-Time Budget Concept

grants.nih.gov/grants/funding/phs398/phs398.html

This Web page provides links to forms needed to complete a PHS 398 grant application.

Administrative Requirements: Enforcement Actions, Suspension, Termination, and Withholding of Support

grants.nih.gov/grants/policy/nihgps_2001/part_iia_7.htm#suspension terminationandwitholding

This NIH Web page provides detailed reporting requirements for investigators once a grant has been awarded. The page provides the NIH grants policy statement; details on monitoring, which includes different types of reporting; progress reports as part of noncompeting continuations, requests, financial reports, unobligated balances, and actual expenditures; invention reporting; reporting to the office of research integrity; and lobbying disclosure. Also included are instructions on record retention, auditing, repercussions for noncompliance, closing out a grant, and appealing a grant decision.

Funding Opportunities and Notices: NIH Guide for Grants and Contracts

grants.nih.gov/grants/guide/index.html

This is a searchable Web site for different types of funding, where grant information is listed by number, title, or key word.

NIH Grants Policy Guidance and Policy

grants.nih.gov/grants/policy/policy.htm

This NIH Web page includes links to the grants policy statements, policy resources, general policy notices, other guidance resources, grant awards and NIH appropriations, and other related links.

NIH Grants Policy Statement Part II: Terms and Conditions of NIH Grant Awards

Subpart A: General

grants.nih.gov/grants/policy/nihgps_2003/NIHGPS_part4.htm

This NIH Web page provides information on completing the preaward process, which occurs after the peer review is completed. Included on this site is information relating to just-in-time procedures, funding principles, eligibility, cost analysis, an overview of terms and conditions of the NIH grants and cooperative agreements, and a detailed description of the public policy requirements and objectives. Also described on this page is policy related to the ethical and safe conduct in science and organizational operations. This section includes the standards of conduct, financial conflict of interest policy, debarment and suspension policy, drug-free workplace policy, health and safety regulations and guidelines, the NIH Guidelines for Research Involving Recombinant DNA Molecules and Human Gene Transfer Research, and NIH guidelines for research using human embryonic stem cells.

Subpart B: Terms and Conditions for Specific Types of Grants, Grantees, and Activities

grants.nih.gov/grants/policy/nihgps_2003/NIHGPS_part9.htm

This NIH Web page includes terms and conditions that are in addition to or elaborate and highlight the standard requirements and terms and conditions in subpart A. This section includes construction grants, individual fellowships and training grants, modular applications and awards, conference grants, consortium agreements, foreign institution grants, federal institution grants, for-profit organizations, and research patient care costs.

PHS Noncompeting Grant Progress Report, Form 2590

grants.nih.gov/grants/funding/2590/2590.htm

This NIH Web page provides links to progress reporting forms (PHS 2590) for noncompeting grants.

NIH Data Sharing Policy

grants.nih.gov/grants/policy/data_sharing

Administrative Requirements for NIH Grants: Changes in Project and Budget

grants.nih.gov/grants/policy/nihgps_2001/part_iia_5.htm#ChangesinProject andBudget

This Web page outlines the requirements for rebudgeting within and between budget categories to meet unanticipated needs and for making other postaward changes.

Small Business Funding Opportunities

grants.nih.gov/grants/funding/sbir.htm#sol

This Web page provides links for all of the information required for submission of small business innovative research grants, including announcements, submission information, policy guidelines, and other resources.

Exploratory/Developmental Grant Applications

grants.nih.gov/grants/guide/pa-files/PA-98-004.html

This program announcement notifies the extramural research community that National Institute on Drug Abuse (NIDA) accepts exploratory/developmental grant applications that fall within its program interests.

NIDA Small Grants Program

www.nih.gov/grants/guide/pa-files/PAR-97-038.html

This program provides research support of up to $50,000 per year (direct costs) for up to two years. This award is not renewable.

NIH Office of Acquisition Management and Policy—Division of Financial Advisory Services

oamp.od.nih.gov/dfas/dfas.asp

The mission of the Division of Financial Advisory Services is to provide quality financial advice and services to ensure the appropriate funding and reimbursement of contracts and grants.

U.S. Department of Health and Human Services Grant Application

grants1.nih.gov/grants/funding/phs398/phs398.html

This page has downloadable instructions and forms for PHS 398.

Department of Health and Human Services: Steps to File a Domestic Federalwide Assurance

www.dhhs.gov/ohrp/assurances/assurances_index.html#domestic

Direct Cost Limitations—Revised Notice

grants.nih.gov/grants/guide/notice-files/NOT-OD-05-004.html

This notice is for applications that include consortium and contractual facilities and administrative costs.

NIH Competing and Noncompeting Research Grants, Fiscal Years 1999–2005

grants1.nih.gov/grants/award/research/rgmechact9905.pdf

FORMS, FORMS, AND MORE FORMS!

Columbia University—Project Administration

www.columbia.edu/cu/opg/projadm/project.html

Northwestern University—NIH Forms Available for Download
www.northwestern.edu/orsp/forms.html#NIH

BUDGETS

Budget Justification Page—Modular Research Grant Application
grants.nih.gov/grants/funding/phs398/modbudgetsample_same.pdf
grants.nih.gov/grants/funding/phs398/modbudgetsample_variation.pdf

Links to Information for Calculating Person-Months

grants1.nih.gov/grants/policy/person_months_faqs.htm

Salary Cap Summary

grants.nih.gov/grants/policy/salcap_summary.htm

This Web page lists the salary caps for executive-level positions from 1990 to 2007.

The Academic Scientists Toolkit

nextwave.sciencemag.org/feature/cdctoolkit.shtml

This Web page provides links to job and grant resources.

Pilot Study to Shorten Review Cycle for New Investigator R01 Applications

grants.nih.gov/grants/guide/notice-files/NOT-OD-06-013.html

The pilot described in this notice is designed to shorten the time to the next review for some new investigators who are not successful in a R01 grant submission and are readily able to address the concerns raised and issues identified in the summary statement. Under carefully defined circumstances for this pilot, new investigators will be able to resubmit amended applications for the next review meeting, rather than waiting a full cycle (which conceivably would take up to nine months). This will shorten the time for the next consideration of the resubmission application by four months.

Addendum to Institutional Clinical and Translational Science Award RFA

grants.nih.gov/grants/guide/notice-files/NOT-RM-06-008.html

This notice is an addendum to RFA-RM-06-002, "Institutional Clinical and Translational Science Award," which was released in the *NIH Guide for Grants and Contracts* on October 12, 2005, at grants.nih.gov/grants/guide/rfa-files/RFA-RM-06-002.html. It clarifies requirements for the T32 component of CTSA Research Education, Training, and Career Development activities to ensure their compatibility with the NIH Roadmap Predoctoral Clinical Research Training Program (T32), posted at grants.nih.gov/grants/guide/rfa-files/RFA-RM-05-015.html.

NIH Research Training and Research Career Opportunities: Extramural Training Mechanisms

grants2.nih.gov/training/extramural.htm

This Web page provides lists of various types of award programs, including National Research Service Awards, Career Development Awards, and Selected Programs for Special Populations and others.

HUMAN SUBJECTS

Office for Human Research Protections Homepage

www.hhs.gov/ohrp/

This site provides general guidance on human subject protection and the government regulations that apply for any grant funded research.

Human Subject Protection

www.hhs.gov/ohrp/humansubjects/guidance/45cfr46.htm

This Web page provides the complete text for the Code of Federal Regulations Title 45, Part 46, Protection of Human Subjects.

Guidance on Research Involving Coded Private Information or Biological Specimens

www.hhs.gov/ohrp/humansubjects/guidance/cdebiol.pdf

This document applies to research involving coded private information or human biological specimens that is conducted or supported by the DHHS. This document provides guidance as to when research using coded private information or specimens is or is not research involving human subjects; reaffirms the policy that under certain limited conditions, research involving coded information or specimens is not human research; clarifies the distinction between (a) research involving coded private information or specimens that does not involve human subjects and (b) human subjects research that is exempt from the requirements of the HHS regulations; and references pertinent requirements of the HIPAA Privacy Rule that may be applicable to research involving coded private information or specimens.

NIH Instructions to Reviewers for Evaluating Research Involving Human Subjects in Grant and Cooperative Agreement Applications

grants1.nih.gov/grants/peer/hs_review_inst.pdf

Office for Human Research Protections Policy Guidance: Exemptions

www.hhs.gov/ohrp/policy/index.html#exempt

This Web page has links to exemptions for public benefit and service programs and exempt research and research that may undergo expedited review.

Summary of the HIPAA Privacy Rule

www.hhs.gov/ocr/privacysummary.pdf

NIH Guidelines for Inclusion of Women and Minorities as Subjects in Clinical Research

grants.nih.gov/grants/guide/notice-files/NOT-OD-02-001.html

This Web page describes the 2001 amendment to the policy regarding the inclusion of women and minorities in clinical research. The complete amended policy address is grants.nih.gov/grants/funding/women_min/women_min.htm.

grants.nih.gov/grants/funding/women_min/guidelines_amended_10_2001.htm

This is the policy implementation page of the inclusion of women and minorities as participants in research involving human subjects. Included is the link to the complete copy of the amendment.

NIH Revitalization Act of 1993 (Section 492B of Public Law 103-43)

grants.nih.gov/grants/guide/notice-files/NOT-OD-02-001.html

NIH Policy for Data and Safety Monitoring: NIH Guide for Grants and Contracts

grants.nih.gov/grants/guide/notice-files/not98-084.html

This Web page explains all sections of the policy related to the safety monitoring and oversight of clinical trials.

Required Education in the Protection of Human Research Participants

grants.nih.gov/grants/guide/notice-files/NOT-OD-00-039.html

This Web page includes the year 2000 initiatives designed to strengthen government oversight of medical research. The announcements also remind institutions of their responsibility to oversee their clinical investigators and institutional review boards (IRBs).

NIH Inclusion of Children Policy Implementation

grants.nih.gov/grants/funding/children/children.htm

This is the policy implementation page of the inclusion of children as participants in research involving human subjects.

The Belmont Report

www.hhs.gov/ohrp/humansubjects/guidance/belmont.htm

A 1979 report on the Ethical Principles and Guidelines for the Protection of Human Subjects of Research by the National Commission for the Protection of Human Subjects of Biomedical and Behavioral Research.

OER Human Subjects Web Site

grants.nih.gov/grants/policy/hs/index.htm

This site provides, in one place, DHHS and NIH requirements and resources for the extramural community involved in human subject research in their roles as applicants/grantees, contractors, peer reviewers, and institutional officials.

Human Subject Regulation Decision Charts

www.hhs.gov/ohrp/humansubjects/guidance/decisioncharts.htm

The basic human subject decision charts developed by OHRP are very useful for an investigator in determining if their project involves human subjects. While it may seem obvious, this question may be confusing when involving research with secondary data files. In addition, the charts are useful in helping investigators prepare protocols for submission to Institutional Review Boards.

OHRP Special Protections for Children as Research Subjects

www.hhs.gov/ohrp/children/

NIH SITES

NIH OER Human Subjects

grants.nih.gov/grants/funding/phs398/HumanSubjects.doc

This Web site provides access to a Word document titled "Supplemental Instructions for preparing the Human Subjects Section of a Research Plan." In its entirety, it is one of the most comprehensive instructional documents, providing an overview of policy, sample vignettes, and step-by-step detailed information on the requirements for research involving human subjects.

HIPAA Privacy Rule: Information for Researchers

privacyruleandresearch.nih.gov/

This Web page provides information on the HIPAA privacy rule and the guidelines for human subjects research in international research.

Awards Data: Success Rates by Institute

grants1.nih.gov/grants/award/success/Success_ByIC.cfm

NIH Enterprise (Employee) Directory

ned.nih.gov/

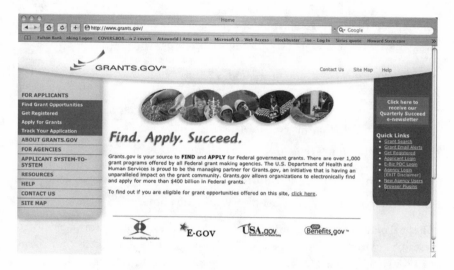

Figure A.1. Snapshot of Grants.gov Home Page

Grants.gov homepage

www.grants.gov

This Web site allows organizations to electronically find and apply for more than $400 billion in federal grants and is the single access point for more than 1,000 grant programs offered by all federal grant making agencies.

NIH Funding Opportunities and Notices: NIH Guide for Grants and Contracts

grants1.nih.gov/grants/guide/index.html

This is the official publication for the NIH medical and behavioral research grant policies, guidelines, and funding opportunities.

NIH Funding Mechanisms

grants2.nih.gov/grants/funding/phs398/instructions2/p3_general_info _mechanisms.htm

NIH Grant Application Forms and Instructions

grants1.nih.gov/grants/forms.htm

Standard Due Dates for Competing Applications

grants1.nih.gov/grants/funding/submissionschedule.htm

NIH Policy on Late Submission of Grant Applications

grants1.nih.gov/grants/guide/notice-files/NOT-OD-05-030.html

Revised NIH Policy on Submission of a Revised (Amended) Application

grants2.nih.gov/grants/guide/notice-files/NOT-OD-03-041.html

NIH Scientific Review Group Roster Index

era.nih.gov/roster/index.cfm

Appeals of Initial Scientific Peer Review

grants2.nih.gov/grants/guide/notice-files/not97-232.html

National Cancer Institute Howard Temin Award Program Announcement

grants1.nih.gov/grants/guide/pa-files/PAR-03-104.html

The goal of the Howard Temin Award is to bridge the transition from a mentored research environment to an independent basic cancer research career for scientists who have demonstrated unusually high potential during their initial stages of training and development. This special award is aimed at fostering the research careers of outstanding junior scientists in basic research who are committed to developing research programs directly relevant to the understanding of human biology and human disease as it relates to the etiology, pathogenesis, prevention, diagnosis, and treatment of human cancer. The major objective of the award is to sustain and advance the early research careers of the most promising M.D.s and Ph.D.s while they consolidate and focus their independent research programs and obtain their own research grant support. To achieve this objective, the Howard Temin Award offers candidates up to five years to gain additional skills and knowledge in human cancer research during a period of one to three years in a mentored environment, followed by transition to the equivalent of a junior faculty position to develop an independent research program.

The National Academies Press

www.nap.edu

This Web site lists publications of the National Academies, the Advisors to the nation on science, engineering, and medicine.

NIH Strategic Research Plan to Reduce and Ultimately Eliminate Health Disparities

ncmhd.nih.gov/our_programs/strategic/index.asp

Ruth L. Kirschstein National Research Service Award (NRSA) Research Training Grants and Fellowships

grants.nih.gov/training/nrsa.htm

NIH Grants Policy Statement (12/03): Insurance Requirements

grants.nih.gov/grants/policy/nihgps_2003/NIHGPS_Part10.htm

Ruth L. Kirschstein National Research Service Award (NRSA) Stipend and Other Budgetary Levels Effective for Fiscal Year 2006

grants2.nih.gov/grants/guide/notice-files/NOT-OD-06-026.html

grants.nih.gov/grants/policy/nihgps_2003/NIHGPS_Part10.htm#_Toc54600187

National Research Service Awards Guidelines

grants.nih.gov/grants/policy/nihgps_2001/part_iib_3.htm

Special Program Considerations for the Kirschstein National Research Service Award

grants1.nih.gov/grants/policy/nihgps_2003/NIHGPS_Part11.htm

NIH Loan Repayment Programs

www.lrp.nih.gov/

This Web site provides links to the different types of loan forgiveness programs offered by NIH, depending on type of research and length of commitment.

Ruth L. Kirschstein National Research Service Award Short-Term Institutional Research Training Grants (T35)

grants.nih.gov/grants/guide/pa-files/PA-05-117.html

Awarded to eligible institutions to develop or enhance research training opportunities for individuals interested in careers in biomedical and behavioral research. Many of the NIH Institutes and Centers use this grant mechanism exclusively to support intensive, short-term research training experiences for students in health professional schools during the summer. In addition, the Short-Term Institutional Research Training Grant may be used to support other types of Pre-doctoral and postdoctoral training in focused, often emerging, and scientific areas relevant to the mission of the funding Institute or Center at the NIH.

Change in Standing Receipt Dates for NIH/AHRQ/NIOSH

grants.nih.gov/grants/guide/notice-files/NOT-OD-07-001.html

The purpose, effective January 2007, informs the research community of a change in standard receipt dates and will apply to both paper and electronic applications.

National Science Foundation Science and Engineering Statistics

www.nsf.gov/statistics/

This Web page has links to publications, data, and analyses about the nation's science and engineering resources.

U.S. Department of Health and Human Services: Poverty Guidelines, Research, and Measurement

aspe.hhs.gov/poverty/index.shtml

NIH Black Scientists Association

bsa.od.nih.gov/

The NIH Black Scientist Association is composed of scientists, physicians, technologists, and science administrators at NIH.

Requirement for Instruction in the Responsible Conduct of Research in National Research Service Award Institutional Training Grants—1992

grants1.nih.gov/grants/guide/notice-files/not92-236.html

U.S. Department of Health and Human Services Office of Research Integrity

ori.dhhs.gov/

The Office of Research Integrity (ORI) promotes integrity in biomedical and behavioral research supported by the U.S. Public Health Service (PHS) at about 4,000 institutions worldwide. ORI monitors institutional investigations of research misconduct and facilitates the responsible conduct of research (RCR) through educational, preventive, and regulatory activities.

Sigma Xi Postdoctoral Survey

postdoc.sigmaxi.org

This survey is designed to improve training and research environment by surveying postdoctorates to provide a better understanding of their experiences.

NIH Grant Support Mechanisms

grants2.nih.gov/grants/guide/notice-files/not94-003.html

This Web page provides a list of NIH activity codes.

SAMHSA Model Programs: Effective Substance Abuse and Mental Health Programs for Every Community

www.modelprograms.samhsa.gov

This Web site provides information on evidence-based program (model programs) designed to prevent or reduce substance abuse and other related high-risk behaviors. The site serves as a resource for anyone interested in learning about and/or implementing these programs.

Guide to Preventive Services

www.thecommunityguide.org

This Web site provides links to evidence-based recommendations for programs and policies to promote population health. Topics covered include alcohol, obesity, and diabetes, among others.

The Cochrane Collaboration

www.cochrane.org

The Cochrane Collaboration provides reviews of health care interventions and promotes the search for evidence through clinical trials and other studies of interventions. This Web site provides links to these reviews.

The Community of Science

www.cos.com

This Web site is a resource for hard-to-find scientific information and other projects across all disciplines. It provides methods for finding funding, experts and collaborators and promoting your own research.

Central Contractor Registration

www.ccr.gov

All prospective vendors/contractors must be registered prior to award of any contract or purchase agreement.

D&B Small Business Solutions

smallbusiness.dnb.com

Link to getting a DUNS number

smallbusiness.dnb.com/manage-business-credit/get-duns-details.asp

A DUNS number is required to submit a grant to NIH. This Web site provides instructions on obtaining the DUNS number for your corporation.

National Youth Anti-Drug Media Campaign: Publications

www.mediacampaign.org/publications/index.html

Completing Grants Application Demonstration

www.grants.gov/images/Application_Package.swf

This interactive Web page with audio takes you through the grant application process.

Appendix: NIH Institutes, Centers, and Their Web Sites

Jennifer N. Lapin

The following material provides a complete listing of the NIH institutes, including their homepage Web site addresses, a URL linking you to their mission statement, additional links to their research and funding pages, and personnel contact information. Where applicable, multiple contacts are listed. In some cases, the only contact information available are email addresses.

NATIONAL INSTITUTES OF HEALTH

Homepage: www.nih.gov/
Mission statement: www.nih.gov/about/index.html#mission.htm

NATIONAL INSTITUTE ON AGING

Homepage: www.nia.nih.gov/
Mission statement: www.nia.nih.gov/AboutNIA/
Contact: Biology of Aging Program (BAP)

National Institute on Aging
Gateway Building, Suite 2C231
7201 Wisconsin Avenue, MSC 9205
Bethesda, MD 20892-9205
Phone: (301) 496-6402
Email: bapquery@nia.nih.gov

Contact: Behavioral and Social Research Program (BSR)
National Institute on Aging
Gateway Building, Suite 533
7201 Wisconsin Avenue, MSC 9205
Bethesda, MD 20892-9205
Phone: (301) 496-3131
Email: bsrquery@nia.nih.gov

Contact: Geriatrics and Clinical Gerontology Program (GCG)
National Institute on Aging
Gateway Building, Suite 3C307
7201 Wisconsin Avenue, MSC 9205
Bethesda, MD 20892-9205
Phone: (301) 496-6761
Email: gcgquery@nia.nih.gov

Contact: Neuroscience and Neuropsychology of Aging Program (NNA)
National Institute on Aging
Gateway Building, Suite 350
7201 Wisconsin Avenue, MSC 9205
Bethesda, MD 20892-9205
Phone: (301) 594-7676
Email: nnaquery@nia.nih.gov

NATIONAL INSTITUTE ON ALCOHOL ABUSE AND ALCOHOLISM

Homepage www.niaaa.nih.gov/
Mission statement: www.niaaa.nih.gov/AboutNIAAA/OrganizationalInformation/
Mission.htm
Research and Funding Homepage www.niaaa.nih.gov/ResearchInformation/
ExtramuralResearch/default.htm
Contact: Ernestine Vanderveen, Ph.D.
Division of Basic Research, NIAAA
6000 Executive Boulevard, Suite 402, MSC 7003
Bethesda, MD 20892-7003
Phone: (301) 443-2531
Fax: (301) 594-0673
Email: tvanderv@willco.niaaa.nih.gov

Contact: Harold I. Perl, Ph.D.
> Division of Clinical and Prevention Research, NIAAA
> 6000 Executive Boulevard, Suite 505, MSC 7003
> Bethesda, MD 20892-7003
> Phone: (301) 443-0788
> Fax: (301) 443-8774
> Email: hperl@willco.niaaa.nih.gov

Contact: Vivian B. Faden, Ph.D.
> Division of Biometry and Epidemiology, NIAAA
> 6000 Executive Boulevard, Suite 514, MSC 7003
> Bethesda, MD 20892-7003
> Phone: (301) 594-6232
> Fax: (301) 443-8614
> Email: vfaden@willco.niaaa.nih.gov

NATIONAL INSTITUTE OF ALLERGY AND INFECTIOUS DISEASES

Homepage: www3.niaid.nih.gov/
Planning and Priorities: www3.niaid.nih.gov/about/overview/planningpriorities/
Research and Funding Homepage: www3.niaid.nih.gov/researchFunding/
Contact: Dr. Milton Hernandez
> Office of Scientific Training and Manpower Development
> Solar Building, Room 3C21
> Bethesda, MD 20892
> Phone: (301) 496-7291
> Fax: (301) 402-0369
> Email: mh35c@nih.gov

NATIONAL INSTITUTE OF ARTHRITIS AND MUSCULOSKELETAL AND SKIN DISEASES

Homepage: www.niams.nih.gov/
Mission Statement: www.niams.nih.gov/an/index.htm
Contact: Richard W. Lymn, Ph.D.
> Research Training Officer
> National Institute of Arthritis and Musculoskeletal and Skin Diseases
> Building 45, Room 5AS-49E
> Bethesda, MD 20892-6500
> Phone: (301) 594-5128
> Fax: (301) 480-4543
> Email: richard_w_lymn@nih.gov

NATIONAL INSTITUTE OF BIOMEDICAL IMAGING AND BIOENGINEERING

Homepage: www.nibib.nih.gov/
Mission Statement: www.nibib.nih.gov/About/MissionHistory
Funding Homepage: www.nibib.nih.gov/FundingMain
Contact: info@nibib.nih.gov

NATIONAL INSTITUTE OF CHILD HEALTH AND HUMAN DEVELOPMENT

Homepage: www.nichd.nih.gov/
Mission Statement: www.nichd.nih.gov/about/nichd_does.cfm
Funding Homepage: www.nichd.nih.gov/funding/funding.htm
Contact: Steven L. Klein, Ph.D.
  Developmental Biology, Genetics & Teratology Branch
  Building 6100, Room 4B01 MSC 7510
  Bethesda, MD 20892-7510
  Phone: (301) 496-5541
  Fax: (301) 480-0303
  Email: KleinS@Exchange.nih.gov

NATIONAL INSTITUTE ON DEAFNESS AND OTHER COMMUNICATION DISORDERS

Homepage: www.nidcd.nih.gov/
Mission Statement: www.nidcd.nih.gov/about/learn/mission.asp
Research Homepage: www.nidcd.nih.gov/research/
Funding Homepage: www.nidcd.nih.gov/funding/
Contact: Daniel A. Sklare, Ph.D.
  Division of Human Communication
  Executive Plaza South, Room 400C-13
  6120 Executive Blvd., MSC 7180
  Bethesda, MD 20892-7180
  Phone: (301) 496-1804
  Fax: (301) 402-6251
  Email: Daniel_Sklare@nih.gov

NATIONAL INSTITUTE OF DENTAL AND CRANIOFACIAL RESEARCH

Homepage: www.nidcr.nih.gov/
Mission Statement: www.nidcr.nih.gov/AboutNIDCR/MissionStatement.htm
Funding Homepage: www.nidcr.nih.gov/Funding
Research Homepage: www.nidcr.nih.gov/Research

Contact: Dr. James A. Lipton
          Assistant Director for Training and Career Development
          Natcher Building, Room 4AN.18J
          Bethesda, MD 20892-6402
          Phone: (301) 594-2618
          Fax: (301) 480-8319
          Email: liptonj@de45.nidcr.nih.gov

NATIONAL INSTITUTE OF DIABETES AND DIGESTIVE AND KIDNEY DISEASES

Homepage: www.niddk.nih.gov/
Mission Statement: www.niddk.nih.gov/welcome/mission.htm#mission
Research and Funding Homepage: www.niddk.nih.gov/fund/fund.htm
Contact: Ronald Margolis, Ph.D.
          Division of Diabetes, Endocrinology, and Metabolic Diseases
          45 Center Drive, Room 5AN-12J, MSC 6600
          Bethesda, MD 20892-6600
          Phone: (301) 594-8819
          Fax: (301) 480-3503
          Email: margolisr@extra.niddk.nih.gov
Contact: Judith Podskalny, Ph.D.
          Division of Digestive Diseases and Nutrition
          45 Center Drive, Room 6AN-12E, MSC 6600
          Bethesda, MD 20892-6600
          Phone: (301) 594-8876
          Fax: (301) 480-8300
          Email: podskalnyj@ep.niddk.nih.gov
Contact: Charles Rodgers, Ph.D.
          Division of Kidney, Urologic, and Hematologic Diseases
          45 Center Drive, Room 6AS-19J MSC 6600
          Bethesda, MD 20892-6600
          Phone: (301) 594-7717
          Fax: (301) 480-3510
          Email: rodgersc@ep.niddk.nih.gov

NATIONAL INSTITUTE ON DRUG ABUSE

Homepage: www.nida.nih.gov/
Mission Statement: www.nida.nih.gov/about/aboutnida.html
Research and Funding Homepage: www.nida.nih.gov/researchers.html

Contact: Andrea Baruchin, Ph.D.
　　　　　Office of Science Policy and Communications
　　　　　6001 Executive Boulevard, Room 5230
　　　　　Bethesda, MD 20892-9591
　　　　　Phone: (301) 443-6071
　　　　　Fax: (301) 443-6277
　　　　　Email: ab47j@nih.gov

NATIONAL INSTITUTE OF ENVIRONMENTAL HEALTH SCIENCES

Homepage: www.niehs.nih.gov/
Mission Statement: www.niehs.nih.gov/external/intro.htm
Research and Funding Homepage: www.niehs.nih.gov/dert/
Contact: Dr. Carol Shreffler
　　　　　Division of Extramural Research and Training
　　　　　P.O. Box 12233 MD EC-23
　　　　　Research Triangle Park, NC 27709
　　　　　Phone: (919) 541-1445
　　　　　Fax: (919) 541-5064
　　　　　Email: shreffl1@niehs.nih.gov

NATIONAL INSTITUTE OF GENERAL MEDICAL SCIENCES

Homepage: www.nigms.nih.gov/
Research and Funding Homepage: www.nigms.nih.gov/Research/
Contact: National Institute of General Medical Sciences
　　　　　45 Center Drive MSC 6200
　　　　　Bethesda, MD 20892-6200
　　　　　Phone: (301) 496-7301

NATIONAL LIBRARY OF MEDICINE

Homepage: www.nlm.nih.gov/about/index.html
Functional Statement: www.nlm.nih.gov/about/functstatement.html)
Funding and Research Homepage: www.nlm.nih.gov/grants.html
Contact: National Library of Medicine
　　　　　8600 Rockville Pike
　　　　　Bethesda, MD 20894
　　　　　888-FIND-NLM (888-346-3656)

NATIONAL INSTITUTE OF MENTAL HEALTH

Homepage: www.nimh.nih.gov/
Mission Statement: www.nimh.nih.gov/about/nimh.cfm
Research and Funding Homepage: www.nimh.nih.gov/researchfunding/index .cfm
Contact: National Institute of Mental Health (NIMH)
    Public Information and Communications Branch
    6001 Executive Boulevard, Room 8184, MSC 9663
    Bethesda, MD 20892-9663
    Phone: (301) 443-4513 (local)
        (866) 615-6464 (toll-free)
    Email: nimhinfo@nih.gov

NATIONAL INSTITUTE OF NEUROLOGICAL DISORDERS AND STROKE

Homepage: www.ninds.nih.gov/
Mission Statement: www.ninds.nih.gov/about_ninds/mission.htm
Research and Funding Homepage: www.ninds.nih.gov/funding/index.htm
Contact: Robert Finklestein, Ph.D.
    Director, Division of Extramural Research
    NIH/NINDS
    Neuroscience Center, Room 3307
    6001 Executive Blvd MSC 9531
    Bethesda, MD 20892-9531
    Email: rf45c@nih.gov
    Phone: (301) 496-9428
Contact: Emmeline Edwards, Ph.D.
    Deputy Director, Extramural Research Program
    NIH/NINDS
    Neuroscience Center, Room 3305
    6001 Executive Blvd MSC 9531
    Bethesda, MD 20892-9531
    Phone: (301) 496-9428
    Email: ee48r@nih.gov

NATIONAL INSTITUTE OF NURSING RESEARCH

Homepage: ninr.nih.gov/ninr/
Mission Statement: ninr.nih.gov/ninr/research/diversity/mission.html
Research and Funding Homepage: ninr.nih.gov/ninr/research.html
Phone: (301) 496-0207

NATIONAL CENTER FOR COMPLEMENTARY AND ALTERNATIVE MEDICINE

Homepage: nccam.nih.gov/
Mission Statement: nccam.nih.gov/about/ataglance/
Research and Funding Homepage: nccam.nih.gov/research/nccamfunds.htm
Contact: NCCAM Clearinghouse
    P.O. Box 7923
    Gaithersburg, MD 20898
    Email: info@nccam.nih.gov
    Phone: (888) 644-6226

NATIONAL CENTER FOR RESEARCH RESOURCES

Homepage: www.ncrr.nih.gov/
Mission Statement: www.ncrr.nih.gov/about_ncrr/mission.asp
Research and Funding Homepage: www.ncrr.nih.gov/rsrch_funding.asp
Contact: Office of Science Policy and Public Liaison
    National Center for Research Resources
    National Institutes of Health
    One Democracy Plaza, Room 984
    6701 Democracy Boulevard, MSC 4874
    Bethesda, MD 20892-4874
    Telephone: (301) 435-0888
    Fax: (301) 480-3558
    Email: info@ncrr.nih.gov

NATIONAL EYE INSTITUTE

Homepage: www.nei.nih.gov/
Mission Statement: www.nei.nih.gov/about/mission.asp
Research and Funding Homepages: www.nei.nih.gov/funding/, www.nei.nih
.gov/funding/app.asp
Contact: Maria Y. Giovanni, Ph.D.
    National Eye Institute, NIH
    EPS Suite 350
    6120 Executive Blvd. MSC 7164
    Bethesda, MD 20892-7164
    Phone: (301) 496-0484 / (301) 402-0528
    Email: myg@nei.nih.gov

NATIONAL HEART, LUNG, AND BLOOD INSTITUTE

Homepage: www.nhlbi.nih.gov/index.htm
Mission Statement: www.nhlbi.nih.gov/about/org/mission.htm
Research and Funding Homepage: www.nhlbi.nih.gov/funding/index.htm
Contact: NHLBI Health Information Center
    Attention: Web Site
    P.O. Box 30105
    Bethesda, MD 20824-0105
    Phone: (301) 592-8573
    Email: nhlbiinfo@nhlbi.nih.gov

NATIONAL CANCER INSTITUTE

Homepage www.cancer.gov/
Mission Statement www.cancer.gov/aboutnci/overview/mission
Research and Funding www.cancer.gov/researchandfunding
Contact: Dr. Lester S. Gorelic or Dr. Andrew Vargosko
    National Cancer Institute
    Office of the Deputy Director for Extramural Sciences
    Office of Centers, Training and Resources
    Executive Plaza North, Room 520, MSC 7390
    Bethesda, MD 20892-7390
    Phone: (301) 496-8580
    Fax: (301) 402-4472
    Email: lg2h@nih.gov or av8b@nih.gov

Lawrence M. Scheier, Ph.D.
President, LARS Research Institute
11735 Glowing Sunset Lane
Las Vegas, NV 89135
Phone: (702) 228-6631
Fax: (702) 228-1051
Cell: (702) 630-7584
and
Adjunct Associate Professor
Washington University School of
  Medicine
Department of Psychiatry
40 N. Kingshighway, Suite 4
St. Louis, MO 63108
Phone: (314) 286-2252
Fax: (314) 286-2265
Email: scheier@cox.net or scheier@
  larsri.org
Web: www.larsri.org

William L. Dewey, Ph.D.
Professor, Department of Pharma-
  cology
Virginia Commonwealth University
1112 East Clay Street
P.O. Box 980613
Richmond, VA 23298-0613

Phone: (804) 827-0375
Home: (804) 747-9989
Fax: (804) 827-1548
Email: wdewey@hsc.vcu.edu

William J. Bukoski, Ph.D.
Senior Scientist, Office of the Director
Division of Epidemiology, Services and
  Prevention Research
National Institute on Drug Abuse
6001 Executive Boulevard
Room 5153, MSC 9589
Bethesda, MD 20892-9589
Phone: (301) 402-1526
Fax: (301) 443-2636
Email: bb75h@nih.gov

Wilson M. Compton, M.D., M.P.E.
Director, Division of Epidemiology,
  Services and Prevention Research
National Institute on Drug Abuse
6001 Executive Boulevard
Room 5153, MSC 9589
Bethesda, MD 20892-9589
Phone: (301) 443-6504
Fax: (301) 443-2636
Email: wcompton@nida.nih.gov

Linda B. Cottler, Ph.D., M.P.H.
Professor of Epidemiology and
Director, Epidemiology and
  Prevention Research Group
Department of Psychiatry
Washington University School of
  Medicine
40 N. Kingshighway, Suite 4
St. Louis, MO 63108
Phone: (314) 286-2252
Fax: (314) 286-2265
Email: cottler@epi.wustl.edu
Web: www.epi.wustl.edu

Thomas N. Ferraro, Ph.D.
Associate Professor
University of Pennsylvania
Departments of Psychiatry and
  Pharmacology
Center for Neurobiology and
  Behavior
School of Medicine
Philadelphia, PA 19104-3403
Phone: (215) 573-4581
Fax: (215) 573-2041
Email: tnf@mail.med.upenn.edu
Web: http://www.med.upenn.
  edu/ins/faculty/ferraro.htm

Mark R. Green, Ph.D.
Deputy Director, Office of
  Extramural Affairs
National Institute on Drug Abuse,
  NIH, DHHS
6101 Executive Blvd., Suite 220,
  MSC 8401
Bethesda, MD 20892-8401
Phone: (301) 435-1431
Fax: (301) 443-0538
Email: mgreen1@nida.nih.gov or
  mg388g@nih.gov

Kenneth W. Griffin, Ph.D., M.P.H.
Associate Professor, Division of
  Prevention and Health Behavior
Department of Public Health
Weill Medical College of Cornell
  University
411 East 69th Street, KB207
New York, NY 10021
Phone: (212) 746-1270
Fax: (212) 746-8390
Email: kgriffin@med.cornell.edu
Web: www.med.cornell.edu/
  public.health

William B. Hansen, Ph.D.
President, Tanglewood Research
420-A Gallimore Dairy Road
Greensboro, NC 27409
Phone: (336) 662-0090 ext. 101
Fax: (336) 662-0099
Email: billhansen@tanglewood.net
Web: www.tanglewood.net

Jeffrey A. Hoffman, Ph.D.
President and CEO, Danya
  International Inc.
8737 Colesville Road, Suite 1100
Silver Spring, MD 20910
Phone: (301) 565-2142
Fax: (301) 565-3710
Email: jhoffman@danya.com
Web: www.danya.com

Michelle R. Hoot, B.S.
Department of Pharmacology and
  Toxicology
Virginia Commonwealth University
P. O. Box 980524
Richmond, VA 23298-0524
Phone: (804) 828-5596
Fax: (804) 827-1548
Email: hootmr@vcu.edu

Dan R. Hoyt, Ph.D.
Chair and Professor, Department of
  Sociology
University of Nebraska-Lincoln
732 Oldfather Hall
Lincoln, NE 68588-0325
Phone: (402) 472-6040
Fax: (402) 472-6070
Email: dhoyt2@unlnotes.unl.edu

Valerie L. Johnson, Ph.D.
Associate Research Professor
Rutgers, The State University
  of New Jersey
Center of Alcohol Studies
607 Allison Rd
Piscataway, NJ 08854
Phone: (732) 445-2424
Fax: (732) 445-3500
Email: vjohnson@rci.rutgers.edu

Jenny N. Karp, M.P.H., C.H.E.S.
Vice President, International
  Public Health
Social Solutions International Inc.
8(a) and Woman-Owned
18303 Wickham Road
Olney, MD 20832
Phone: (202) 249-2305
Fax: (301) 570-4772
Email: jnkarp@socialsolutions.info
Web: www.socialsolutions.info

Karol L. Kumpfer, Ph.D.
Professor, Department of Health
  Promotion and Education
1901 E. South Campus Drive, Room
  2103-B
University of Utah
Salt Lake City, UT 84112
Phone: (801) 581-7718
Fax: (801) 583-7979

Email: Karol.Kumpfer@health.utah.edu
Web: www.strengtheningfamilies
  program.org

Jennifer N. Lapin, Ph.D.
Assessment Data Research Analyst
Office of Assessment
School District of Philadelphia
440 North Broad Street
Philadelphia, PA 19131
Phone: (215) 400-5826
Fax: (215) 400-4255
Email: jnlapin@phila.k12.pa.us

Frances R. Levin, M.D.
Kennedy-Leavy Professor of Clinical
  Psychiatry
Department of Psychiatry
College of Physicians and Surgeons
Columbia University
New York State Psychiatric Institute
1051 Riverside Drive
New York, NY 10032
Phone: (212) 543-5896
Fax: (212) 543-6018
Email: frl2@columbia.edu

Michelle A. Lewis, M.S.
Assistant Director of Grants
  Administration
New York University
College of Nursing
246 Greene Street
New York, NY 10003
Phone: (212) 998-5300
Fax: (212) 995-3143
Email: lewismichellea@verizon.net

Kelly Munly, M.S.
Research Associate, Danya
  International, Inc.
8737 Colesville Road, Suite 1200

Silver Spring, MD 20910
Phone: (240) 645-1097
Fax: (301) 565-3710
Email: kmunly@danya.com

David M. Murray, Ph.D.
Professor and Chair, Division of
    Epidemiology
College of Public Health
The Ohio State University
B222 Starling Loving Hall
320 West 10th Avenue
Columbus, OH 43210
Phone: (614) 293-2928
Fax: (614) 293-3937
Email: dmurray@cph.osu.edu

Ida K. Namur, B.S.
Research Associate, Social Solutions
    International, Inc.
18303 Wickham Road
Olney, MD 20832
Phone: (301) 774-0897
Fax: (301) 570-4772
Email: inamur@socialsolutions.info
Web: www.socialsolutions.info

Susanna Nemes, Ph.D.
President and CEO, Social Solutions
    International, Inc.
18303 Wickham Road
Olney, MD 20832
Phone: (301) 774-0897
Fax: (301) 570-4772
Email: snemes@socialsolutions.info
Web: www.socialsolutions.info

Robert J. Pandina, Ph.D.
Professor and Director, Center
    of Alcohol Studies
Rutgers, The State University of New
    Jersey

607 Allison Rd
Piscataway, NJ 08854
Phone: (732) 445-2518
Fax: (732) 445-3500
Email: rpandina@rci.rutgers.edu

Mary Ann Pentz, Ph.D.
Professor, Preventive Medicine
Director, Center for Prevention
    Policy Research
University of Southern California
Keck School of Medicine
Institute for Prevention Research
Department of Preventive Medicine
1000 South Fremont Avenue, Unit 8
Alhambra, CA 91803
Phone: (626) 457-6691
Fax: (626) 457-6695
Email: pentz@usc.edu

Alan W. Stacy, Ph.D.
Professor, Preventive Medicine
Director, Transdisciplinary Drug
    Abuse Prevention Research Center
Institute for Prevention Research
Department of Preventive Medicine
University of Southern California
1000 S. Fremont Ave.
Building A Room 4216
Alhambra, CA 91803
Phone: (626) 457-6636
Fax: (626) 457-4012
Email: astacy@usc.edu
Web: http://tprc.usc.edu/

Julia Franklin Summerhays, M.S.
Associate Instructor, Department of
    Health Promotion and Education
Administrator, Research Facilitation
    Team
College of Health and Center for
    Rehabilitation Research
University of Utah

1901 E. South Campus Drive, Room 2220
Salt Lake City, UT 84112
Phone: (801) 581-7289
Email: jfranklin.summerhays@health
.utah.edu

Steven Sussman, Ph.D.
Professor, Department of Preventive
Medicine
Transdisciplinary Prevention Research
Center
Institute for Health Promotion and
Disease Prevention Research
Keck School of Medicine
University of Southern California
1000 S. Fremont Avenue, Unit 8,
Building A-5, Suite #5228
Alhambra, CA 91803-4737
Phone: (626) 457-6635
Cell: (626) 376-0389
Fax: (626) 457-4012
Email: ssussma@usc.edu

Mark Swieter, Ph.D.
Chief, Training and Special Projects
Review Branch
Office of Extramural Affairs
NIDA/NIH/DHHS

6101 Executive Blvd
Rm. 209, MSC 8401
Bethesda, MD 20892-8401
Phone: (301) 435-1389
Fax: (301) 443-0538
Email: ms80x@nih.gov

Jennifer B. Unger, Ph.D.
Associate Professor of Preventive
Medicine
Institute for Health Promotion and
Disease Prevention Research
University of Southern California Keck
School of Medicine
1000 S. Fremont, Box 8
Alhambra, CA 91803
Phone: (626) 457-4052
Email: unger@usc.edu

Jennifer Weil, Ph.D.
Vice President, Substance Abuse
Research
Social Solutions International Inc
18303 Wickham Road, Olney MD 20832
Phone: (301) 774-0897
Fax: (301) 570-4772
Email: jweil@socialsolutions.info
Web: www.socialsolutions.info